LABORATORY

Case Book

MEDICINE

An Introduction to Clinical Reasoning

LABORATORY MEDICINE
Case Book

An Introduction to Clinical Reasoning

Jana Raskova, MD
Professor of Pathology and Laboratory Medicine
Robert Wood Johnson Medical School
Piscataway, New Jersey

Stephen M. Shea, MD, FRCP
Professor of Pathology and Laboratory Medicine
Robert Wood Johnson Medical School
Piscataway, New Jersey

Frederick C. Skvara, MD
Associate Professor of Pathology and Laboratory Medicine
Robert Wood Johnson Medical School
Piscataway, New Jersey

Nagy H. Mikhail, MD
Assistant Professor of Pathology and Laboratory Medicine
Robert Wood Johnson Medical School
Piscataway, New Jersey

Appleton & Lange
Stamford, Connecticut

Copyright © 1997 by Appleton & Lange
A Simon & Schuster Company

97 98 99 00 01 / 10 9 8 7 6 5 4 3 2 1

Prentice Hall International (UK) Limited, *London*
Prentice Hall of Australia Pty. Limited, *Sydney*
Prentice Hall Canada, Inc., *Toronto*
Prentice Hall Hispanoamericana, S.A., *Mexico*
Prentice Hall of India Private Limited, *New Delhi*
Prentice Hall of Japan, Inc., *Tokyo*
Simon & Schuster Asia Pte. Ltd., *Singapore*
Editora Prentice Hall do Brasil Ltda., *Rio de Janeiro*
Prentice Hall, *Upper Saddle River, New Jersey*

ISBN: 0-8385-5574-8
ISSN: 1090-9435

Senior Editor: John P. Butler
Managing Editor, Development: Gregory R. Huth
Production Editor: Jennifer Sinsavich
Production Editor: Lisa M. Guidone
Designer: Janice Barsevich Bielawa

PRINTED IN THE UNITED STATES OF AMERICA

CONTENTS

Laboratory Medicine Case Book: An Introduction to Clinical Reasoning was conceived as a response to the needs of medical students taking a course in pathology and laboratory medicine at the Robert Wood Johnson Medical School. It became clear to us that the greatest challenge for the student is to make effective use of the concepts of basic science in a clinical context. When the student first encounters patients with real problems, he or she often feels less than prepared. To integrate a variety of information to arrive at a diagnosis is an art rather than a science—the art known as clinical reasoning. The first aim of this book has been to lay a foundation for the development of this skill. With this in mind, we have compiled 30 cases, covering a variety of major disease processes.

Each case is presented as a diagnostic problem, and the student is guided through it by a series of multiple choice questions. These questions explore abnormal laboratory, radiologic, and morphologic findings as they relate to the clinical history and presentation. Questions also probe the student's understanding of the structural and functional changes underlying disease processes as well as the student's skill in interpreting laboratory data. In most cases, the questions leave the diagnosis open until the end of the case, where a complete description is provided of all images and figures, along with justified answers to the questions. A list of final diagnoses and a summary conclude the case. A section entitled "Lab Tips" describes and explains one or two relevant and useful laboratory procedures.

Our cases are crafted to stimulate the reader's curiosity and to encourage the reader to consult reference texts. Cases also provide feedback on the reader's performance. This feature makes the book suitable for the review of pathology, pathophysiology, and laboratory medicine. In addition, cases may serve as a vehicle providing a clinical context for the study of preclinical disciplines.

Although it is not the aim of this book to address treatment or patient management, we believe that its focus on diagnostic methodology will make it helpful to the students in the clinical years and beyond.

We hope that students find *Laboratory Medicine Case Book: An Introduction to Clinical Reasoning* useful, interesting, and even fun.

Jana Raskova, MD
Stephen M. Shea, MD, FRCPath
Frederick C. Skvara, MD
Nagy H. Mikhail, MD
Piscataway, New Jersey
January 1997

LABORATORY MEDICINE

Case Book

An Introduction to Clinical Reasoning

▶ **Clinical History and Presentation**

A 66-year-old man was brought to the emergency room from his home after he was found to be unresponsive. His blood sugar was 28 mg/dL, and he regained consciousness after administration of dextrose. The patient was diagnosed at another hospital 3 months ago as having diabetes mellitus and was started on insulin. At the same time, his chest x-ray revealed a mass in the left lung which on further work-up was diagnosed as bronchogenic carcinoma. Since then, the patient has had three cycles of chemotherapy, the latest one 6 days ago. Physical examination on this admission revealed a confused and lethargic man. Blood pressure was 150/90 mm Hg, temperature was 98.8° F, respiratory rate was 26 per minute, and heart rate was 92 beats per minute. Pertinent physical findings included decreased breath sounds on the left side, marked weakness of both legs, and a "puffy" appearance of the face.

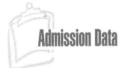

Admission Data

TABLE 1–1. HEMATOLOGY		
WBC	8.14 thousand/μL	(3.6–11.2)
Neut	88.6%	(44–88)
Lymph	8.2%	(12–43)
Mono	1.7%	(2–11)
Eos	1.5%	(0–5)
RBC	3.18 million/μL	(4.0–5.8)
Hgb	9.9 g/dL	(12.6–17.0)
HCT	30.4%	(42–52)
MCV	95.4 fL	(80–102)
MCH	31.2 pg	(27–35)
Plts	205 thousand/μL	(130–400)

TABLE 1–2. CHEMISTRY		
Glucose	28 mg/dL	(65–110)
BUN	25 mg/dL	(7–24)
Creatinine	1.2 mg/dL	(0.7–1.4)
Uric acid	8.1 mg/dL	(3.0–8.5)
Cholesterol	150 mg/dL	(150–240)
Calcium	8.5 mg/dL	(8.5–10.5)
Protein	5.5 g/dL	(6–8)
Albumin	2.7 g/dL	(3.7–5.0)
LDH, Total	537 U/L	(100–225)
LDH_1	23%	(17–27)
LDH_2	37%	(28–38)
LDH_3	18%	(18–28)
LDH_4	11%	(5–15)
LDH_5	11%	(6–13)
Alk Phos	194 U/L	(30–120)
AST	30 U/L	(0–55)
GGTP	247 U/L	(0–50)
Bilirubin	0.6 mg/dL	(0.0–1.5)

TABLE 1–3. ELECTROLYTES

Na	142 mEq/L	(134–143)
K	2.6 mEq/L	(3.5–4.9)
Cl	86 mEq/L	(95–108)
CO_2	53 mEq/L	(21–32)

TABLE 1–4. ARTERIAL BLOOD GASES

pH	7.54	(7.35–7.45)
PCO_2	49 mmHg	(32–46)
PO_2	52 mmHg	(74–108)
HCO_3	43 mEq/L	(21–29)
Base excess	+18 mEq/L	(−2 − +2)
O_2 saturation	89%	(92–96)

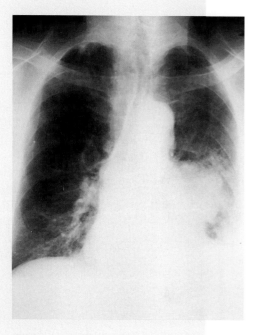

FIGURE 1–1. Patient's chest x-ray (3 months previously).

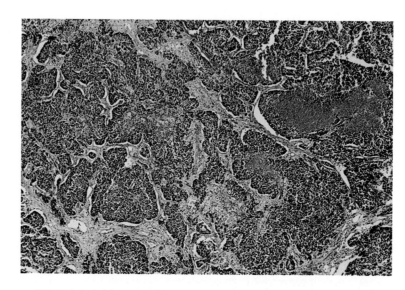

FIGURE 1–2. Left lung mass. Hematoxylin–eosin stain. Original magnification ×12.

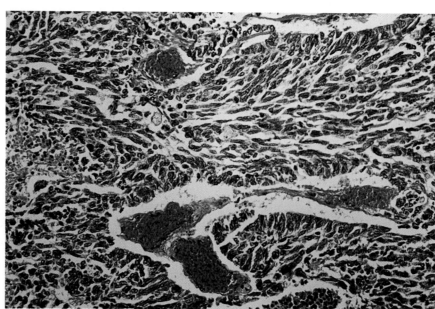

FIGURE 1–3. Left lung mass. Hematoxylin–eosin stain. Original magnification ×50.

▶ **Questions**

On the basis of the preceding information, you can best conclude the following:

1. The patient's abnormal CBC is best explained by which of the following conditions?
   a. profound post-chemotherapy myelosuppression
   b. a septic state
   c. vitamin B_{12} deficiency
   d. aplastic anemia
   e. changes compatible with anemia of chronic disease and lymphopenia

2. The primary acid-base disturbance is:
   a. respiratory acidosis
   b. metabolic alkalosis
   c. metabolic acidosis
   d. respiratory alkalosis

3. Hypokalemia in this patient could be caused by all of the following EXCEPT:
   a. osmotic diuresis of hyperglycemia
   b. hemolytic blood sample
   c. increased production of aldosterone
   d. vomiting
   e. diarrhea

4. The most likely cause of increased serum levels of lactate dehydrogenase (LDH), alkaline phosphatase (Alk Phos), and gamma glutamyl transferase (GGTP) is:
   a. extrahepatic biliary obstruction
   b. the presence of malignancy and possible liver involvement
   c. myocardial infarction
   d. disease of muscle

5. The histologic diagnosis of the patient's lung cancer as depicted in Figures 1–2 and 1–3 is:
   a. squamous cell carcinoma
   b. adenocarcinoma
   c. small cell (oat cell) carcinoma
   d. bronchioloalveolar carcinoma

▶ Clinical Course

The patient's glycemia stabilized and his electrolyte abnormalities were corrected by appropriate replacement therapy. In addition to an MRI (magnetic resonance imaging) scan of the brain, which was normal, the following studies were performed:

TABLE 1–5. ENDOCRINE STUDIES (DAY 3)

Test	Patient Result	Reference Range
Serum ACTH (7 AM)	314.0 pg/mL	0.0–100.0 pg/mL
Serum Cortisol (7 AM)	51.0 μg/dL	5.0–25.0 μg/dL
Serum Cortisol (4 PM)	45.2 μg/dL	2.5–12.5 μg/dL
Serum Aldosterone	13.7 ng/dL	0.0–12.0 ng/dL

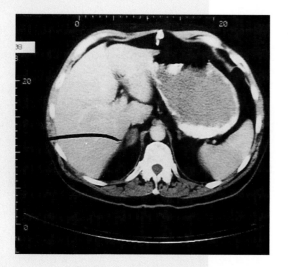

FIGURE 1–4. CT scan of abdomen.

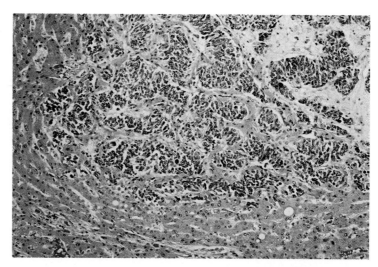

FIGURE 1–5. Patient's liver. Hematoxylin–eosin stain. Original magnification ×31.

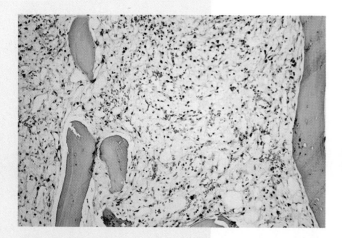

FIGURE 1–6. Bone marrow at autopsy (15 days post-chemotherapy). Hematoxylin–eosin stain. Original magnification ×31.

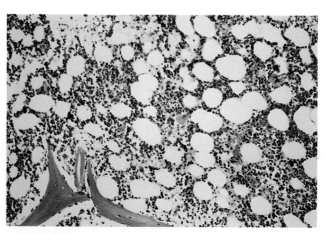

FIGURE 1–7. Normal bone marrow biopsy. Hematoxylin–eosin stain. Original magnification ×31.

TABLE 1–6. HEMATOLOGY STUDIES

Test	Reference Range	Day 3	Day 6	Day 7	Day 8
WBC	3.6–11.2 thousand/μL	6.02	0.83	0.65	0.84
neut	44.0–88.0%	97.00	96.00	25.00	5.00
lymph	12.0–43.0%	3.00	2.00	71.00	88.00
mono	2.0–11.0%	0.00	2.00	4.00	7.00
Hgb	12.6–17.0 g/dL	9.30	7.60	7.50	8.40
HCT	42.0–52.0%	28.20	22.00	22.10	24.30
MCV	80–102 fL	95.00	90.20	93.20	93.90
Plts	130–400 thousand/μL	187.00	96.00	66.00	66.00

As seen in the above table, the patient's hematologic status deteriorated, and he died in septic shock on day 9 (15 days after his last cycle of chemotherapy). Several pertinent findings from the autopsy are shown in Figures 1–5 and 1–6.

▶ Questions

6. This patient's endocrine abnormalities may indicate all of the following EXCEPT:
   a. diabetes is likely due to his hypercortisolism
   b. hypercortisolism is due to the primary adrenal problem
   c. ectopic production of ACTH by the tumor
   d. electrolyte abnormalities are due to increased aldosterone production

7. Identify the INCORRECT statement:
   a. small cell carcinoma of the lung is usually not associated with a history of cigarette smoking
   b. small cell carcinoma of the lung best responds to chemotherapy and radiation therapy
   c. small cell carcinoma of the lung most often starts in the central or hilar lung region
   d. small cell carcinoma of the lung tends to metastasize widely

8. The most common lung cancer in women and nonsmokers is:
   a. small cell carcinoma
   b. adenocarcinoma
   c. squamous cell carcinoma
   d. large cell carcinoma

9. The most common type of lung cancer associated with ectopic hormone production is:
   a. small cell carcinoma
   b. adenocarcinoma
   c. squamous cell carcinoma
   d. large cell carcinoma

10. The most common site of metastatic lesions for all types of bronchogenic carcinoma is:
    a. brain
    b. bone
    c. adrenal gland
    d. liver

11. All of the following statements are correct EXCEPT:
    a. paraneoplastic syndromes may present as the earliest manifestation of an occult neoplasm
    b. hypercalcemia is probably the most common paraneoplastic syndrome
    c. most patients with advanced malignant disease present with some paraneoplastic syndrome
    d. ectopic production of ACTH is the most common endocrinopathic paraneoplastic syndrome

NOTES

▶ Figure Descriptions

Figure 1–1. Patient's chest x-ray (3 months previously).

The chest x-ray shows an irregular left lung mass which the radiologist interpreted as likely due to a primary lung cancer with possible adjacent pneumonia.

Figure 1–2. Left lung mass (patient). Hematoxylin–eosin stain. Original magnification ×12.

The normal architecture of the lung is gone. Instead, one sees sheets of darkly staining cells, areas of necrosis, and fibrosis. No glandular or squamous differentiation is apparent at this magnification.

Figure 1–3. Left lung mass(patient). Hematoxylin–eosin stain. Original magnification ×50.

In this photomicrograph, we can better appreciate the nature of the tumor cells. They are small with little apparent cytoplasm, the nuclei are oval and spindle-shaped, and mitoses are easily found. A focus of necrosis is also present. These are features of small cell carcinoma of the lung.

Figure 1–4. CT scan of abdomen.

This CT scan shows bilateral adrenal gland hyperplasia with the right adrenal gland appearing larger than the left gland at this level.

Figure 1–5. Liver. Hematoxylin–eosin stain. Original magnification ×31.

This photomicrograph shows the edge of a tumor nodule (upper right) with infiltration by clumps of tumor cells between the adjacent hepatic cords. The tumor cells have a spindled appearance, with little cytoplasm, and are consistent with metastatic small cell carcinoma of the lung.

Figure 1–6. Bone marrow at autopsy (15 days post chemotherapy). Hematoxylin–eosin stain. Original magnification ×31.

Immediately apparent in this photomicrograph is the marked hypocellularity of the marrow, which is a consequence of the chemotherapy. The marked depletion in marrow hematopoietic elements is reflected in the patient's peripheral blood cell count. No evidence of tumor is present. If the patient had survived, his bone marrow eventually would have recovered the appearance seen in Figure 1–7.

Figure 1–7. Normal bone marrow. Hematoxylin–eosin stain. Original magnification ×31.

The marrow is normocellular with adequate numbers of fat cells and a heterocellular hematopoietic cell population.

► Answers

1. **(e)** The CBC shows a normocytic normochromic anemia and lymphopenia. Cells of myelomonocytic origin and platelets are within the normal range, which rules out myelosuppression and a septic state. Vitamin B_{12} deficiency leads to a macrocytic anemia. Aplastic anemia is characterized by a pancytopenia which is not present here.

2. **(b)** The primary disturbance is partly compensated metabolic alkalosis (increased pH, HCO_3, and P_{CO_2}).

3. **(b)** Hemolyzed blood specimens give artificially elevated levels of serum potassium. The more severe the hemolysis, the more pronounced the increase in the potassium level. All other options (osmotic diuresis, increased aldosterone production, diarrhea and vomiting) lead to the loss of potassium.

4. **(b)** Increase in total LDH levels, with a nonspecific isoenzyme pattern, is seen in about 50% of patients with carcinoma, particularly in advanced stages. An increase in serum GGTP levels is seen in a variety of carcinomas, including lung cancer, even in the absence of liver metastases. Serum alkaline phosphatase may be produced by neoplasms such as lung cancer, without involvement of the liver. Extrahepatic biliary obstruction would lead to an increase in serum bilirubin and a much greater increase in alkaline phosphatase than seen here. Finally, this group of enzymes is not appropriate for the diagnosis of myocardial infarction or diseases of muscle.

5. **(c)** The microscopic appearance of the tumor is characteristic of small cell ("oat cell") carcinoma of the lung. *See descriptions of Figures 1–2 and 1–3.*

6. **(b)** The hypercortisolism in this patient is due to ectopic production of ACTH by the tumor. Cortisol inhibits glucose uptake in most tissues, which leads to hyperglycemia and diabetes mellitus. The increased ACTH is most likely being produced by the lung tumor, and not by an enlarged pituitary gland (ie, the MRI of the brain was normal), and it induces bilateral adrenal gland hyperplasia. The electrolyte abnormalities are typical of hyperaldosteronism and increased levels of aldosterone were documented.

7. **(a)** Small cell carcinoma of the lung is strongly associated with a history of cigarette smoking. Only 1% of tumors occur in nonsmokers. This type of cancer originates in the central or hilar region, metastasizes early and widely, and initially responds well to chemotherapy and/or radiation therapy.

8. **(b)** Adenocarcinoma of the lung is the most common primary lung cancer in women and nonsmokers.

9. **(a)** The most common type of lung cancer associated with ectopic hormone production is a small cell carcinoma. The tumor cells are considered to originate from the neuroendocrine cells of the bronchial epithelium.

10. (**c**) The adrenals are the most common metastatic site for primary lung cancers and are involved in over 50% of the cases. They are followed by the liver (30–50%), brain (20%), and bone (20%).

11. (**c**) Only about 10% of patients with advanced malignancies present with paraneoplastic syndromes. Hypercalcemia is the most common paraneoplastic syndrome. Of the paraneoplastic endocrinopathies, a Cushing's syndrome due to ectopic production of ACTH is the most common. A paraneoplastic syndrome sometimes presents as the first manifestation of an occult neoplasm.

▶ Final Diagnosis and Synopsis of Case

- Small Cell Carcinoma of the Left Lung With Metastasis to the Liver and Ectopic ACTH Secretion, Resulting in Bilateral Adrenal Gland Hyperplasia
- Diabetes Mellitus
- Hyperaldosteronism
- Metabolic Alkalosis
- Septic Shock Due to Bone Marrow Suppression by Chemotherapy

A 66-year-old man was diagnosed 3 months prior to his death as having a small cell carcinoma of the lung. The patient's first clinical symptom, an elevated blood sugar level, was most likely due to a paraneoplastic Cushing's syndrome caused by the ACTH-induced hypercortisolism. His hypokalemic metabolic alkalosis was most likely also due to a paraneoplastic endocrinopathy and only speculation can be made about his increasing leg weakness belonging to this same category. The patient underwent three cycles of chemotherapy. Several days after the last cycle, he developed a severe hypoglycemic episode. The cause of this hypoglycemic episode is unclear, but it could be related to poor control of his diabetes. The patient died of sepsis secondary to a profound myelosuppression following his last cycle of chemotherapy.

LAB TIPS

Serum ACTH Measurement

Because of the instability of ACTH in plasma due to degradation by plasma proteases, plasma for ACTH determination should be frozen immediately after collection and placed in a plastic vial, since ACTH will adsorb to glass. The preferred method of analysis is radioimmunoassay. The circadian variation of ACTH roughly parallels that of cortisol, with afternoon levels about 50% lower than morning levels. *See the table below for diagnostic usefulness of serum ACTH measurements.*

Serum Cortisol Measurement

The problem with cortisol assays has always been a lack of specificity, since a number of other compounds will cross-react with some of the reagents used in the assays. Currently, the best procedures are immunoassays and high-performance liquid chromatography. Serum cortisol levels are most useful when measured as part of an adrenal stimulation or suppression test.

Erythrocyte Hemolysis

While there are a number of disease processes that can lead to the abnormal lysis of red blood cells, hemolysis can also occur during the collection of blood for laboratory analysis. Since a number of the intracellular components of erythrocytes exist in concentrations much greater than their extracellular levels, the hemolysis of a significant amount of the cells in a sample can cause a falsely elevated level for certain analytes. Elevated levels of potassium, lactate dehydrogenase, aspartate aminotransferase, and alanine aminotransferase, are among a number of substances that can be found in hemolyzed blood specimens.

SERUM ACTH MEASUREMENTS

Disease	Serum ACTH Levels	Serum Cortisol Levels
Primary adrenal insufficiency	Increased	Decreased
Secondary adrenal insufficiency	Normal or decreased	Decreased
Adrenal Cushing's (adenoma/carcinoma)	Decreased	Normal or increased
Pituitary Cushing's	Markedly increased	Increased
Ectopic ACTH-secreting tumors	Markedly increased	Increased

NOTES

▶ **Clinical History and Presentation**

A 38-year-old black man presented with severe generalized joint pain of one day's duration. The patient denied fever, chills, night sweats, vomiting, or weight loss. He stated that he had had similar episodes for the last 20 years. Physical examination revealed a well-developed, obese male in mild distress. His oral temperature was 98° F, heart rate was 76 beats per minute, respiratory rate was 20 per minute, and blood pressure was 123/64 mmHg. The lungs were clear to auscultation and percussion and the abdomen was soft and non-tender. The painful joints were neither swollen, warm, nor tender to palpation.

Admission Data

TABLE 2–1. HEMATOLOGY

WBC	11 thousand/μL	(3.6–11.2)
Neut	60%	(44–88)
Lymph	35%	(12–43)
Mono	3%	(2–11)
Eos	2%	(0–5)
RBC	2.54 million/μL	(4.4–5.8)
Hgb	8.4 g/dL	(14.0–17.0)
HCT	25.7%	(40.0–49.0)
MCV	101.2 fL	(80–94)
MCH	33.1 pg	(27.0–32.0)
MCHC	32.7 g/dL	(32.0–36.5)
Plts	312 thousand/μL	(130–400)

TABLE 2–2. CHEMISTRY

Glucose	89 mg/dL	(65–110)
BUN	13 mg/dL	(7–24)
Creatinine	0.9 mg/dL	(0.7–1.4)
Uric Acid	8.8 mg/dL	(3.0–8.5)
Cholesterol	117 mg/dL	(150–240)
Protein	6.8 g/dL	(6.0–8.0)
Albumin	4.5 g/dL	(3.7–5.0)
LDH	624 U/L	(100–225)
Alk Phos	108 U/L	(30–120)
AST	16 U/L	(0–55)
GGTP	25 U/L	(0–50)
Bilirubin	1.8 mg/dL	(0.0–1.5)
Direct Bilirubin	0.32 mg/dL	(0.02–0.18)

TABLE 2–3. URINALYSIS

Color	Amber	(Yellow)
Clarity	Clear	(Clear)
Bile	Neg	(Neg)
Urobilinogen	2+	(Neg)

TABLE 2–4. SPECIAL HEMATOLOGY

Reticulocytes	17.2%	(0.1–2.0)
Vitamin B$_{12}$	228 pg/mL	(225–1000)
Folate	11.4 μg/mL	(2.0–19.7)
Schilling I	21.1%	(>9.0%)

NOTES

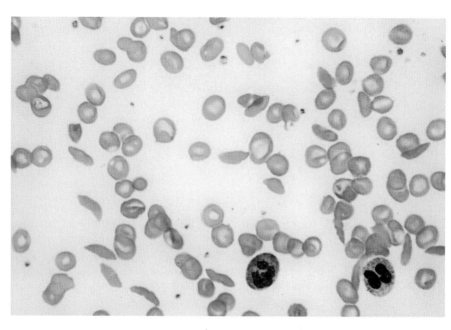

FIGURE 2–1. Peripheral blood smear on admission. Wright/Giemsa stain. Original magnification ×630.

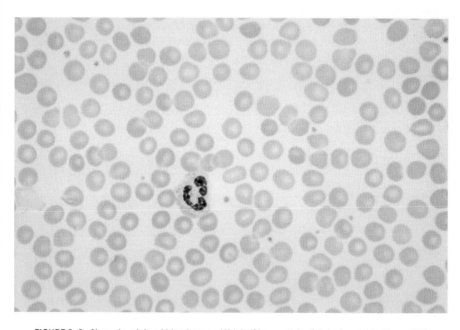

FIGURE 2–2. Normal peripheral blood smear. Wright/Giemsa stain. Original magnification ×630

▶ **Questions**

On the basis of the preceding information, you can best conclude the following:

1. The peripheral blood smear shown in Figure 2–1 is compatible with:
   a. iron deficiency anemia
   b. spherocytosis
   c. sickle cell anemia
   d. a normal smear

2. In confirming this patient's diagnosis, the most useful test at this time would be:
   a. hemoglobin electrophoresis
   b. serum protein electrophoresis
   c. a computerized axial tomography (CAT) scan of one of the painful joints
   d. synovial fluid examination
   e. a routine x-ray of one of the painful joints

3. The elevated serum bilirubin in this patient is most likely due to:
   a. hepatocellular injury
   b. extrahepatic biliary obstruction
   c. chronic hemolysis
   d. intrahepatic biliary obstruction

▶ Clinical Course

The patient was transfused with packed red blood cells and begun on an analgesic for his bone pain. While the bone pain responded well to this therapy, the patient began to complain of chest and abdominal pain. Additional studies were performed and can be seen below. His hemoglobin level stabilized, eventually climbing to 9.0 g/dL, the analgesics were tapered, and he was discharged on day 17 after admission, to be followed as an out-patient.

TABLE 2–5. HEMATOLOGY

Test	Admission	Day 2	Day 8	Day 16	Day 17
Hgb	8.4 g/dL	7.9 g/dL	7.3 g/dL	8.7 g/dL	9.0 g/dL
HCT	25.7%	23.9%	22.7%	27.1%	28.0%

TABLE 2–6. SICKLE CELL PREPARATION TEST

Hgb solubility:	Turbid	(Clear)

TABLE 2–7. ALKALINE HEMOGLOBIN ELECTROPHORESIS

−				+
Patient			■	
Control		■	■	■ ■
Origin	▲		▲	
	A_2, C, E, O		S, D, G	F A

TABLE 2–8. CARDIAC ENZYMES

CK	46 U/L	(0–160)
CK MM	100%	(96–100)
CK MB	0%	(0–4)
LDH	550 U/L	(100–225)
LDH$_1$	34%	(17–27)
LDH$_2$	39%	(28–38)
LDH$_3$	14%	(18–28)
LDH$_4$	5%	(5–15)
LDH$_5$	8%	(5–15)

TABLE 2–9. ELECTROLYTES

Na	142 mEq/L	(134–143)
K	4.9 mEq/L	(3.5–4.9)
Cl	104 mEq/L	(95–108)
CO_2	27 mEq/L	(21–32)

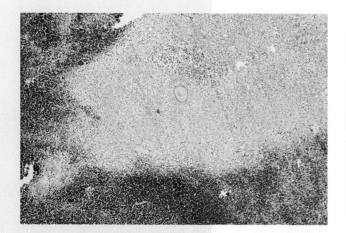

FIGURE 2–3. Spleen from another patient with this disease. Hematoxylin–eosin stain. Original magnification ×12.

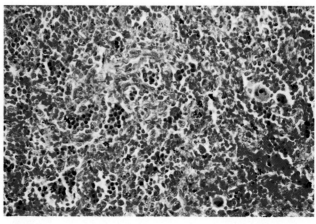

FIGURE 2–4. Spleen from another patient with this disease. Hematoxylin–eosin stain. Original magnification ×78.

▶ **Questions**

4. The patient's joint pain is most likely due to:
   a. formation of pannus
   b. hemorrhage into the joint
   c. degenerative arthritic changes
   d. vaso-occlusive complications of the patient's underlying condition

5. The abnormal red blood cell morphology seen in Figure 2–1 is due to:
   a. total lack of synthesis of the β-globin chain
   b. unusual sensitivity of the red blood cell to complement-mediated lysis
   c. vitamin B_{12} deficiency
   d. substitution of valine for glutamic acid at the 6th position of the β-globin chain
   e. deficiency of spectrin protein

6. Which of the following is the LEAST likely long-term complication of this condition?
   a. cholelithiasis
   b. splenomegaly
   c. salmonella osteomyelitis
   d. systemic iron overload
   e. bone infarction

7. The photomicrograph in Figure 2–3 shows:
   a. splenic infarction
   b. abscess
   c. leukemic infiltrate
   d. lesion typical of sarcoidosis
   e. Hodgkin's disease

8. The photomicrograph in Figure 2–4 shows:
   a. splenic infarction
   b. extramedullary hematopoiesis
   c. acute myelogenous leukemia
   d. passive congestion of spleen
   e. Hodgkin's disease

9. In this patient, the lactate dehydrogenase isoenzyme study is most consistent with:
   a. myocardial infarction
   b. hepatocellular injury
   c. red blood cell hemolysis
   d. myopathy
   e. pulmonary infarction

10. The patient's hemoglobin electrophoresis indicates the presence of:
    a. Hgb F
    b. Hgb A_{1c}
    c. Hgb S
    d. Hgb SC
    e. Hgb A_2

NOTES

▶ Figure Descriptions

Figure 2–1. Peripheral blood smear on admission. Wright/Giemsa stain. Original magnification ×630.

In addition to a decrease in the number of erythrocytes, this photomicrograph shows a number of sickled cells. The platelets and leukocytes appear normal.

Figure 2–2. Normal peripheral blood smear. Wright/Giemsa stain. Original magnification ×630.

The red blood cells are relatively uniform in size and shape, and appear to be normochromic. A polymorphonuclear leukocyte is present near the center of the image.

Figure 2–3. Spleen from another patient with this disease. Hematoxylin–eosin stain. Original magnification ×12.

This photomicrograph shows a large, pale area of infarction bordered by congested red pulp.

Figure 2–4. Spleen from another patient with this condition. Hematoxylin–eosin stain. Original magnification ×78.

The increased red cell destruction that occurs in sickle cell anemia may eventually lead to extramedullary hematopoiesis in the spleen, as seen in this image of the red pulp. Note the small groups of normoblasts (ie, irregular collections of cells with small, dark nuclei and scanty cytoplasm) in the sinusoids. Several megakaryocytes can also be identified.

▶ Answers

1. **(c)** This peripheral blood smear is characteristic of sickle cell anemia *(see description of Figure 2–1).* It shows irreversibly sickled cells (ISC). The red blood cells are not microcytic or hypochromic, there are no spherocytes, and the smear is definitely abnormal.

2. **(a)** Detection of HbS by hemoglobin electrophoresis confirms the diagnosis of sickle cell anemia. The examination of synovial fluid or radiological examination of the joints may be informative, but would not confirm the diagnosis of sickle cell anemia. Protein electrophoresis is not contributory, since the underlying problem is a hemoglobinopathy.

3. **(c)** This patient has a predominantly unconjugated hyperbilirubinemia. Although the direct bilirubin fraction is also elevated, it represents less than 18% of the total bilirubin. The causes of predominantly unconjugated hyperbilirubinemia (ie, conjugated bilirubin is less than 20% of the elevated level of total bilirubin) are limited to hemolysis, impaired hemoglobin formation, hereditary diseases of bilirubin transport into the hepatocytes, or defects of bilirubin conjugation.

4. **(d)** In sickle cell anemia, vaso-occlusive crises, which represent painful episodes of ischemic necrosis, primarily affect bones, lung, liver, brain, penis, and spleen. Formation of pannus (inflammatory synovium) or hemorrhage into the joint are not features of sickle cell anemia. Secondary degenerative arthritis may occur as a result of repeated bone infarcts in the vicinity of joints.

5. **(d)** Sickle cell anemia is a hereditary hemoglobinopathy resulting from a point mutation on the globin gene. This is associated with substitution of valine for glutamic acid at the sixth position of the β-globin chain. This changes HbA to HbS. A lack of synthesis of α- or β-globin chains is characteristic of thalassemia; spectrin is deficient in hereditary spherocytosis; unusual sensitivity of red blood cells to complement-mediated lysis is a feature of paroxysmal nocturnal hemoglobinuria; and deficiency of Vitamin B_{12} leads to megaloblastic anemia.

6. **(b)** Splenomegaly is not a feature of sickle cell anemia. Upon deoxygenation, HbS molecules undergo aggregation and polymerization, leading to sickling of the red cells. Because of their inelasticity and propensity to adhere to the capillary endothelium, sickle cells tend to occlude small blood vessels, resulting in foci of tissue hypoxia and infarction. Late in the course of this disease, these repeated episodes of vaso-occlusion in the spleen lead to progressive scarring and shrinkage in the spleen size (autosplenectomy). Cholelithiasis is very common, due to increased bilirubin production. Salmonella osteomyelitis and other infections are due to an increased susceptibility of these patients to infections. Systemic iron overload occurs due to repeated transfusions. Infarctions of bones are a direct consequence of vaso-occlusive episodes.

7. **(a)** The photomicrograph (Figure 2–3) shows a large, pale area of infarction with adjacent congested red pulp.

8. **(b)** The photomicrograph (Figure 2–4) shows extramedullary hematopoiesis in the spleen. In acute myelogenous leukemia, the sinusoids would be distended with numerous large myeloblasts. In passive congestion of the spleen, the cords appear thickened due to the deposition of collagen, sinuses appear dilated, and excessive hemosiderin deposition may be present. Tumor nodules of Hodgkin's disease would be easily identified.

NOTES

9. (c) LDH_1 and LDH_2 are present mainly in the myocardium, kidney, and red blood cells. LDH_3 is found primarily in the lung. LDH_4 and LDH_5 are present primarily in the skeletal muscle and liver. The increased LDH_1 and LDH_2 and the absence of an "LDH flip," combined with the normal CK-MB fraction seen in this patient, are consistent with chronic hemolysis.

10. (c) The patient's hemoglobin electrophoretic pattern indicates the presence of hemoglobin S (see Lab Tips).

▶ Final Diagnosis and Synopsis of Case

• Sickle Cell Anemia

This was a case of a young black man with sickle cell disease who presented with multiple veno-occlusive crises that affected primarily his bones and joints. In this case, the diagnosis of sickle cell disease, rather than trait, was based on clinical findings, a positive hemoglobin solubility test, and the hemoglobin electrophoresis, which showed that hemoglobin S was the only hemoglobin present. The presence of unconjugated hyperbilirubinemia, increased serum lactate dehydrogenase, and anemia are due to the premature sequestration and lysis of the abnormal erythrocytes.

LAB TIPS

Sickle Cell Hemoglobin Solubility Test (Sickle Cell Preparation)

When a reducing agent (sodium hydrosulfite) is added to a buffered solution of lysed red blood cells, hemoglobin S, if present, polymerizes to form a turbid solution. The test is predominantly used to screen for hemoglobin S. It will not differentiate between sickle cell trait (AS), sickle cell disease (SS), or when hemoglobin S is combined with hemoglobin C (SC). A positive test should be followed by hemoglobin electrophoresis. False positives are due to increased numbers of Heinz bodies (post-splenectomy), lipemia, abnormal γ-globulins, polycythemia, and increased numbers of nucleated red blood cells. False negatives are due to severe anemia (HbS < 7–8 g/dL), high levels of HbF (young infants), presence of plenothiazine, and deteriorated reagents.

Hemoglobin Electrophoresis

The first step in the electrophoretic separation of hemoglobin is an alkaline electrophoresis on cellulose acetate media. Hemoglobin has a negative charge at an alkaline pH and migrates toward the anode. The amino acid substitution alters the electrophoretic mobility. Some abnormal hemoglobins will migrate together (eg, S, D and G; C, E, and O). If abnormal hemoglobins are found during alkaline electrophoresis, they can usually be separated by running an acid electrophoresis on citrate agar.

HEMOGLOBIN ELECTROPHORESIS IN REPRESENTATIVE HEMOGLOBINOPATHIES

	Alkaline Electrophoresis (Cellular Acetate) − ... +				**Acid Electrophoresis (Citrate Agar)** + ... −				
	Origin	A₂, C, E, O	S, D, G	F	A	C	S	Origin	A, D, G, E, O	F
Normal adult					■				■	
Normal newborn				■	■				■	■
Sickle cell trait			■		■		■		■	
Sickle cell disease			■				■			
SC disease		■	■			■	■			
E trait		■			■				■	

The width of the band is roughly proportional to the relative amounts of hemoglobin.

▶ **Clinical History and Presentation**

A 28-year-old man was admitted to the hospital with chief complaints of nausea, vomiting, and abdominal pain. Additional symptoms included polyuria, polydipsia, and postural dizziness. The patient had a 10-year history of diabetes mellitus and multiple urinary tract infections. Physical examination revealed a pale, thin, severely dehydrated, and somewhat confused male. Blood pressure was 145/70 mmHg while sitting, heart rate was 110 beats per minute, respiration rate was 36 per minute, and oral temperature was 98.4 ° F. His chest was clear and his abdomen was soft with no organomegaly.

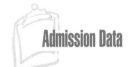

Admission Data

TABLE 3–1. HEMATOLOGY

WBC	14.3 thousand/μL	(3.6–11.0)
Neut	88%	(44–88)
Lymph	7%	(12–43)
Mono	5%	(2–11)
RBC	5.53 million/μL	(4.4–5.8)
Hgb	16.5 g/dL	(14.0–17.0)
HCT	49.3%	(40.0–49.0)
Plts	373 thousand/μL	(130–400)

TABLE 3–2. URINALYSIS

Color	Dark yellow	(Yellow)
Clarity	Hazy	(Clear)
Glucose	4+	(Neg)
Protein	4+	(Neg)
Blood	Neg	(Neg)
RBC casts	Neg	(Neg)
Granular casts	Pos	(Neg)
WBC	2/HPF	(0–5)
Ketones	3+	(Neg)
Bacteria	1+	(Neg)

TABLE 3–3. CHEMISTRY

Glucose	479 mg/dL	(65–110)
BUN	29 mg/dL	(7–24)
Creatinine	2.0 mg/dL	(0.7–1.4)
Uric acid	10.6 mg/dL	(3.0–8.5)
Calcium	10.2 mg/dL	(8.5–10.5)
Protein, total	10.3 g/dL	(6.0–8.0)
Albumin	6.1g/dL	(3.7–5.0)
LDH	333 U/L	(100–225)
Alk Phos	131 U/L	(30–120)
AST	15 U/L	(0–55)
GGTP	27 U/L	(0–50)
Amylase	30 U/L	(23–85)

TABLE 3–4. MICROBIOLOGY

Urine Culture—Negative

TABLE 3–5. ELECTROLYTES

Na	132 mEq/L	(134–143)
K	5.9 mEq/L	(3.5–4.9)
Cl	89 mEq/L	(95–108)

TABLE 3–6. ARTERIAL BLOOD GASES

pH	6.94	(7.35–7.45)
PCO_2	13 mmHg	(32–46)
PO_2	150 mmHg	(74–135)
HCO_3	3 mEq/L	(21–29)
O_2 saturation	98%	(92–96)
Base excess	−27 mEq/L	(−2–+2)

TABLE 3–7. OTHER TESTS

Patient's glycosylated hemoglobin— 16.9%	
Reference values:	
Normal (nondiabetics)	(4.0–7.0)
Diabetics—good control	(<9.0)
Diabetics—poor control	(>12.0)

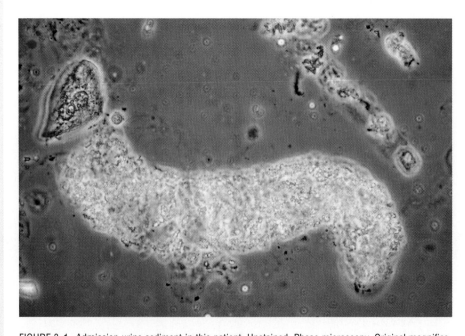

FIGURE 3–1. Admission urine sediment in this patient. Unstained. Phase microscopy. Original magnification ×125.

▶ Questions

On the basis of the preceding information you can best conclude the following:

1. This patient's hyperkalemia is most likely due to:
   a. osmotic diuresis
   b. increased respiratory rate
   c. ketoacidosis
   d. excess insulin

2. The abnormal urine sediment shown in Figure 3–1 most likely indicates:
   a. renal parenchymal disease
   b. lower urinary tract infection
   c. lower urinary tract hemorrhage
   d. transitional cell carcinoma of the urinary bladder
   e. urolithiasis

3. All of the following statements about glycosylated hemoglobin (hemoglobin A_{1c}) are true, EXCEPT:
   a. it is the product of a nonenzymatic glycosylation of protein
   b. it is the product of a slow and irreversible process
   c. it reflects the state of diabetic control during the preceding few months
   d. measurement of glycosylated hemoglobin is an obsolete test, no longer widely used

4. The patient's history of multiple episodes of urinary tract infection may be due to:
   a. impaired leukocyte function
   b. poor blood supply to tissues
   c. defects in migration and chemotaxis of leukocytes
   d. a defect in phagocytosis
   e. all of the above

5. The LEAST likely correct statement about the abnormalities found in this patient is:
   a. dehydration in this patient is mostly due to osmotic diuresis
   b. osmotic diuresis contributes to low serum sodium and chloride levels
   c. upon treatment of this patient's acute problem, he will need a potassium supplement
   d. an increase in the white blood cell count is virtually indicative of an underlying infection
   e. an increase in the total serum protein is not incompatible with the concurrent finding of proteinuria

6. Which of the following is the best interpretation of the patient's admission blood gas values?
   a. uncompensated metabolic acidosis
   b. acute respiratory acidosis
   c. fully compensated metabolic acidosis
   d. compensated respiratory acidosis

7. Which of the following statements about the urinalysis findings in this patient is correct?
   a. the glucosuria per se does not signify intrinsic renal damage
   b. the ketonuria is a typical finding in diabetic ketoacidosis and does not per se indicate intrinsic renal damage
   c. the degree of proteinuria in this patient would be best evaluated by a 24-hour quantitative analysis
   d. the presence of granular casts in this patient may be indicative of an intrinsic renal problem
   e. all of the above statements are correct

► Clinical Course

The patient was admitted to the intensive care unit and begun on intravenous fluid therapy and an insulin drip. Blood glucose levels and serum electrolytes were closely monitored. Within 24 hours, the patient's condition improved considerably and he became fully alert. On the third hospital day, he was transferred out of the intensive care unit. Six days later the patient's general condition was greatly improved and he was discharged.

TABLE 3–8. URINALYSIS—DAY 3

Color	Dark yellow	(Yellow)
Clarity	Hazy	(Clear)
Protein	4+	(Neg)
Blood	Neg	(Neg)
WBC	2/HPF	(0–5)
Bacteria	1+	(Neg)
Granular casts	Pos	(Neg)

TABLE 3–9. HEMATOLOGY—DAY 3

WBC	5.98 thousand/μL	(3.6–11.0)
RBC	4.3 million/μL	(4.4–5.8)

TABLE 3–10. CHEMISTRY—DAY 3

Glucose	131 mg/dL	(65–110)
BUN	12 mg/dL	(7–24)
Creatinine	1.1 mg/dL	(0.7–1.4)

TABLE 3–11. ELECTROLYTES—DAY 3

Na	137 mEq/L	(134–143)
K	3.7 mEq/L	(3.5–4.9)
Cl	106 mEq/L	(95–108)
CO_2	23 mEq/L	(21–32)

TABLE 3–12. ARTERIAL BLOOD GASES—DAY 3

pH	7.38	(7.35–7.45)
PCO_2	34 mmHg	(32–46)
PO_2	100 mmHg	(74–108)
HCO_3	22 mEq/L	(21–29)
O_2 saturation	94%	(92–96)

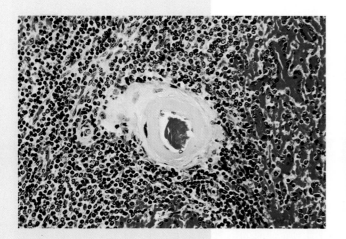

FIGURE 3–2. Splenic arteriole from another patient with this disease and hypertension. Hematoxylin–eosin stain. Original magnification ×78.

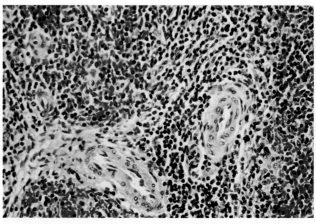

FIGURE 3–3. Normal splenic arteriole. Hematoxylin–eosin stain. Original magnification ×78.

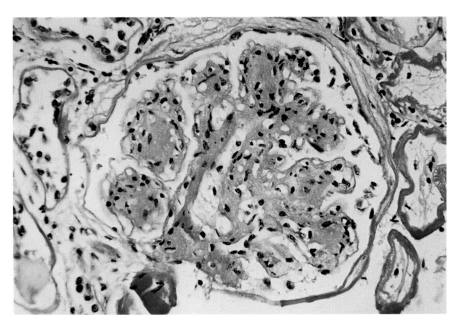

FIGURE 3–4. Renal biopsy in another patient with this disease. PAS stain. Original magnification ×78.

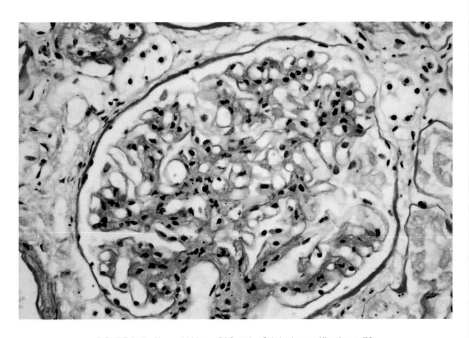

FIGURE 3–5. Normal kidney. PAS stain. Original magnification ×78.

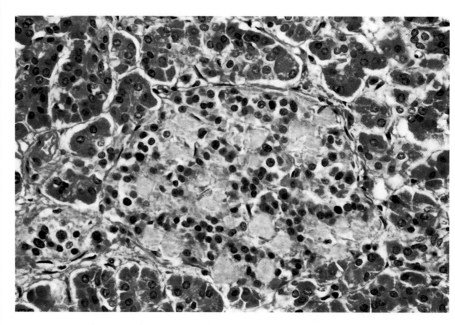

FIGURE 3–6. Pancreas in another patient with this disease. Hematoxylin–eosin stain. Original magnification ×100.

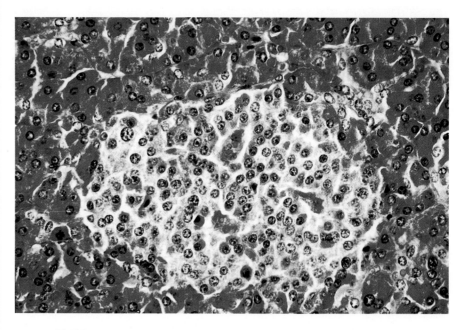

FIGURE 3–7. Normal pancreas. Hematoxylin–eosin stain. Original magnification ×100.

▷ Questions

8. The lesion depicted in Figure 3–2 represents:
    a. atherosclerosis
    b. hyaline arteriolosclerosis
    c. hyperplastic arteriolosclerosis (onion skinning)
    d. polyarteritis nodosa
    e. leukocytoclastic angiitis

9. The PAS (periodic acid-Schiff) positive material in Figure 3–4 represents:
    a. a mesangial cell proliferation
    b. an amyloid deposition
    c. acellular hyalin masses
    d. necrotic glomerular epithelium
    e. a wire-loop lesion

10. The changes noted in the islet of Langerhans seen in Figure 3–6 are most likely due to:
    a. an associated plasma cell dyscrasia
    b. deposition of amyloid
    c. ketoacidosis
    d. atherosclerosis

11. All of the following lesions are typically seen in the kidneys of diabetic patients EXCEPT:
    a. diffuse glomerulosclerosis
    b. nodular glomerulosclerosis
    c. renal microvascular disease
    d. benign nephrosclerosis
    e. renal cell carcinoma

12. Identify the correct statement about the abdominal pain with which this patient presented:
    a. it is a relatively frequent finding in diabetic patients with ketoacidosis
    b. it usually resolves upon the treatment of diabetic ketoacidosis
    c. it may be due to gastric stasis and distention resulting from metabolic abnormalities
    d. all of the above statements are correct

13. The most likely pathogenesis of this patient's condition is:
    a. delayed insulin secretion
    b. insulin resistance
    c. reduction in the beta-cell mass
    d. none of the above

▶ Figure Descriptions

Figure 3–1. Admission urine sediment in this patient. Unstained. Phase microscopy. Original magnification ×125.

The large, curved structure in the center of the photomicrograph is a granular cast. These are relatively common and can be found in a number of glomerular and tubular diseases and are frequently seen in chronic renal failure. The "granules" may represent products of cellular degradation or aggregation of serum proteins.

Figure 3–2. Splenic arteriole from another patient with this disease and hypertension. Hematoxylin–eosin stain. Original magnification ×78.

This photomicrograph is from a patient who had long-standing diabetes mellitus and hypertension. The arteriolar wall shows a homogeneous, smooth eosinophilic band of material directly beneath the endothelium. Termed hyaline arteriolosclerosis, it is found in patients with diabetes mellitus, hypertension, and in aged individuals.

Figure 3–3. Normal splenic arteriole. Hematoxylin–eosin stain. Original magnification ×78.

For comparison, here are portions of a normal splenic arteriole.

Figure 3–4. Renal biopsy in another patient with this disease. Periodic acid-Schiff (PAS) stain. Original magnification ×78.

This is a glomerulus from another patient with diabetes mellitus. Note the ovoid, pink masses in the mesangium of the glomerular lobules and the patent capillary loops peripheral to these masses. This is known as nodular glomerulosclerosis or Kimmelstiel-Wilson disease and is almost specific for diabetes mellitus.

Figure 3–5. Normal kidney. Periodic acid-Schiff (PAS) stain. Original magnification ×78.

Here the mesangium of the glomerular lobules does not show acellular masses of PAS-positive material and there are numerous open, delicate capillary loops.

Figure 3–6. Pancreas from another patient with this disease. Hematoxylin–eosin stain. Original magnification ×100.

A number of changes can occur in the pancreatic islets of patients with diabetes mellitus. In addition to a reduction in the number and size of islets, beta cells may be degranulated, islets may become fibrotic, and, as seen in this photomicrograph from another patient, the islets may be replaced by amyloid deposits. The actual material is the polypeptide amylin and it appears as irregular, acellular masses within the islet. Note also that the number of islet cells has been reduced, probably reflecting the decrease in the number of beta cells.

Figure 3–7. Normal pancreas. Hematoxylin–eosin stain. Original magnification ×100.

Note the even distribution of cells throughout the islet and the absence of any amorphous material. While the hematoxylin–eosin stain does not allow us to definitively identify the different islet cell types, we can see, based on differential stain absorption, that several types of cells are present within this islet.

▶ Answers

1. (c) The hyperkalemia in diabetic ketoacidosis is due to the movement of intracellular potassium to the extracellular compartment. Osmotic diuresis by itself leads to hypokalemia. An increased respiratory rate may lead to a diminished P_{CO_2}, but is without effect on potassium levels. Excess insulin would tend to cause a hypokalemia due to the movement of potassium into cells.

2. (a) The granular casts seen in this urinary sediment result from the disintegration of cells as they become trapped in the renal tubules within a protein matrix. This might be a result of parenchymal renal damage. It does not occur with lower urinary tract infection or hemorrhage, stones, or bladder carcinoma. All of these, however, may cause hematuria.

3. (d) The measurement of non-enzymatically glycosylated ("glycated") hemoglobin (hemoglobin A_{1c}) is a test regularly used to monitor diabetic control. Glycosylation is a slow and irreversible process that occurs throughout the life of the red blood cell in hyperglycemic persons and reflects the average degree of hyperglycemia in the preceding few months.

4. (e) Each of the listed mechanisms (impaired leukocyte function such as chemotaxis, migration, phagocytosis, and microbial killing), and a poor blood supply, all consequences of diabetes, would contribute to urinary tract and other infections.

5. (d) This patient had diabetic ketoacidosis, a major acute complication of insulin-dependent diabetes (IDDM). It may have occurred due to cessation of insulin therapy or because of physical (infection, surgery, etc) or emotional stress. The increased white blood cell count alone is not indicative of infection; it is a feature of diabetic acidosis. Infection, however, should be ruled out in the presence of specific symptoms or findings. Glycosuria produces osmotic diuresis and electrolyte loss and leads to severe dehydration. Increase in total serum protein is a reflection of an intravascular volume depletion and does not reflect the actual protein status. Therefore, the seemingly increased total serum protein level is compatible with actual protein loss via the urine. The increase in serum potassium is due to severe acidosis. In fact, this patient had an actual total body deficit of potassium (due to urinary potassium loss) and needed potassium supplementation upon correction of his acidosis.

6. (a) The patient had an acidosis, as the pH is reduced. Since the P_{CO_2} is also reduced, this was a metabolic acidosis. With an acute respiratory acidosis, the pH would be reduced, but the P_{CO_2} would be increased. In a fully compensated metabolic acidosis the pH would be within the normal range, though the P_{CO_2} would still be decreased. In a compensated respiratory acidosis, the pH would also be within the normal range though the P_{CO_2} would still be increased. The "base excess," calculable from blood gas values, was -27 mEq/L, indicating a metabolic acidosis.

7. (e) All of the statements are correct. Glycosuria occurs when the normal renal threshold for glucose reabsorption is exceeded (it roughly corresponds to serum glucose of about 180 mg/dL). Ketonuria occurs in many situations (starvation, dehydration, etc), but a severe ketonuria (4+), usually accompanied by the presence of ketones in plasma, is most often due to severe metabolic acidosis such as diabetic ketoacidosis. Glycosuria and ketonuria are not necessarily indicative of renal damage. The heavy proteinuria would be best evaluated by a 24-hour urine measurement, since the degree of urine concentration in random specimens may influence results. The presence of granular casts may be indicative of intrinsic renal damage, since granular casts result from the disintegration of the cellular material as it passes through the renal tubules. They are seen in renal parenchymal diseases, but occasional granular casts may be seen in normal urine.

8. (**b**) The lesion shown in Figure 3–2 is that of hyaline arteriolosclerosis, an arteriolar lesion often seen in hypertension. It can also be found in diabetes mellitus, usually in patients with longstanding diabetes. Hyperplastic arteriolosclerosis, in which the onion skin appearance of the arteriole wall is quite prominent (due to the reduplication, in concentric layers, of the smooth muscle cells of the vessel wall) is associated with malignant hypertension. Inflammation with neutrophils is the characteristic finding in both polyarteritis nodosa (medium and small arteries), and leukocytoclastic angiitis (venules, capillaries, and arterioles). Atherosclerosis is primarily a disease of elastic arteries. *(See description of Figure 3–2).*

9. (**c**) The nodules seen in some of the glomeruli in patients with diabetes mellitus are acellular hyaline masses at the glomerular periphery. As its name implies, in mesangial cell proliferation one finds hypercellularity of the mesangium, not seen here. The deposition of amyloid in the kidney is seen in the glomeruli (usually not in a nodular configuration), interstitium, and vessels, but it is not a feature of diabetes. The glomerular wire-loop lesion seen in systemic lupus erythematosus refers to a peculiar thickening of the glomerular capillary wall and is not seen here. *(See description of Figure 3–4).*

10. (**b**) The deposition of amyloid, in the form of a variety of amyloid derived from amylin, may occur in insulin–dependent diabetes mellitus (IDDM). However, it is more characteristic of non-insulin-dependent diabetes mellitus (NIDDM). Plasma cell dyscrasias cause widespread deposition of a different amyloid, derived from immunoglobulin light chains or light chain fragments, and does not significantly affect the islets. Atherosclerosis and ketoacidosis do not specifically affect the islets.

11. (**e**) Renal microvascular disease (hyaline arteriolosclerosis), which is also a feature of benign nephrosclerosis, and the diffuse and nodular glomerulosclerosis are all features of renal lesions in diabetes. Renal cell carcinoma is not associated with diabetic kidney disease.

12. (**d**) All of the statements are correct. The abdominal pain occurs as one of the presenting symptoms, together with nausea, vomiting, and polyuria, in patients with diabetic ketoacidosis. It usually resolves upon improvement of the metabolic acidosis. The pain is most likely due to gastric stasis and distention.

13. (**c**) This patient suffers from Type I diabetes mellitus (IDDM). This form of diabetes results from a severe, or absolute, lack of insulin due to a reduction in the beta cell mass. Other choices listed (delayed insulin secretion and insulin resistance) characterize the pathogenesis of Type II diabetes mellitus (NIDDM), not that of IDDM.

► Final Diagnosis and Synopsis of Case

- Diabetes Mellitus (Type I) With Diabetic Ketoacidosis
- Diabetic Nephropathy

A 28-year-old man with Type I diabetes mellitus presented with typical symptoms and findings of diabetic ketoacidosis. Based on his glycosylated hemoglobin level, we assumed poor control of his diabetes. The precipitating cause of this episode of ketoacidosis, however, remained unclear. The patient responded well to fluid and electrolyte replacement and to insulin and was discharged to be followed as an out-patient. This case also explored, through material obtained from other patients, some of the typical morphological findings of diabetes mellitus.

LAB TIPS

Glucose Tolerance Test

The oral glucose tolerance test in non-pregnant individuals consists of giving the patient a 75 g load of glucose over a 5-minute period and measuring the blood glucose level before the ingestion and 2 hours after the ingestion. In pregnancy, the load is 100 g of glucose, and samples are drawn before the ingestion, at 1 hour, 2 hours, and 3 hours following the glucose load. The following table is one system of interpretation of this test.

GLUCOSE TOLERANCE TEST

Classification	Fasting	1 Hour	2 Hour	3 Hour
Normal	<110 mg/dL	—	and <140 mg/dL	—
Impaired glucose tolerance	<110 mg/dL	—	and 140–199 mg/dL	—
Diabetes	≥ 140 mg/dL	—	and ≥ 200 mg/dL	—
Normal (pregnancy)	<105 mg/dL	—	—	—
Gestational diabetes	105 mg/dL	or >190 mg/dL	or >165 mg/dL	or >145 mg/dL

Microscopic Examination of Urine Sediment

Visual examination of the urine sediment is an important aid in the diagnosis of a number of diseases. The first morning urine sample will often yield the most formed elements for analysis. The urine should be examined fresh as lysis of cells and casts can occur within several hours of collection. Since many of the elements present in urine have a low refractive index, microscopic visualization is enhanced by the use of subdued brightfield illumination or by means of optical staining techniques (ie, darkfield, phase contrast, differential interference contrast, polarized light). Polarized light is especially useful to distinguish crystals and fibers from cellular or protein cast material. The formed elements that can be seen in urinary sediment include cells (epithelial cells lining the upper and lower urinary tract, leukocytes, erythrocytes), casts (matrix, inclusion, pigment, cell), crystals (normal and abnormal, drugs), artifacts (clothing fibers, spermatozoa, starch granules, oil droplets), organisms (bacteria, fungi, parasites), fat bodies, protein fibers, etc.

(Continued)

Lab Tips (continued)

Percutaneous Renal Biopsy

The objective of this procedure is to obtain a core of kidney tissue containing both cortex and medulla that can be processed for examination by light microscopy, immunofluorescence, and electron microscopy. A local anesthetic is applied to the biopsy site (angle formed by the lowest palpable rib and the lateral edge of the sacrospinal muscle) and along the biopsy tract, a small skin incision is made, and the biopsy needle is inserted along the previously anesthetized tract into the kidney. The specimen is placed on a saline-soaked gauze pad and transported to the laboratory, where it is placed in the appropriate solutions for the above requested examinations. This procedure can provide valuable information on the state of the glomeruli and tubules. It is especially useful in the diagnosis of glomerulonephritis, diabetic renal disease, and the involvement of the kidney in systemic lupus erythematosus and amyloidosis. It is not performed in patients with renal tumors, severe hypertension, uremia, or a single kidney. While it is a relatively safe procedure, complications may occur and include infection, bleeding, and hematoma formation.

► **Clinical History and Presentation**

A 45-year-old woman presented with a complaint of severe headache, fever, nausea, vomiting, and photophobia for the preceding 4 days. Three days prior to the onset of these symptoms, she had a flu-like illness with a sore throat. There was no other pertinent medical or surgical history and she was on no medications at the time. Physical examination revealed an obese female, fully oriented, with an oral temperature of 102.3 ° F. Blood pressure was 128/74 mmHg, and heart rate was 130 beats per minute. Pertinent findings included mild neck stiffness on forward flexion and a petechial rash involving the back and both lower posterior extremities. The neurological examination did not show any motor or sensory deficit. A lumbar puncture was performed, and the patient was admitted to the hospital.

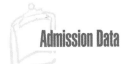 **Admission Data**

TABLE 4–1. HEMATOLOGY		
WBC	12.83 thousand/µL	(4.5–11.0)
Neut	83.7%	(44–88)
Lymph	7.3%	(12–43)
Mono	5.4%	(2–11)
Eos	2.6%	(0–5)
RBC	4.98 million/µL	(3.9–5.0)
Hgb	13.8 g/dL	(12.0–15.0)
HCT	42.6%	(36.0–44.0)
MCV	85.6 fL	(79.0–96.0)
MCH	27.8 pg	(26.0–32.0)
Plts	381 thousand/µL	(150–400)

TABLE 4–2. URINALYSIS		
pH	6.0	(5.0–7.50)
Protein	Neg	(Neg)
Glucose	Neg	(Neg)
Ketone	Neg	(Neg)
Bile	Neg	(Neg)
Occult blood	1+	(Neg)
Color	Light amber	(Yellow)
Clarity	Slightly cloudy	(Clear)
WBC	5–9/HPF	(0–5)
RBC	5–9/HPF	(0–2)
Epith. cells	20–29/HPF	(0)
Bacteria	3+	(Neg)
Mucus	1+	(Neg)
Urobilinogen	Neg	(Neg)

TABLE 4–3. CHEMISTRY

Glucose	96 mg/dL	(65–110)
BUN	11 mg/dL	(7–24)
Creatinine	1.0 mg/dL	(0.7–1.4)
Uric acid	5.1 mg/dL	(3.0–7.5)
Cholesterol	198 mg/dL	(150–240)
Calcium	8.6 mg/dL	(8.5–10.5)
Protein	6.9 g/dL	(6.0–8.0)
Albumin	3.6 g/dL	(3.7–5.0)
LDH	157 U/L	(100–225)
Alk Phos	70 U/L	(30–120)
AST	8 U/L	(0–55)
GGTP	50 U/L	(0–50)
Bilirubin	0.5 mg/dL	(0.0–1.5)

TABLE 4–4. MICROBIOLOGY

Blood culture—Pending
CSF culture—Pending
Urine culture—Pending
Throat culture—Pending

TABLE 4–5. ELECTROLYTES

Na	134 mEq/L	(134–143)
K	4.1 mEq/L	(3.5–4.9)
Cl	102mEq/L	(95–108)
CO_2	20 mEq/L	(21–32)

TABLE 4–6. CEREBROSPINAL FLUID

Color	Colorless	(Colorless)
Clarity	Clear	(Clear)
WBC	105/μL	(0–10)
Lymph	75%	(0–10)
Neut	15%	(0)
RBC	20/μL	(0)
Glucose	63 mg/dL	(40–80)
Protein, total	53 mg/dL	(15–45)
VDRL	Non-reactive	(Non-reactive)

TABLE 4–7. SEROLOGY

Lyme disease antibodies—Pending

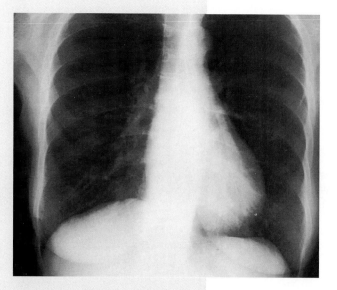

FIGURE 4–1. Patient's chest x-ray, A-P view.

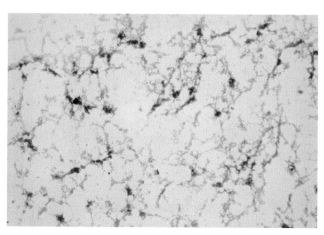

FIGURE 4–2. Cerebrospinal fluid. Gram stain. Original magnification ×197.

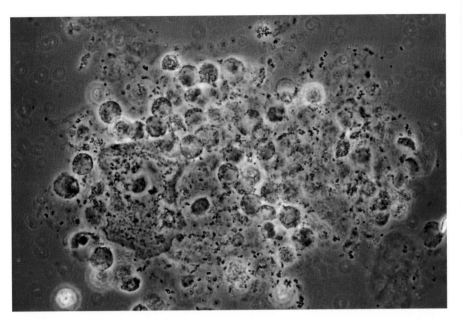

FIGURE 4–3. Admission urine sediment. Unstained. Phase microscopy. Original magnification ×125.

▶ Questions

On the basis of the preceding information, you can best conclude the following:

1. The urinalysis and the urine sediment in this patient are best characterized as:
   a. diagnostic of glomerulonephritis
   b. diagnostic of a coagulopathy
   c. diagnostic of renal tubular and/or interstitial disease
   d. suggestive of urinary tract inflammation or infection

2. All of the following statements about this patient's cerebrospinal fluid are correct EXCEPT:
   a. the cerebrospinal fluid glucose level is within the normal range in relation to the blood glucose level
   b. the number and proportion of white blood cells are characteristic of a pyogenic infection
   c. the Gram stain does not show any organisms
   d. the findings are consistent with aseptic meningitis

3. The chest x-ray in Figure 4–1 is most consistent with:
   a. tuberculosis
   b. lobar pneumonia
   c. pulmonary abscess
   d. no pulmonary pathology

4. The hematological data in this patient suggest:
   a. leukocytosis with an absolute neutrophilia
   b. leukocytosis with a relative lymphocytopenia
   c. leukocytosis with an absolute lymphocytopenia
   d. all of the above
   e. none of the above

NOTES

▶ Clinical Course

The patient was initially started on antibiotics which were later discontinued upon negative culture results. She was treated symptomatically and her condition gradually improved. By the sixth day of hospitalization, her CBC and urinalysis had returned to normal, her headache had subsided, the rash had disappeared, and her oral temperature was 98.6 ° F. A CT scan of the head was normal and the patient was discharged 7 days after admission.

TABLE 4–8. TEST RESULTS

Microbiology (Day 1 Through Week 6)	
Blood culture	No growth in 5 days
Throat culture	Normal flora
Cerebrospinal fluid cultures	No growth in 5 days
	No fungus isolated in 3 weeks
	No acid–fast bacilli isolated in 6 weeks
Urine culture	24 hour culture—Gram–negative rods (5000 colony–forming units/mL)
Serology (Day 2)	
Lyme disease antibodies	Negative

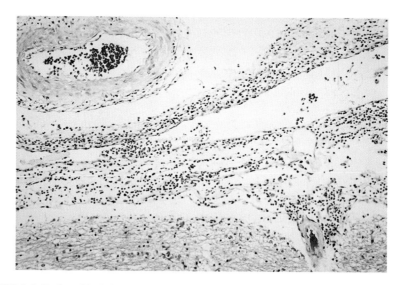

FIGURE 4–4. Portion of brain from another patient with this condition. Hematoxylin–eosin stain. Original magnification ×31.

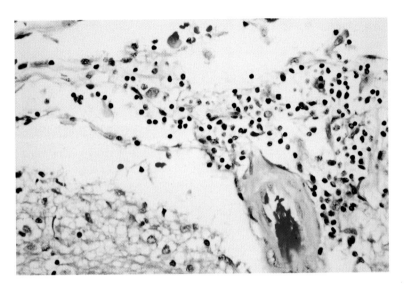

FIGURE 4–5. Portion of brain from another patient with this condition. Hematoxylin–eosin stain. Original magnification ×100.

▶ Questions

5. All of the following statements about the CNS problem this patient was diagnosed as having are correct EXCEPT:
   a. it usually affects patients under age 30
   b. it is usually a self-limited illness
   c. it usually leads to impairment of consciousness
   d. cerebrospinal fluid abnormalities may persist for several weeks in patients who are otherwise asymptomatic

6. Symptoms and clinical findings related to the CNS problem such as this patient experienced are known to be caused by:
   a. fungal infection
   b. viral infection
   c. sarcoidosis
   d. systemic lupus erythematosus
   e. all of the above

7. All of the following statements concerning this patient's condition are correct EXCEPT:
   a. the urinary tract infection was the primary cause of her central nervous system problem
   b. the patient most likely had aseptic viral meningitis
   c. her elevated temperature and skin rash were most likely due to the same etiology as her central nervous system problem
   d. in most instances, patients recover completely from this central nervous system problem

8. The microscopic appearance of the brain of another patient (Figures 4–4 and 4–5) shows:
   a. the presence of bacterial organisms
   b. the presence of an acute inflammatory cell infiltrate
   c. changes characteristic of a pyogenic process
   d. none of the above

▶ Figure Descriptions

Figure 4–1. Chest x-ray, PA.

The admission chest x–ray, as seen here, is essentially normal. There is no evidence of pneumonia, cardiac disease, or tumor.

Figure 4–2. Cerebrospinal fluid. Gram stain. Original magnification ×197.

In adults, one may find up to 5 leukocytes (lymphocytes/monocytes)/µL of cerebrospinal fluid. This patient's cerebrospinal fluid white blood cell count was elevated, mainly due to lymphocytes (normal–appearing lymphocytes). There are no microorganisms present in this photomicrograph.

Figure 4–3. Urine sediment, unstained. Phase microscopy. Original magnification ×125.

Several squamous epithelial cells, a number of white blood cells, and various bacteria can be seen in this photomicrograph of the patient's urinary sediment.

Figure 4–4. Portion of brain from another patient with aseptic meningitis. Hematoxylin–eosin stain. Original magnification ×31.

This image is from another patient with aseptic meningitis. The subarachnoid space is widened due to fluid and a cellular infiltrate, which extends into the Virchow-Robin space, but does not involve the cerebral cortex.

Figure 4–5. Portion of brain from another patient with aseptic meningitis. Hematoxylin–eosin stain. Original magnification ×100.

At higher power, we can see that the cellular infiltrate is composed of small round cells morphologically identical to lymphocytes, and of macrophages. Since acute inflammatory cells and bacterial organisms are not present, the histological picture is consistent with aseptic meningitis.

▶ Answers

1. **(d)** This patient did not have any genitourinary tract symptoms, but presented with red blood cells, white blood cells, epithelial cells, and bacteria in the urine. While the absence of casts did not exclude glomerulonephritis and tubular and interstitial disease, the findings were not sufficient in themselves for the diagnosis of any of these diseases. In coagulopathies one would expect to see mostly red blood cells in the urine and clinically, the patient did not have any symptoms of a coagulopathy. The culture results will have shown whether the patient had a bacteriuria or just an aseptic pyuria.

2. **(b)** The cerebrospinal fluid was obtained relatively late in the patient's symptomatology, a fact that should always be considered in the interpretation of the results. The glucose level was normal; the white blood cells were increased with a predominance of mononuclear cells; some red blood cells were present and there was a slight elevation of the spinal fluid protein. The Gram stain did not show any microorganisms. Such results are consistent with aseptic meningitis. In a typical pyogenic infection, the spinal fluid white blood cell count is likely to be much higher (ie, thousands), the cerebrospinal fluid glucose level would be decreased, and the protein level would be increased to over 100 mg/dL.

3. **(d)** The chest x-ray did not show any pathological pulmonary changes (such as infiltrates, lymphadenopathy, abscess, etc).

4. (**d**) This patient had a mild leukocytosis. There was a relative decrease in the lymphocyte proportion and also an absolute decrease in lymphocyte number (patient had about 935 lymphocytes/μL. Lymphopenia is defined as <1500 lymphocytes/μL). The patient had over 10,000 neutrophils/μL, which exceeds a normal neutrophil count ($<8,000/\mu$L).

5. (**c**) Aseptic or viral meningitis in the majority of cases does not cause an impairment of consciousness. More than 90% of patients are below age 30; the disease is an acute and self-limited illness. CSF abnormalities are most pronounced following 4–6 days of illness, but the cerebrospinal fluid white blood cell count may remain increased for several weeks after the patient recovers.

6. (**e**) Aseptic meningitis is an acute illness characterized by meningeal symptoms, fever, cerebrospinal fluid pleocytosis, and bacteriologically sterile cultures. It may be caused by a virus (viral meningitis) or by other agents, such as fungi, rickettsia, protozoa, etc, and also by non-infectious causes (sarcoidosis, systemic lupus erythematosus, etc).

7. (**a**) The absence of a significant growth of bacteria (ie, $>10^5$ colony-forming units/mL) in the urine culture coupled with the lack of any genitourinary symptoms makes the diagnosis of sepsis with secondary involvement of the central nervous system unlikely. The overall presentation, including the skin rash and the course of the disease, is compatible with an aseptic viral meningitis. Patients usually recover without any consequences and are entirely well within 2 weeks.

8. (**d**) The microscopic appearance of the brain (Figures 4–4 and 4–5) shows the presence of a cellular infiltrate composed of lymphocytes and some macrophages. No bacterial organisms, neutrophils, or necrosis are present.

▶ Final Diagnosis and Synopsis of Case

• Aseptic Viral Meningitis

This patient presented with a prodromal "flu-like" illness followed by an intense headache, fever, nausea, vomiting, and photophobia without any impairment of consciousness. There were signs of meningeal irritation (ie, neck stiffness), and a rash on both legs. The cerebrospinal fluid analysis showed lymphocytic pleocytosis, slightly increased protein, and a normal glucose level. Bacterial cultures were negative and the CT scan of the brain was normal. An additional abnormal finding was the presence of white blood cells, red blood cells, epithelial cells, and bacteria in her urine. On admission, the urine bacterial culture, however, did not support a diagnosis of a urinary tract infection, and the repeated urinalysis was normal. The patient was treated symptomatically, the antibiotics were discontinued after negative bacterial cultures of the cerebrospinal fluid and blood were obtained. The patient recovered without any sequelae.

   This was a typical course of uncomplicated aseptic meningitis, most likely due to a virus. A viral etiology is likely because of the prodromal symptoms. The organism, however, has not been identified in this case. It should be remembered that there are also non-viral causes of aseptic meningitis, such as intracranial infections located near meninges (ie, mastoiditis, otitis media, etc); drug-induced meningitis; meningitis associated with systemic diseases such as sarcoidosis, etc. This patient was generally in good health; the CT scan of her brain was normal and she had no other signs or symptoms to support any other cause of her meningitis.

LAB TIPS

Cerebrospinal Fluid Analysis

For the laboratory results to be meaningful, the lumbar puncture must be performed carefully and the specimens labeled accurately. While the most important role of a lumbar puncture is in the diagnosis of infective meningitides (ie, bacterial, fungal, mycobacterial, and amebic), it also plays a role in diagnosing malignancy, subarachnoid hemorrhage, multiple sclerosis, and demyelinating disorders. By ruling out a number of the above entities, it can help support a diagnosis of viral meningitis. To perform the puncture, the patient is placed on the side with the neck flexed and the knees drawn up as far as possible (ie, a fetal position), the lumbar area is thoroughly cleaned, and the needle is inserted between the 3rd and 4th lumbar vertebrae into the subarachnoid space. If the opening pressure is normal and there is no marked fall in pressure when 1–2 mL of fluid is removed, then 10–20 mL of cerebrospinal fluid may be slowly removed. The fluid is collected in three sterile tubes. The first tube collected is used for chemistry and immunology studies, the second tube is used for microbiologic studies, and the third tube is used for a cell count and differential.

The fluid is examined grossly for color and turbidity. A microscopic examination is performed to determine the number and types of cells present (ie, red blood cells, neutrophils, lymphocytes, plasma cells, eosinophils, monocytes, macrophages, and malignant cells). Chemical analysis allows measurement of total protein, albumin, IgG, myelin basic protein, C-reactive protein, glucose, lactate, enzymes, and tumor markers. Immunologic studies for antibodies or antigens can also be performed if clinically indicated in a particular case. Finally, microscopic examinations (ie, Gram stain, acid-fast stain, etc) and cultures for organisms are an important part of the laboratory evaluation of cerebrospinal fluid.

5

Chapter

A 58-Year-Old
Confused Man
With Abdominal
Pain and
Vomiting

▶ **Clinical History and Presentation**

A 58-year-old man was brought to the emergency room after he was found to be confused and complaining of abdominal pain and vomiting. The patient was known to have abused alcohol for thirty years and has been previously hospitalized for a variety of alcohol-related problems. The patient also had familial hyperlipidemia. The presenting pain was described as "dull," and had been increasing in intensity over the previous three days. The patient's wife stated that he had had a poor appetite and chronic diarrhea. On physical examination, he was confused and combative. His temperature was 99.9° F, heart rate was 84 beats per minute, blood pressure was 116/70 mmHg, and respiratory rate was 20 per minute. The skin and sclerae were icteric. Examination of the chest was unremarkable except for mild gynecomastia. There was tenderness in the right upper quadrant of the abdomen and a grossly enlarged liver was palpable. Bowel sounds were normal and the rectal examination showed a small amount of stool positive for occult blood. The extremities showed palmar erythema and asterixis.

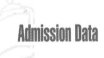 **Admission Data**

TABLE 5–1. HEMATOLOGY (SPECIMEN LIPEMIC)		
WBC	4.72 thousand/μL	(3.6–11.2)
Neut	52.4%	(44–88)
Lymph	29.1%	(12–43)
Eos	2.7%	(0–5)
Baso	1.2%	(0–2)
RBC	3.26 million/μL	(4.0–5.8)
Hgb	13.6 g/dL	(12.6–17.0)
HCT	36.6%	(42.0–52.0)
MCV	112.1 fL	(80.0–102.1)
MCH	41.6 pg	(27.0–35.0)
MCHC	37.1 g/dL	(30.7–36.7)
Plts	152 thousand/μL	(130–140)

NOTES

TABLE 5–2. CHEMISTRY (SPECIMEN LIPEMIC)

Glucose	147 mg/dL	(65–110)
BUN	4 mg/dL	(7–24)
Creatinine	0.6 mg/dL	(1.7–2.4)
Uric acid	7.2 mg/dL	(3.0–8.5)
Cholesterol	880 mg/dL	(150–240)
Calcium	8.2 mg/dL	(8.5–10.5)
Protein	5.9 g/dL	(6.0–8.0)
Albumin	2.8 g/dL	(3.7–5.0)
LDH	207 U/L	(100–225)
Alk Phos	233 U/L	(30–120)
AST	258 U/L	(0–55)
GGTP	2846 U/L	(0–50)
Bilirubin, total	5.5 mg/dL	(0.0–1.5)
Bilirubin, direct	0.32 mg/dL	(0.02–0.18)
ALT	73 U/L	(8–30)
Amylase	89 U/L	(23–85)

TABLE 5–3. COAGULATION (SPECIMEN LIPEMIC)

PT	14.5 sec	(11–14)
aPTT	26.0 sec	(22–31)

TABLE 5–4. TOXICOLOGY

ETOH	353.4 mg/dL	(0)

TABLE 5–5. ELECTROLYTES (SPECIMEN LIPEMIC)

Na	129 mEq/L	(134–143)
K	3.0 mEq/L	(3.5–4.9)
Cl	95 mEq/L	(95–108)
CO_2	22 mEq/L	(21–32)

TABLE 5–6. SEROLOGY

HAAb (Hepatitis A antibody)	Neg
HCAb (Hepatitis C antibody)	Neg
HBcAb (Hepatitis B core antibody)	Neg
HBsAg (Hepatitis B surface antigen)	Neg
HBsAb (Hepatitis B surface antibody)	Neg

TABLE 5–7. URINALYSIS

pH	6.5	(5.0–7.5)
Protein	Neg	(Neg)
Glucose	Neg	(Neg)
Bile	Trace	(Neg)
Occult blood	Neg	(Neg)
Color	Straw	(Yellow)
Clarity	Clear	(Clear)
Urobilinogen	Neg	(Neg)
WBC	6/HPF	(0–5)
RBC	0/HPF	(0–5)
Bacteria	Neg	(Neg)

NOTES

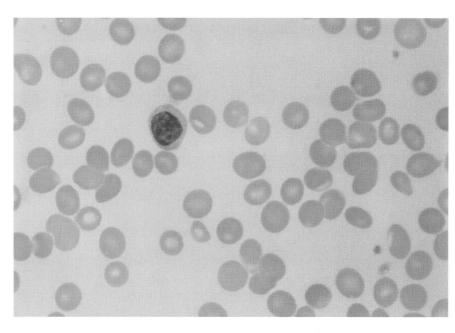

FIGURE 5–1. Admission peripheral blood smear. Wright/Giemsa stain. Original magnification ×252.

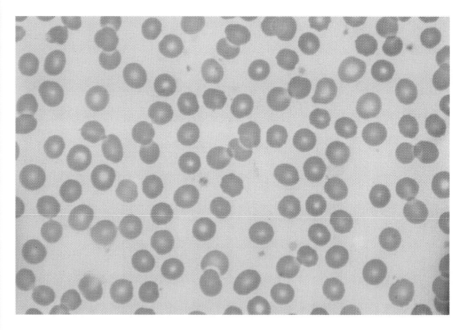

FIGURE 5–2. Normal peripheral blood smear. Wright/Giemsa stain. Original magnification ×252.

▶ **Questions**

On the basis of the preceding information, you can best conclude the following:

1. The LEAST likely problem to be considered in this patient is:
   a. gastritis
   b. alcoholic hepatitis
   c. hyperlipidemia
   d. acute alcoholic intoxication
   e. pyelonephritis

2. The patient's serum sodium and potassium were decreased. These findings may be attributable to:
   a. vomiting
   b. diarrhea
   c. liver cirrhosis
   d. all of the above
   e. none of the above

3. The patient's blood urea nitrogen level was low. This finding can be attributed to which of the following:
   a. malnutrition
   b. liver damage
   c. impaired protein synthesis
   d. all of the above
   e. none of the above

4. The patient's abnormal red blood indices and findings depicted in Figure 5–1, considered in conjunction with his other laboratory findings, are most compatible with:
   a. chronic blood loss
   b. iron deficiency
   c. liver disease
   d. none of the above

5. Identify the INCORRECT statement:
   a. the increase in serum bilirubin in this patient is most likely due to extrahepatic biliary obstruction
   b. the normal serum level of lactate dehydrogenase (LDH) does not exclude the presence of liver damage
   c. the pattern of the increase in the serum levels of "liver" enzymes is suggestive of hepatocyte injury
   d. the blood urea nitrogen level corroborates the evidence of hepatocyte injury
   e. the patient's urinalysis does not exclude the presence of hepatocyte injury

▶ Clinical Course

The patient was admitted, placed on seizure precautions and treated for acute alcohol withdrawal symptoms. He was given intravenous fluids and his electrolyte abnormalities were corrected. During his hospital stay he underwent additional studies. The results of these studies are shown below (blood chemistries, abdominal ultrasound (Figure 5–3), liver biopsy (Figures 5–5 and 5–6), and endoscopy (Figure 5–7)). The patient also underwent endocrinologic evaluation for his hyperlipidemia (results are not shown here) and an arrangement was made for him to enter an alcoholic rehabilitation program. He was also begun on medication for his gastric problem.

TABLE 5–8. CHEMISTRY

	Reference Range	Day 2	Day 4	Day 7
BUN	7–24 mg/dL	3.0	7.0	11.0
Calcium	8.5–10.5 mg/dL	7.6	9.6	9.1
Albumin	3.7–5.0 g/dL	3.6	3.5	3.6
GGTP	0–50 U/L	2462	2335	1458
Bilirubin, total	0.0–1.5 mg/dL	3.1	1.2	0.9
Electrolytes				
Potassium	3.5–4.9 mEq/L	3.4	4.5	4.4

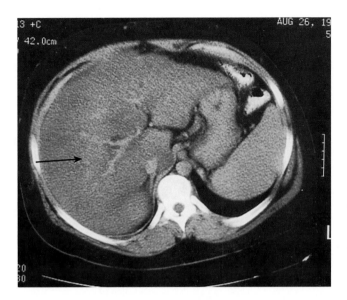

FIGURE 5–3. Abdominal CT scan.

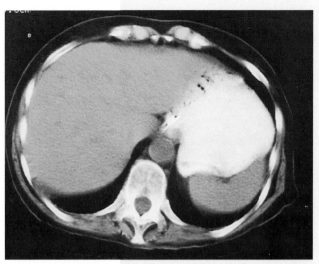

FIGURE 5–4. Normal abdominal CT scan.

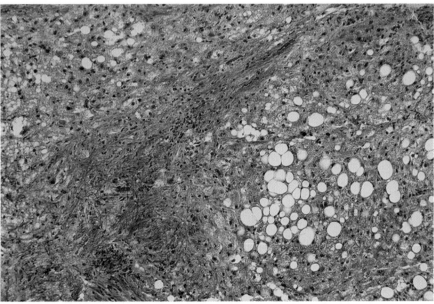

FIGURE 5–5. Liver biopsy. Trichrome stain. Original magnification ×31.

NOTES

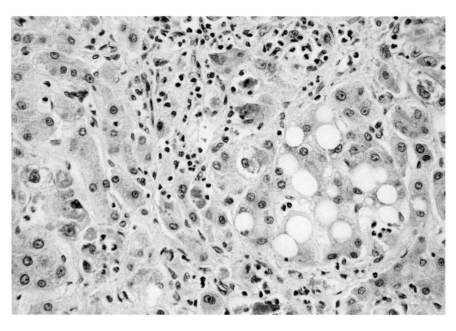

FIGURE 5–6. Liver biopsy, high power. Hematoxylin–eosin stain. Original magnification ×78.

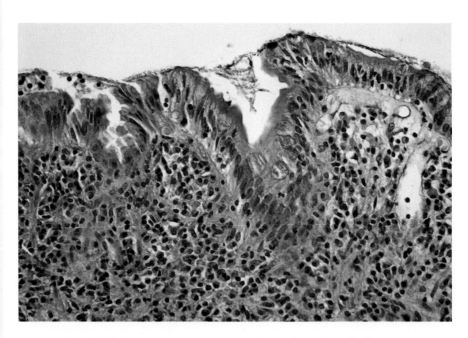

FIGURE 5–7. Gastric biopsy. Hematoxylin–eosin stain. Original magnification ×78.

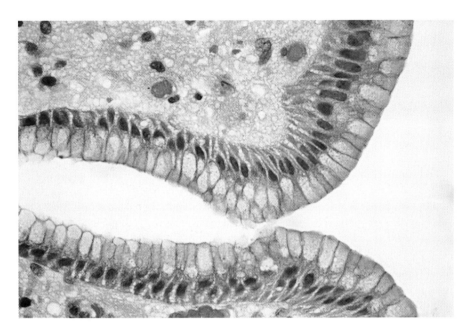

FIGURE 5–8. Normal gastric mucosa. Hematoxylin–eosin stain. Original magnification ×125.

▶ Questions

6. The microscopic appearance of the patient's liver, as shown in Figures 5–5 and 5–6 is best interpreted as being due to which of the following?
   a. cirrhosis due to primary hemochromatosis
   b. cirrhosis due to chronic ethanol ingestion
   c. metastatic adenocarcinoma
   d. acute viral hepatitis due to hepatitis B virus (HBV)
   e. sarcoidosis

7. Because of the patient's elevated "liver" enzyme values, a hepatic virus screen was ordered. It was reported as negative. In general, among adults becoming infected by hepatitis viruses, which of the following infections is most likely to lead to chronic hepatitis?
   a. hepatitis A virus (HAV) infection
   b. hepatitis B virus (HBV) infection
   c. hepatitis C virus (HCV) infection
   d. hepatitis D virus (HDV) infection
   e. hepatitis E virus (HEV) infection

8. Alcoholic hepatitis is most closely associated with which of the following histologic features?
   a. Mallory bodies and acute inflammatory cells
   b. Councilman bodies and chronic inflammatory cells
   c. "ground glass" hepatocytes
   d. hepatocytes with "sanded" nuclei
   e. none of the above

9. The histologic appearance of the gastric biopsy in Figure 5–7 is consistent with:
   a. chronic infection of gastric mucosa
   b. an immunologic disease
   c. chronic ethanol ingestion
   d. cigarette smoking
   e. all of the above

NOTES

▶ Figure Descriptions

Figure 5–1. Admission peripheral blood smear. Wright/Giemsa stain. Original magnification ×252.

The patient's macrocytic anemia is demonstrated in this photomicrograph. Most of the red blood cells are larger than normal and do not show normal central pallor. A normal lymphocyte is also present in the image.

Figure 5–2. Normal peripheral blood smear. Wright/Giemsa stain. Original magnification ×252.

At the same magnification as Figure 5–1, the increased numbers of red blood cells and the relatively smaller size of most of them as compared to the red blood cells in Figure 5–1 may be noted.

Figure 5–3. Abdominal CT scan.

Because of the large amount of fat in the hepatocytes in alcoholic cirrhosis, the liver (arrow) appears darker than the spleen on CT examination. The liver also appears coarser and there is accentuation of the portal veins.

Figure 5–4. Normal abdominal CT scan.

As can be seen in this scan, the liver always appears brighter than the spleen in the normal individual.

Figure 5–5. Liver biopsy. Masson trichrome stain. Original magnification ×31.

In this low power photomicrograph of the patient's liver, a large, blue band of fibrosis extends between the lower left and upper right corners. Additional small bands of fibrosis extend outward, adding to the disruption of the normal liver architecture. Note that fibrosis appears to engulf single hepatocytes. With increased scarring comes destruction of hepatocytes and a regenerative process, resulting in nodules, seen here on the right side of the field. A number of the parenchymal cells show a marked fatty change. These histological findings are consistent with alcoholic cirrhosis.

Figure 5–6. Liver biopsy. Hematoxylin–eosin stain. Original magnification ×78.

In this portion of the patient's liver, the disease is more active and the biopsy provides a good example of alcoholic hepatitis. A number of degenerating hepatocytes are present and contain large eosinophilic inclusions (Mallory bodies). Fibrosis and an inflammatory infiltrate (lymphocytes, macrophages, and neutrophils) accompany these degenerating parenchymal cells. Note a tendency for the neutrophils to accumulate around the cells with Mallory bodies. Fatty change is again noted in hepatocytes.

Figure 5–7. Gastric biopsy. Hematoxylin–eosin stain. Original magnification ×78.

This is an example of chronic gastritis. The mucosal inflammatory infiltrate consists predominantly of lymphocytes and plasma cells. Occasional goblet cells are seen in the lining epithelium.

Figure 5–8. Normal gastric mucosa. Hematoxylin–eosin stain. Original magnification ×125.

No inflammatory cells are present in this photomicrograph of normal gastric mucosa.

▶ **Answers**

1. (**e**) The patient's history, presentation and admission data suggest that he could have had gastritis (blood in stool), alcoholic hepatitis (liver function tests, clinical presentation, icterus), hyperlipidemia (laboratory findings), and acute alcoholic intoxication (ETOH level, confusion and combativeness). The least likely problem is the occurrence of pyelonephritis, since the patient had no complaints pointing to a urinary tract infection, and the urinalysis shows no pyuria or bacteriuria.

2. (**d**) The patient had been vomiting, had diarrhea, and had developed cirrhosis typical of alcohol abuse, with abnormal laboratory findings. All these factors are known to contribute to decreased serum sodium and potassium.

3. (**d**) Urea is produced in the liver and represents the major nonprotein nitrogen containing product of protein catabolism. Several conditions lead to a decrease in blood urea nitrogen levels: liver damage, malnutrition (insufficient protein intake), and impaired protein synthesis and catabolism.

4. (**c**) Iron deficiency and chronic blood loss cause a microcytic hypochromic anemia. Macrocytic, hyperchromic anemias can be caused by pernicious anemia (ie, vitamin B_{12} deficiency), folate deficiency, and liver disease. Alcohol also causes macrocytosis. This patient had evidence of liver disease, which together with alcohol abuse contributed to his macrocytic anemia.

5. (**a**) This patient had hyperbilirubinemia with virtually all bilirubin of unconjugated type, which is not excreted in urine. In the absence of a significant hemolytic anemia, this increase was most likely due to defective hepatic clearance of unconjugated bilirubin. Extrahepatic biliary tract obstruction initially produces an increase in conjugated bilirubin, but eventually the ratio of conjugated to unconjugated bilirubin reaches 1 to 1. This was not the case in this patient. The normal lactate dehydrogenase (LDH) serum level does not exclude the presence of injury to hepatocytes, since liver disease does not produce a marked increase in total LDH. The LDH_5 isoenzyme, however, may be increased without an apparent increase in the total LDH level. The enzymatic pattern (increased AST, GGTP, and alkaline phosphatase) points to liver damage and a low blood urea nitrogen level is also consistent with the damage to the hepatocytes.

6. (**b**) This biopsy shows fatty change and a fibrotic pattern consistent with micronodular cirrhosis. The most likely cause is chronic alcohol ingestion. Hepatitis B can cause cirrhosis only as a consequence of protracted, chronic active hepatitis. Primary hemochromatosis can cause cirrhosis, but one would also expect to see heavy hemosiderin deposition in the cytoplasm of the periportal hepatocytes. There is no evidence of metastatic adenocarcinoma or of the granulomas of sarcoidosis.

7. (**c**) Chronic hepatitis is rare after HAV infection and unknown after HEV infection. HDV can only cause infection in association with HBV, and chronic infection is relatively rare. Hepatitis B causes chronic hepatitis in about 5% of adults (though it will do so in about 90% of neonates). HCV causes chronic hepatitis in about 50% of cases.

8. (**a**) Eosinophilic Mallory bodies consisting largely of cytokeratin filaments form cytoplasmic inclusions in acute alcoholic hepatitis, and when associated with an acute inflammatory response to hepatocyte necrosis, are virtually pathognomonic of alcoholic hepatitis. Similar bodies, however, can be seen in conditions such as hepatocellular carcinoma, Wilson's disease, or primary biliary cirrhosis. Councilman bodies are seen in viral hepatitis and are associated with a chronic inflammatory infiltrate; they were first described in yellow fever. "Ground glass" hepatocytes and hepatocytes with "sanded" nuclei are associated respectively with cytoplasmic hepatitis B surface antigen (HB_sAg) and with hepatitis B core antigen (HB_cAg).

9. (e) This biopsy shows chronic superficial gastritis with a chronic inflammatory infiltrate in the mucosa. This chronic gastritis can be the result of infection with *Helicobacter pylori*, or it may result from an autoimmune disease (pernicious anemia), or from the toxic effects of chronic ethanol ingestion or cigarette smoking. Other biopsies showed acute inflammation and superficial erosions; these can also result from ethanol toxicity, or from the use of non-steroidal anti-inflammatory drugs (NSAID), such as aspirin.

▶ Final Diagnosis and Synopsis of Case

- Alcoholic Liver Disease Manifested as Alcoholic Hepatitis and Micronodular Cirrhosis
- Macrocytic Anemia Secondary to Liver Disease
- Familial Hyperlipidemia
- Gastritis

A 58-year-old man with a long history of alcohol abuse was admitted for investigation of his icterus and abdominal discomfort. His admitting data revealed macrocytic anemia, significantly increased liver enzymes and unconjugated bilirubinemia, which all indicated liver damage. His stool tested positively for occult blood. The patient was also hypokalemic, hyponatremic and his albumin was low. In addition, he had severe hyperlipidemia. During his hospital stay, the patient was stabilized and treated to prevent alcohol withdrawal symptoms. The electrolyte imbalance was corrected by intravenous fluids. The patient underwent a workup for his liver problem, which was diagnosed as alcoholic hepatitis superimposed on micronodular cirrhosis. The source of the gastrointestinal bleeding was identified by endoscopy as a superficial gastritis and the patient was started on appropriate medication. His hyperlipidemia was followed on an outpatient basis. The patient also entered an alcohol rehabilitation program.

LAB TIPS

Lactescent (Lipemic) Serum

When the serum triglyceride level exceeds 400 mg/dL, the specimen will appear milky and the results of certain laboratory tests may be affected. First, the lipid particles increase the turbidity of the sample, which will increase the absorbance of light. This can lead to a false elevation of analyte concentration in tests based on this principle. Second, interference may be due to a chemical interaction of the lipids with the test components. In theory, lactescent plasma or serum may interfere with any tests in which blood is examined without modification, and although it is possible in some cases to correct for the hyperlipidemia, the correction may not be complete. A number of the lab values in our patient may reflect, in part, the influence of his hyperlipidemia.

EFFECTS OF LACTESCENT PLASMA/SERUM ON SELECTED LABORATORY TESTS

Test	Method/Mechanism	Result
Albumin	Bromocresol Green/turbidity	False increase
Calcium	Cresolphthalein/turbidity	False increase
Amylase	Inhibition of amylase activity	False decrease
Urea	Inhibition of uricase/urease activity	False decrease
Creatine kinase	Chemical interference	False decrease
Bilirubin	Chemical interference	False decrease
Protein, total	Chemical interference	False decrease
Sodium	Electrolyte exclusion effect	False decrease
Hemoglobin	Automated cell counter	False increase
MCH and MCHC	False elevation of hemoglobin	False increase

▶ **Clinical History and Presentation**

A 73-year-old man was brought to the emergency room complaining of severe abdominal pain. The pain had begun 2 days previously, was accompanied by nausea and vomiting, and had become progressively worse. The pain was most severe in the epigastrium and radiated to his back, but not to his chest. The patient had no history of peptic ulcer or gallstones. He denied smoking or the consumption of alcohol. He was afebrile on admission. Blood pressure was 115/85 mmHg, heart rate was 92 beats per minute, and respiratory rate was 20 per minute. The sclerae were icteric. The abdomen was extremely tender. Bowel sounds were diminished. Rectal examination revealed normal sphincter tone and stool was negative for occult blood.

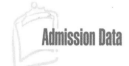 **Admission Data**

TABLE 6–1. HEMATOLOGY		
WBC	13.7 thousand/μL	(3.6–11.2)
Neut	92%	(44–88)
Lymph	3%	(12–43)
Mono	5%	(2–11)
RBC	5.5 million/μL	(4.0–5.6)
Hgb	15.1 g/dL	(12.6–17.0)
HCT	47.2%	(37.2–50.4)
MCV	85.8 fL	(80.5–102.1)
MCH	27.5 pg	(27.0–35.0)
Plts	208 thousand/μL	(130–400)

TABLE 6–2. URINALYSIS		
pH	5	(5.0–7.5)
Protein	Neg	(Neg)
Glucose	1+	(Neg)
Ketones	Neg	(Neg)
Bilirubin	Pos	(Neg)
Occult blood	Neg	(Neg)
Color	Orange	(Yellow)
Clarity	Hazy	(Clear)
Sp. grav	1.019	(1.010–1.035)
WBC	15–19/HPF	(0–5)
RBC	0/HPF	(0–2)
Epith. cells	5–9/HPF	(0)
Casts	Neg	(Neg)
Urobilinogen	Neg	(Neg)

NOTES

TABLE 6–3. CHEMISTRY		
Glucose	184 mg/dL	(65–110)
BUN	21 mg/dL	(7–24)
Creatinine	1.3 mg/dL	(0.7–1.4)
Calcium	9.3 mg/dL	(8.5–10.5)
Protein, total	7.1 g/dL	(6.0–8.0)
Albumin	4.4 g/dL	(3.7–5.0)
LDH	450 U/L	(100–225)
Alk Phos	238 U/L	(30–120)
AST	392 U/L	(0–55)
GGTP	242 U/L	(0–50)
Bilirubin	3.7 mg/dL	(0–1.5)
Bilirubin, direct	2.85 mg/dL	(0.02–0.18)

TABLE 6–4. SPECIAL CHEMISTRY		
Serum amylase	3429 U/L	(23–85)
Serum lipase	216 U/L	(4–24)
Urinary amylase (2 hour timed specimen)	510 U/hr	(3–22)

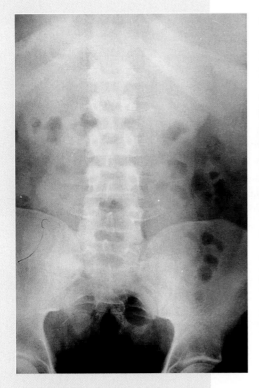

FIGURE 6–1. Admission flat plate of abdomen.

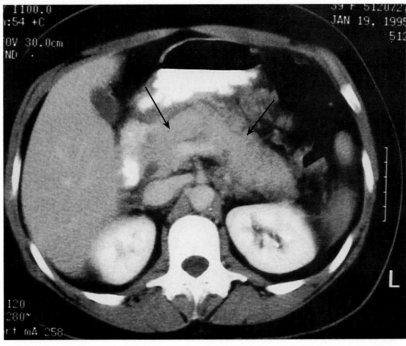

FIGURE 6–2. Abdominal CT in patient.

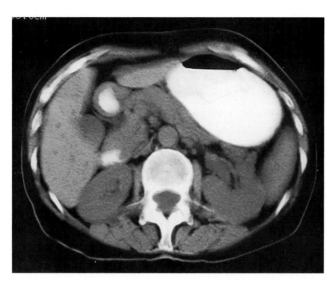

FIGURE 6–3. Normal CT of abdomen.

Questions

On the basis of the preceding information, you can best conclude the following:

1. This patient's abdominal pain is most likely due to:
   a. perforated viscus
   b. myocardial infarction
   c. dissecting aneurysm of the aorta
   d. pancreatitis

2. This patient's serum amylase level is elevated. This increase in serum amylase is known to be associated with any of the following EXCEPT:
   a. cholecystitis
   b. pancreatitis
   c. intestinal infarction
   d. myocardial infarction

3. Identify the INCORRECT statement about bilirubin in the urine of this patient:
   a. it is water soluble
   b. it is not toxic to the tissues
   c. it is one of the consequences of hemolysis
   d. it is the predominant bilirubin fraction in this patient

4. Which of the following statements concerning the laboratory findings in this patient is correct?
   a. the elevated serum amylase and glucose could be due to the same underlying pathological condition
   b. the elevated serum lipase and glucose could be due to the same underlying pathological condition
   c. the changes in levels of liver enzymes and bilirubin are consistent with cholestasis
   d. all of the above
   e. none of the above

▶ Clinical Course

The patient's pain continued and he was treated conservatively for his primary problem. His CBC and chemistries were closely monitored *(see Table 6–5)*. On day 6 of the admission, a gallbladder ultrasound was performed and showed multiple gallstones. He was taken to the operating room on day 10 for a cholecystectomy.

TABLE 6–5. LABORATORY DATA, DAYS 3 TO 12

Test	Reference Range	Day 3	Day 6	Day 10	Day 12
Hematology					
WBC	3.6–11.1 thousand/μL	17.93	12.8	11.9	9.2
Hgb	12.6–17.0 g/dL	14.5	13.5	14.3	12.4
HCT	37.2–50.4%	44.5	40.5	44.2	37.9
Plts	130–400 thousand/μL	178	220	311	214
Chemistry					
Glucose	65–110 mg/dL	122	136	102	134
BUN	7–24 mg/dL	15	17	17	10
Creatinine	0.7–1.4 mg/dL	1.3	1.4	1.4	1.2
Calcium	8.5–10.5 mg/dL	9.0	8.5	9.2	7.6
LDH	100–225 U/L	325	234	241	247
Alk Phos	30–120 U/L	238	185	203	153
AST	0–55 U/L	55	31	33	67
GGTP	0–50 U/L	147	99	108	91
Bilirubin	0.0–1.5 mg/dL	3.0	1.2	0.7	0.6
Bilirubin, direct	0.02–0.18 mg/dL	1.53	0.54	0.31	0.26
Special Chemistry					
Amylase, serum	23–85 U/L	78	106	117	90
Lipase, serum	4–24 U/L	11	27	34	25
Electrolytes					
Sodium	134–143 mEq/L	133	135	131	127
Potassium	3.5–4.9 mEq/L	4.3	2.9	4.5	4.0
Chloride	95–108 mEq/L	96	101	95	94
CO_2	21–32 mEq/L	23	24	26	26

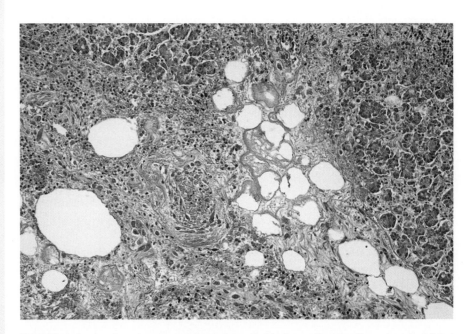

FIGURE 6–4. Portion of pancreas from another patient with this disease. Hematoxylin–eosin stain. Original magnification ×31.

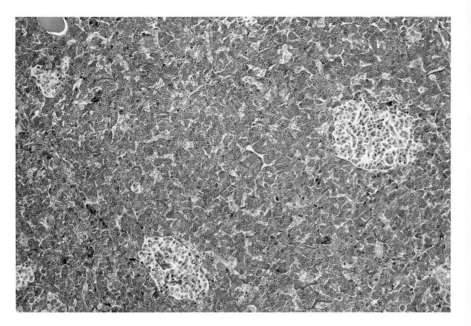

FIGURE 6–5. Normal pancreas. Hematoxylin–eosin stain. Original magnification ×31.

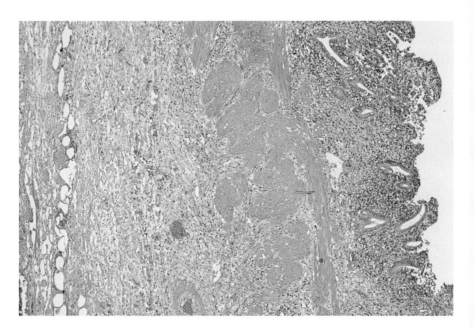

FIGURE 6–6. Portion of patient's gallbladder. Hematoxylin–eosin stain. Original magnification ×12.

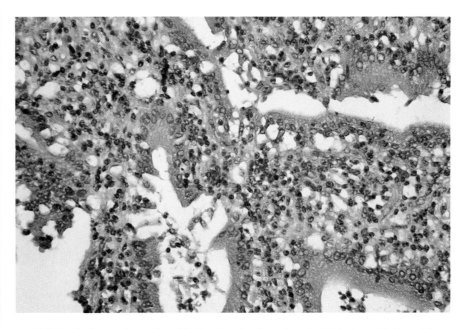

FIGURE 6–7. Portion of patient's gallbladder. Hematoxylin–eosin stain. Original magnification ×78.

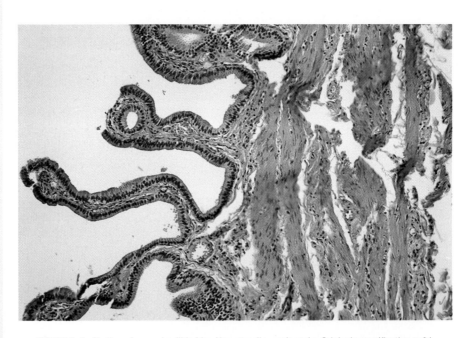

FIGURE 6–8. Portion of normal gallbladder. Hematoxylin–eosin stain. Original magnification ×31.

▶ **Questions**

5. The histologic findings in Figure 6–4 are most consistent with:
   a. pancreatic carcinoma
   b. diabetes mellitus
   c. pancreatic pseudocyst
   d. acute pancreatitis

6. The histologic findings in Figures 6–6 and 6–7 are most consistent with:
   a. cholecystitis
   b. cholecystitis and neoplastic changes
   c. gangrene
   d. normal gallbladder

7. The pathogenesis of the pattern of tissue injury responsible for the patient's primary acute problem for which he was admitted may include:
   a. acinar cell injury by ethanol
   b. duct obstruction with rupture of ductules
   c. activation of hydrolytic enzymes
   d. all of the above
   e. none of the above

8. All of the following statements concerning this patient's metabolic abnormalities are correct EXCEPT:
   a. increased serum total and direct bilirubin are most likely due to cholelithiasis
   b. decreased serum calcium level is due to accelerated gallstone formation
   c. the abnormal liver function enzymes reflect mild cholestasis
   d. the sustained white blood cell elevation most likely reflects an inflammatory rather than an infectious process
   e. the elevated urine bilirubin is consistent with biliary obstruction

9. All of the following statements about the primary acute problem for which this patient was admitted are correct EXCEPT:
   a. it affects less than 10% of patients with gallstones
   b. it may lead to pseudocyst formation
   c. it may lead to shock
   d. it is hereditary
   e. it is not of neoplastic character

NOTES

▶ Figure Descriptions

Figure 6–1. Flat plate of abdomen.

The abdominal flat plate was made to look for the presence of free air in the abdominal cavity secondary to a perforated viscus. The radiograph demonstrates a normal gas pattern, bony structures, and soft tissue outlines. There is no evidence of intra-abdominal free air or fluid.

Figure 6–2. Abdominal CT.

The pancreas (arrows) is diffusely enlarged and not sharply defined. The peripancreatic fat planes have been destroyed by edema and an inflammatory infiltrate. These radiographic findings are consistent with acute pancreatitis.

Figure 6–3. Normal abdominal CT.

In another patient, at a slightly different level, the normal pancreas is easily identified and readily separated from the surrounding structures by the peripancreatic fat planes.

Figure 6–4. Portion of pancreas from another patient. Hematoxylin–eosin stain. Original magnification ×31.

The histologic findings in acute pancreatitis, seen in this photomicrograph from another patient, include fat necrosis, destruction of acinar cells, and an inflammatory infiltrate.

Figure 6–5. Normal pancreas. Hematoxylin–eosin stain. Original magnification ×31.

The acinar cells are intact, fat necrosis is not present, and no inflammatory cells are present. Several normal islets may be seen in the photomicrograph.

Figure 6–6. Portion of gallbladder from patient. Hematoxylin–eosin stain. Original magnification ×12.

This low-power photomicrograph of the gallbladder shows a marked thickening of the gallbladder wall. The thickening is due to fibrosis and inflammation. The mucosa is ulcerated and focally hemorrhagic.

Figure 6–7. Portion of gallbladder from patient. Hematoxylin–eosin stain. Original magnification ×78.

In an area of the gallbladder where the mucosa is still intact, an inflammatory infiltrate, composed mainly of neutrophils, is present. Lymphocytes and macrophages are also present and in other sections were focally predominant. The findings in Figures 6–6 and 6–7 are consistent with a diagnosis of acute and chronic cholecystitis.

Figure 6–8. Normal gallbladder. Hematoxylin–eosin stain. Original magnification ×31.

This photomicrograph is at a higher magnification than Figure 6–6, yet we can easily view the entire gallbladder wall, an indication that it is not thickened. No inflammation is apparent.

▶ Answers

1. (**d**) This patient's acute abdominal pain was due to acute pancreatitis. A perforated duodenal ulcer can be excluded by the absence of free air in the x-ray of the abdomen. While the pain of myocardial infarction or dissecting aneurysm of the aorta can radiate to the abdomen, these conditions are not associated with a rise in serum amylase and serum lipase, as is characteristic of most cases of acute pancreatitis.

2. (**d**) While a rise in serum amylase is characteristic of acute pancreatitis, it can also occur in acute cholecystitis and intestinal infarction. It is not associated with myocardial infarction.

3. (**c**) The patient had predominantly conjugated hyperbilirubinemia due to cholestasis (the total serum bilirubin is increased and the direct (conjugated) fraction is greater than 50% of the total bilirubin level). Conjugated bilirubin is water soluble, nontoxic and, when produced in excess, is excreted by the kidney (in contrast to unconjugated bilirubin). Hemolytic anemia leads to excess production of unconjugated bilirubin, which is not excreted in urine.

4. (**d**) All of the statements are correct. The patient had acute pancreatitis, which causes elevation of serum amylase and lipase. Hyperglycemia is common and is due to multiple factors, including decreased insulin release, increased output of adrenal glucocorticoids, catecholamines, and increased glucagon release. The elevation of liver enzymes and predominantly conjugated hyperbilirubinemia are consistent with cholestasis.

5. (**d**) The photomicrograph shown in Figure 6–4 shows necrosis of pancreatic tissue, with acute inflammation and fat necrosis, as is characteristic of acute pancreatitis. The image does not show neoplastic tissue, the islet changes (amyloid) sometimes seen in diabetes, or the chronic inflammation associated with pancreatic pseudocysts.

6. (**a**) The histologic findings show changes in the gallbladder wall most consistent with cholecystitis. *(See descriptions of Figures 6–6 and 6–7)*. The glandular changes are reactive in nature and not neoplastic. The wall is not necrotic and perforated, which are features of a gangrenous cholecystitis.

7. (**d**) All three of the factors mentioned can contribute to the evolution of acute pancreatitis. Ethanol has been thought to impair the apical secretion of pancreatic enzymes, which can then enter lysosomes and become activated, injuring the parenchymal cells; or injure these cells directly. Ductal obstruction, (eg, cholelithiasis), can lead to rupture of ductules and the escape of activated enzymes into the interstitium.

8. (**b**) Any incorporation of calcium into gallstones, even if sufficient to render them radiopaque, is quantitatively trivial in relation to the sequestration of calcium in calcium soaps characteristic of acute pancreatitis. Moreover, such incorporation would be a slow process, and would not cause an acute hypocalcemia, in contrast with the effect of the calcium sequestration occurring in acute pancreatitis. Leukocytosis is a feature of acute pancreatitis, as is a rise in serum bilirubin, if the pancreatitis is related to biliary tract obstruction. Urinary bilirubin is increased, and urinary urobilinogen is negative in biliary obstruction.

9. (**d**) The patient was admitted with acute pancreatitis. He was also diagnosed to have cholelithiasis. Acute pancreatitis occurs in about 5% of patients with gallstones. One of the complications of acute (but more often of chronic) pancreatitis is a formation of localized collections of pancreatic secretions, called pseudocysts. Acute pancreatitis is an inflammatory, not neoplastic, condition, which may lead to severe systemic complications, such as peripheral vascular collapse and shock. About 5% of patients die of shock during the first week of the clinical course. There is no indication that acute pancreatitis belongs to the group of hereditary disorders.

▶ Final Diagnosis and Synopsis of Case

• Acute Pancreatitis, Secondary to Acute and Chronic Cholecystitis With Cholelithiasis

This case demonstrates acute pancreatitis associated with cholecystitis and cholelithiasis in an elderly male. Biliary tract disease, which was present in this patient, and alcoholism, not a factor here, are associated with 80% of the cases of acute pancreatitis. Typical features of acute pancreatitis seen in this patient included acute abdominal pain, nausea, vomiting, leukocytosis, increased serum and urinary amylase, increased serum lipase, a drop in serum calcium levels, and features of mild cholestasis. This was a relatively mild course of the disease and did not lead to such feared complications as disseminated intravascular coagulation, adult respiratory distress syndrome, acute renal failure, or shock. The patient clinically improved after the surgery (cholecystectomy).

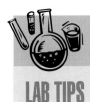

LAB TIPS

Amylase Determination in Serum and Urine

α-amylase is a metalloenzyme that hydrolyzes the α–1,4-glucosidic linkages in polysaccharides. A number of isoenzymes exist and they can be generally separated into those that are synthesized by the acinar cells of the pancreas (pancreatic amylase) and those that are derived from parotid gland, lung, liver, etc, (salivary amylase). Amylase is a relatively small molecule that is easily filtered by the renal glomeruli and partially reabsorbed by the renal tubules. Since it is not absorbed across the normal gastrointestinal mucosa, increased serum activity can be seen when there is decreased renal clearance (ie, renal failure) and in conditions in which there is increased leakage from the acinar cells directly into the blood stream or into the surrounding lymphatics. There are a large number of different methods available for the determination of amylase activity and the units from one method cannot usually be converted into the units of another method.

Within 6–48 hours of the onset of acute pancreatitis, serum amylase activity rises in 80% of patients. It returns to normal levels in 3–5 days if tissue necrosis is limited or the attack is not complicated by pseudocyst formation. The level of activity is not usually correlated with the severity of the disease. Urine amylase activity increases shortly after the rise in serum activity and usually persists slightly longer. Normal serum amylase activity is seen in 20% of patients with acute pancreatitis and activity may be falsely decreased in hyperlipemic states. In addition to acute pancreatitis, amylase activity may be increased in pancreatic carcinoma with obstruction, diabetic ketoacidosis, cholecystitis, peptic ulcer disease, viral hepatitis, lung and ovarian carcinomas, salivary gland inflammations (ie, mumps), ruptured ectopic pregnancy, appendicitis, dissecting aortic aneurysm, renal failure (ie, decreased clearance), and in patients with macroamylasemia (ie, amylase bound to immunoglobulin and thus too large to be cleared by the kidney). Conditions in which activity may be decreased include chronic pancreatitis, congestive heart failure, pregnancy (late), and pleurisy.

Serum Lipase Determination

Since lipase is produced predominantly in the pancreas, it is considered a specific marker for pancreatic disease. Lipase hydrolyzes triglycerides, present in micelles, into monoglycerides. Because of problems in the test procedure, lipase has not been used as often as amylase for the diagnosis of acute pancreatitis. However, with the elucidation of the role of co-lipase, a protein needed for pancreatic lipase activity against micellar triglycerides, and its inclusion in some test kits, the performance of the lipase assay has improved markedly and its use in the diagnosis of pancreatitis should increase.

Lipase activity increases within 12 hours of an attack of acute or chronic pancreatitis, remains elevated for up to 7–10 days, and does not always coincide with the rise in serum amylase activity. When used with amylase activity, the diagnostic sensitivity for acute pancreatitis approaches 100%.

▶ **Clinical History and Presentation**

An 82-year-old woman was brought to the emergency room with a chief complaint of severe shortness of breath and a feeling of heaviness over her anterior chest. Her symptoms had begun approximately four hours previously and were increasing in severity. The patient had a long history of hypertension which had been well controlled by medications. She had had several cerebrovascular accidents which had left her bedridden with contractures of the extremities and neurogenic bladder dysfunction. Recently, she had developed a mild diabetes mellitus which was controlled by diet. Physical examination revealed a pale, anxious woman with severe shortness of breath. Blood pressure was 130/80 mmHg, heart rate was 112 beats per minute, respiratory rate was 36 per minute, and temperature was 99.1 ° F. Pertinent physical findings included bilateral pulmonary rales and multiple contractures of the extremities. A Foley catheter was in place. An electrocardiogram showed changes consistent with anterior ventricular wall ischemia.

Admission Data

TABLE 7–1. HEMATOLOGY

WBC	12.18 thousand/μL	(3.3–10.5)
Neut	75%	(44–88)
Lymph	20%	(12–43)
Mono	5%	(2–11)
RBC	3.19 million/μL	(3.9–5.1)
Hgb	10.0 g/dL	(11.6–15.6)
HCT	29.5%	(35.0–47.0)
MCV	92.2 fL	(83.0–99.0)
MCH	31.4 pg	(27.8–32.6)
MCHC	34 g/dL	(31.0–36.0)
Plts	375 thousand/μL	(130–400)

TABLE 7–2. CHEMISTRY

Glucose	281 mg/dL	(65–110)
BUN	61 mg/dL	(7–24)
Creatinine	1.5 mg/dL	(0.7–1.4)
Uric acid	8.2 mg/dL	(3.0–7.5)
Cholesterol	235 mg/dL	(150–240)
Calcium	8.5 mg/dL	(8.5–10.5)
Protein	6.2 g/dL	(6–8)
Albumin	3.0 g/dL	(3.7–5.0)
LDH	230 U/L	(100–225)
Alk Phos	115 U/L	(30–120)
AST	119 U/L	(0–55)
GGTP	49 U/L	(0–50)
Bilirubin	0.8 mg/dL	(0.0–1.5)

TABLE 7–3. ELECTROLYTES

Na	140 mEq/L	(134–143)
K	3.9 mEq/L	(3.5–4.9)
Cl	99 mEq/L	(95–108)
CO_2	24 mEq/L	(21–32)

TABLE 7–4. CARDIAC ENZYMES

CK	213 U/L	(0–130)
CK MM	97%	(96–100)
CK MB	3%	(0–4)
LDH, total	230 U/L	(100–225)
LDH_1	19%	(17–27)
LDH_2	31%	(28–38)
LDH_3	20%	(18–28)
LDH_4	14%	(10–16)
LDH_5	16%	(6–13)

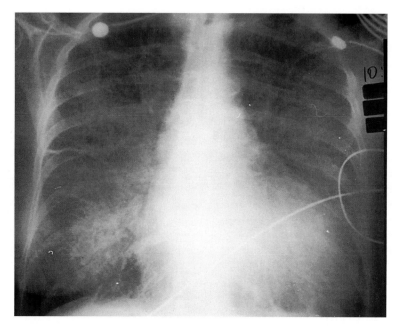

FIGURE 7–1. Chest x-ray on admission.

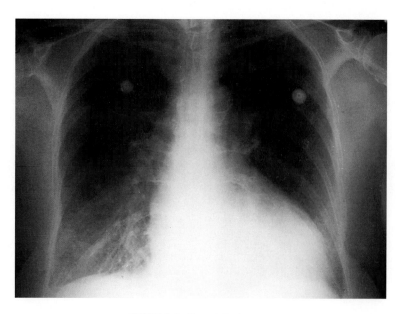

FIGURE 7–2. Normal chest x-ray.

▶ Questions

On the basis of the preceding information, you can best conclude the following:

1. Prior to obtaining laboratory and other admission data, you would consider which of the following to be a cause of her severe dyspnea?
   a. pulmonary embolus
   b. pneumonia
   c. congestive heart failure secondary to hypertensive heart disease
   d. myocardial infarction
   e. all of the above

2. The chest x-ray shows:
   a. right lower lobe pneumonia
   b. a pulmonary abscess
   c. emphysema
   d. pneumothorax
   e. pulmonary edema

3. The microscopic appearance of this patient's lung would LEAST likely show:
   a. widening of alveolar septa
   b. edema fluid in the alveolar spaces
   c. the presence of an acute inflammatory infiltrate in the alveoli
   d. congested capillaries

4. All of the following statements about azotemia in this patient are correct EXCEPT:
   a. it is likely to be related to the left-sided heart failure
   b. it is likely to be due to the reduction in renal perfusion
   c. this type of azotemia is likely to be caused by an increase in cardiac output
   d. a condition leading to this type of azotemia leads to activation of the renin-angiotensin-aldosterone system

5. Results of the cardiac enzymes at this stage of the patient's symptomatology:
   a. exclude the diagnosis of myocardial infarction
   b. confirm the diagnosis of myocardial infarction
   c. confirm the diagnosis of pulmonary embolus
   d. are not conclusive and the test should be repeated

NOTES

▶ Clinical Course

The patient was admitted to the CCU and monitored according to CCU protocol. She required invasive hemodynamic monitoring to maximize cardiac output and mechanical ventilation to maintain adequate oxygenation. She remained virtually anuric and expired 28 hours after admission. Her laboratory data are summarized below. An autopsy was performed.

TABLE 7–5. CHEMISTRY

	18 Hours Post Admission	26 Hours Post Admission	Reference Range
BUN	80 mg/dL	92 mg/dL	7–24 mg/dL
Creatinine	1.9 mg/dL	2.0 mg/dL	0.7–1.4 mg/dL

TABLE 7–6. ELECTROLYTES

	18 Hours Post Admission	26 Hours Post Admission	Reference Range
Na	138 mEq/L	135 mEq/L	134–143 mEq/L
K	5.6 mEq/L	6.8 mEq/L	3.5–4.9 mEq/L
Cl	96 mEq/L	92 mEq/L	95–108 mEq/L

TABLE 7–7. CARDIAC ENZYMES

	18 Hours Post Admission	26 Hours Post Admission	Reference Range
CK	3380 U/L	3532 U/L	0–130 U/L
CK MM	85%	83%	96–100%
CK MB	15%	17%	0–4%
LDH, total	1330 U/L	1410 U/L	100–225 U/L
LDH_1	31%	30%	17–27%
LDH_2	29%	28%	28–38%
LDH_3	18%	18%	18–28%
LDH_4	5%	6%	10–16%
LDH_5	17%	18%	6–13%

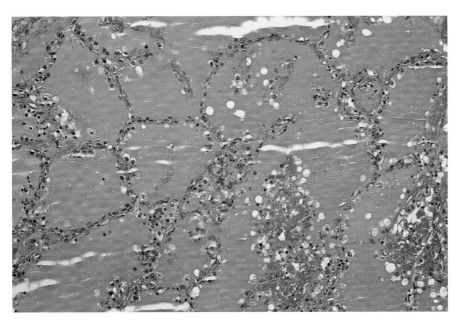

FIGURE 7–3. Portion of right lung. Hematoxylin–eosin stain. Original magnification ×31.

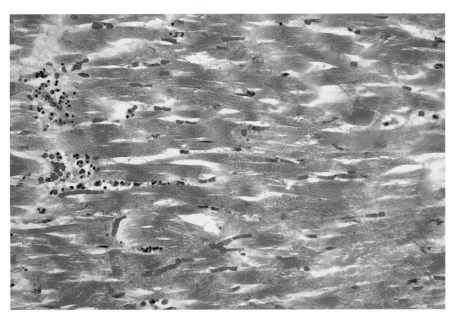

FIGURE 7–4. Left ventricular myocardium. Hematoxylin–eosin stain. Original magnification ×78.

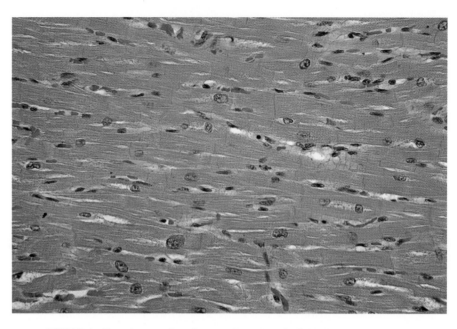

FIGURE 7–5. Normal myocardium. Hematoxylin–eosin stain. Original magnification ×78.

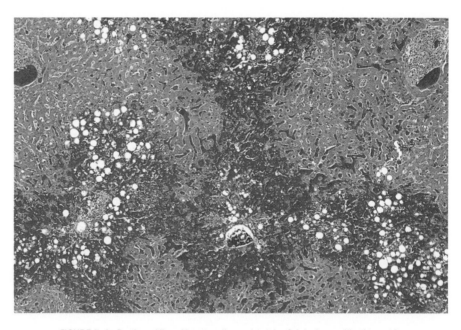

FIGURE 7–6. Portion of liver. Hematoxylin–eosin stain. Original magnification ×12.

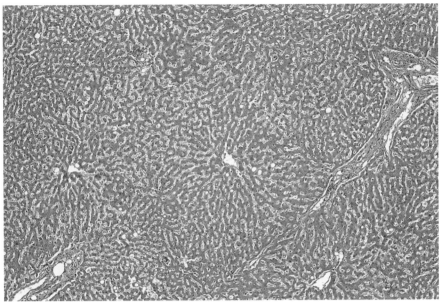

FIGURE 7–7. Normal liver. Hematoxylin–eosin stain. Original magnification ×12.

▶ Questions

6. A microscopic examination (Figure 7–4) of the heart shows all of the following EXCEPT:
   a. changes typical of coagulative necrosis
   b. the presence of acute inflammatory cells
   c. changes consistent with acute myocardial infarction
   d. a scar in the myocardium suggesting an old myocardial infarction

7. In the condition with which this patient presented, one would expect all of the following EXCEPT:
   a. the total serum lactate dehydrogenase (LDH) level to be increased 3–6 hours after the onset of symptoms
   b. the LDH_1 isoenzyme serum level to be higher than LDH_2 isoenzyme level 36 hours after the onset of symptoms
   c. the total serum creatine kinase (CK) level to be maximally increased about 24 hours after the onset of symptoms
   d. the normal serum creatine kinase level 4 days after the onset of symptoms
   e. elevated creatine kinase-MB fraction 8 hours after the onset of symptoms

8. The microscopic appearance of the liver in Figure 7–6 shows:
   a. changes consistent with chronic active hepatitis B infection
   b. changes consistent with cirrhosis
   c. changes consistent with congestion
   d. changes consistent with sarcoidosis
   e. none of the above

9. All of the following statements about this patient's condition are correct EXCEPT:
   a. an increased serum potassium is most likely due to the use of diuretics
   b. the azotemia is due to decreased cardiac output
   c. the cardiac enzyme profile supports the diagnosis of an acute myocardial infarction
   d. the symptoms and post-mortem findings reveal heart failure
   e. microscopic examination of the heart revealed the presence of myocardial infarction

NOTES

▶ Figure Descriptions

Figure 7–1. Chest x-ray on admission.

The chest x-ray shows a haziness in the perihilar regions and the pulmonary vascular markings are not well-defined. These changes are consistent with bilateral pulmonary edema. EKG leads can be seen in the x-ray.

Figure 7–2. Normal chest X-ray.

The perihilar regions appear clear and the vascular markings are fairly sharply defined. EKG leads can be seen in the x-ray.

Figure 7–3. Portion of right lung. Hematoxylin–eosin stain. Original magnification ×31.

Both lungs were large and heavy. The right lung weighed 625 grams, though the average weight of the right lung in an adult female is 450 grams. Sectioning produced large amounts of frothy fluid on the cut surface. This photomicrograph is representative of the histologic findings in both lungs and shows a pale pink-staining fluid filling the alveolar spaces. Scattered macrophages and inflammatory cells are present. The alveolar walls are widened and the capillaries congested. This is the microscopic appearance of pulmonary edema.

Figure 7–4. Left ventricular myocardium. Hematoxylin–eosin stain. Original magnification ×78.

The heart weighed 360 grams, though the average heart weight in an adult female is 250 grams. The changes seen in the myocardial fibers in this photomicrograph represent coagulative necrosis. Myocytes are more eosinophilic and are focally hyalinized, showing loss of striations and disintegration. Of the myocyte nuclei visible, some exhibit karyolysis, pyknosis, and karyorrhexis. A small collection of neutrophils is also present. These are the changes of an acute myocardial infarction of 24–48 hours duration.

Figure 7–5. Normal myocardium. Hematoxylin–eosin stain. Original magnification ×78.

The myocardial fibers are intact with easily visible cross-striations. Myocyte nuclei appear relatively uniform. No inflammatory changes are present.

Figure 7–6. Portion of liver. Hematoxylin–eosin stain. Original magnification ×12.

This is an example of centrilobular hemorrhagic necrosis with blood filling the centrilobular sinusoids and the adjacent necrotic parenchyma. Note the sparing of the portal areas.

Figure 7–7. Normal liver. Hematoxylin–eosin stain. Original magnification ×12.

The centrilobular region is intact with no evidence of significant sinusoidal dilatation. The portal areas are unremarkable.

▶ Answers

1. **(e)** The patient presented with the acute onset of shortness of breath. In view of her medical history (cerebrovascular accidents, immobility, hypertension, and diabetes mellitus), and her age, all four options (pulmonary embolus, pneumonia, myocardial infarction, and cardiac decompensation due to hypertension) should have been considered.

2. **(e)** The chest x-ray reveals bilateral pulmonary edema *(See description of Figure 7–1)*.

3. **(c)** The chest x-ray shows bilateral pulmonary edema. The patient presented with an acute left-sided heart failure due to myocardial infarction. The lung changes in pulmonary edema include edematous widening of the alveolar septa, congested capillaries, and edema fluid in the alveolar spaces. Acute inflammatory cells are not prominent in edema due to heart failure.

4. **(c)** The patient had a left-sided heart failure due to an acute myocardial infarction. Heart failure leads to the decreased cardiac output which, in turn, leads to decreased kidney perfusion. This leads to the activation of the renin-angiotensin-aldosterone system.

5. **(d)** The patient's symptoms had begun about 6 hours before the cardiac enzyme profile was done. There is an increase in the total creatine kinase, but the creatine kinase-MB isoenzyme level is within the normal range. The LDH level is mildly elevated and the isoenzyme pattern is normal. These findings were not yet diagnostic of anything and should have been repeated, since it was relatively early in the course of the disease.

6. **(d)** The patient died about 32 hours after the onset of the myocardial infarction and her heart showed changes typical of this stage of myocardial injury. Coagulative necrosis with preserved outlines of myofibers was evident; acute inflammatory cells (neutrophils) were present and would have become more prominent if the patient had lived another day. Scar tissue would appear in an infarction after about six weeks and would be characterized by fibrous tissue replacing necrotic myocytes. It was not present at 32 hours post-infarct.

7. **(a)** In acute myocardial infarction the serum LDH becomes elevated about 12–24 hours after the onset of symptoms, reaches a peak of 36–48 hours and falls to normal 5–10 days after the onset of the infarction. Out of five LDH isoenzymes, LDH_1 elevation is considered most typical for acute myocardial infarction, especially when the LDH_1 value is higher than that of the LDH_2 isoenzyme. The total serum creatine kinase level begins to rise 4–6 hours after the onset of the infarction and reaches a peak in about 24 hours. It returns to normal by the 3rd day after the onset of symptoms. The creatine kinase-MB fraction (found predominantly in cardiac muscle) should be elevated 8 hours after the onset of symptoms. *(See Lab Tip)*

8. **(c)** The morphologic appearance of the liver is characteristic of a passive congestion resulting from heart failure. The central hepatocytes became necrotic, the central vein and vascular sinusoids are distended with blood *(See description of Figure 7–6)*. There is no piecemeal necrosis, characteristic of chronic active hepatitis B infection; no fibrous septa surrounding islands of parenchymal cells, characteristic of cirrhosis; and there are no granulomas, characteristic of sarcoidosis.

9. **(a)** The increased serum potassium in this patient was not likely to be caused by the diuretics used to treat the patient's pulmonary edema, but was more likely due to the retention of potassium. This patient had a pre-renal azotemia, caused by a decreased cardiac output and her glomerular filtration rate was greatly reduced, which leads to oliguria or anuria. The cardiac enzyme profile (increased creatine kinase with increase in the MB isoenzyme and increase in LDH with LDH_1 greater than LDH_2) is typical of an acute myocardial infarction. Her lung edema and liver congestion are characteristic of heart failure. The morphological appearance of the section of the heart reveals the presence of a myocardial infarction *(See description of Figure 7–4)*.

NOTES

▶ Final Diagnosis and Synopsis of Case

- Acute Myocardial Infarction With Congestive Heart Failure (Pulmonary Edema, Prerenal Azotemia, Acute and Chronic Passive Congestion of Liver, Cardiogenic Shock)
- Atherosclerosis
- Diabetes Mellitus

This was a case of a painless presentation of an acute myocardial infarction. The incidence of painless infarction is greater in elderly patients, and especially in those with diabetes mellitus. The patient's chief complaint was sudden onset of breathlessness and a feeling of chest "heaviness." The patient was elderly with a long history of atherosclerosis leading to several cerebrovascular accidents, which left her bedridden with contractures of the extremities and a dysfunctional bladder. She was also diabetic and mildly hypertensive. In spite of all her medical problems, she appeared to be well controlled by medications until the day of admission. Her presentation clearly indicated an acute change in her status. The initial work-up and physical examination pointed to an acute myocardial infarction with left ventricular failure. Her cardiac enzymes on admission were elevated, but the pattern was nonspecific. The EKG showed ST-segment elevation in precordial leads V_1-V_4, suggesting transmural ischemia. Physical examination and chest x-ray were consistent with the diagnosis of pulmonary edema. Repeat cardiac enzyme profiles confirmed the diagnosis of a myocardial infarction. The patient was oliguric and later anuric, which most likely reflected the decreased cardiac output and led to prerenal azotemia and potassium retention. In spite of aggressive management, she developed cardiogenic shock and died. The post-mortem findings are consistent with heart failure and show a large acute myocardial infarction, with a mild neutrophilic infiltrate.

LAB TIPS

Cardiac Panel

The precise components of the cardiac panel and the timing of samples often vary among different institutions. With the increasing availability of thrombolytic therapy, early diagnosis of a myocardial infarction is extremely important, as these agents should be given as soon as possible after the infarct. Maximum benefit from these enzyme determinations comes from serial measurements over time, and a commonly used schedule allows for separate specimens to be collected on admission, at 24 hours, and at 48 hours.

CARDIAC PANEL

Component	Normal Serum Levels	Significance in Acute Myocardial Infarction
Creatine kinase, total (CK) {creatine phosphokinase (CPK)	0–130 U/L	Starts to increase 4–6 hours post-infarct; peaks at 24–36 hours; returns to normal levels by 3rd day; not specific since it can be increased in a number of other conditions
CK–MB (significant levels present only in myocardium)	0–4% of total CK	Begins to rise 4 to 6 hours post-infarct; peaks at 18–24 hours; returns to normal levels by 3rd day; very specific and sensitive for AMI
Lactate dehydrogenase, total (LDH)	100–225 U/L	Starts to rise 12–18 hours post-infarct; peaks 36–48 hours; may remain elevated for up to two weeks; not specific
LDH_1 (highest concentration is in myocardium)	17–27% of total LDH (usually less than LDH_2)	More significant than total LDH; useful when patients present 2 to 3 days post-infarct when CK and CK–MB will be normal; LDH_1 will often be higher than LDH_2 (ie "flipped pattern")
Cardiac troponin–T[a]	0–0.1 ng/mL	Rises 4–6 hours post-infarct; may stay elevated for up to 2 weeks; highly specific and sensitive

[a]A regulatory protein complex in myocardium that can be detected by monoclonal antibodies.

A 60-Year-Old Woman With Fever, Cough, and Low Back Pain

▶ Clinical History and Presentation

A 60-year-old woman presented with fever and a productive cough of approximately two months' duration. She also complained of fatigue and low back pain. Physical examination revealed an alert and oriented woman. Blood pressure was 120/90 mmHg, heart rate was 90 per minute and regular, temperature was 102.2° F, and respiratory rate was 23 per minute. Examination of the lungs revealed bilateral rales. The rest of the physical examination was unremarkable. Sputum was obtained for Gram stain and culture (Figure 8–1). A chest x-ray (Figure 8–2) was obtained. The patient was given a two week course of antibiotics and was advised to schedule a follow-up visit after two weeks.

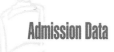

Admission Data

TABLE 8–1. HEMATOLOGY		
WBC	12.0 thousand/μL	(3.3–11.0)
Neut	76%	(44–88)
Band	12%	(0–10)
Lymph	8%	(12–43)
Mono	2%	(2–11)
Eos	1%	(0–5)
Baso	1%	(0–2)
Nucleated RBC	5%	(0)
RBC	3.1 million/μL	(3.9–5.0)
RETIC	1.1%	(0.5–1.5)
Hgb	8.5 g/dL	(11.6–15.6)
HCT	25.6%	(37.0–47.0)
MCV	82.6 fL	(79.0–99.0)
MCH	27.5 pg	(26.0–32.6)
MCHC	32.2 g/dL	(31.0–36.0)
Plts	188 thousand/μL	(130–400)

NOTES

TABLE 8–2. CHEMISTRY

Glucose	97 mg/dL	(65–110)
Creatinine	1.5 mg/dL	(0.7–1.4)
BUN	28 mg/dL	(7–24)
Uric acid	7 mg/dL	(3.0–8.5)
Cholesterol	200 mg/dL	(150–240)
Calciuim	11.4 mg/dL	(8.5–10.5)
Protein	9.8 g/dL	(6–8)
Albumin	3.2 g/dL	(3.7–5.0)
LDH	265 U/L	(100–250)
Alk Phos	190 U/L	(0–120)
AST	30 U/L	(0–55)
GGTP	40 U/L	(0–50)
Biluribin	0.4 mg/dL	(0.0–1.5)
Bilirubin, direct	0.13 mg/dL	(0.02–0.18)

TABLE 8–3. ELECTROLYTES

Na	137 mEq/L	(134–143)
K	3.5 mEq/L	(3.5–4.9)
Cl	99 mEq/L	(95–108)
CO_2	25 mEq/L	(21–32)

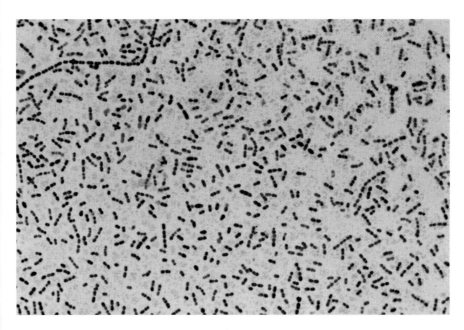

FIGURE 8–1. Culture of sputum. Gram stain. Original magnification ×315.

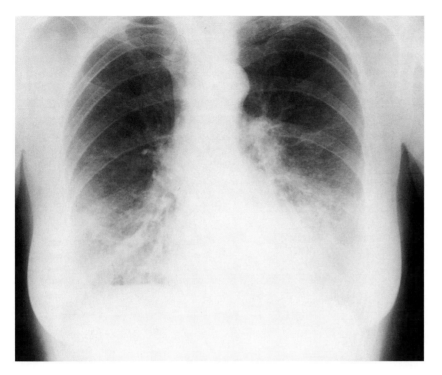

FIGURE 8–2. Admission chest x-ray.

▶ Questions

On the basis of the preceding information, you can best conclude the following:

1. Based on the patient's presentation and laboratory findings, it can be LEAST likely concluded that:
   a. this patient may be a chronic bleeder, most likely from the gastrointestinal tract
   b. this patient has an infectious process affecting the lung
   c. this patient could have a pathological process involving bone
   d. the increase of BUN and creatinine in this patient are not diagnostic of a primary renal problem

2. Which of the following tests would best help you to further investigate this patient's anemia?
   a. x-ray of the upper gastrointestinal tract
   b. serum folate level determination
   c. serum vitamin B12 level determination
   d. review of blood smear and reticulocyte count

3. The Gram stain of the culture of this patient's sputum (Figure 8–1):
   a. shows Gram positive cocci
   b. shows Gram negative bacilli
   c. shows the presence of fungi
   d. none of the above

4. The chest x-ray depicted in Figure 8–2 is most consistent with:
   a. bronchopneumonia
   b. massive pleural effusion
   c. sarcoidosis
   d. congestive heart failure

▶ Clinical Course

During the patient's follow-up visit two weeks later, she stated that the fever was gone and her chest was cleared. She did, however, still suffer from lower back pain, which had increased in intensity since her last visit. She also complained of pain in her rib cage. Her laboratory work-up and her skull x-ray are shown below. Following these results, an additional, special work-up was performed, and the patient was referred to an oncologist for treatment.

TABLE 8–4. HEMATOLOGY

WBC	3.4 thousand/μL	(3.3–11.0)
Neut	9%	(44–88)
Lymph	27%	(12–43)
Mono	4%	(2–11)
Eos	0%	(0–5)
Baso	0%	(0–2)
RBC	3.2 million/μL	(3.9–5.0)
Hgb	8.6 g/dL	(11.6–15.6)
HCT	26.1%	(37.0–47.0)
MCV	81.5 fL	(79.0–99.0)
MCH	26.8 pg	(26.0–32.6)
MCHC	32.9 g/dL	(31.0–36.0)
RETIC	1%	(0.5–1.5)
Plts	110 thousand/μL	(130–400)

TABLE 8–5. URINALYSIS

pH	6	(5.0–7.5)
Protein	3+	(Neg)
Glucose	Neg	(Neg)
Ketone	Neg	(Neg)
Occult blood	Neg	(Neg)
Color	Yellow	(Yellow)
Clarity	Clear	(Clear)
Sp. grav	1.050	(1.010–1.055)
WBC	3/HPF	(0–5)
RBC	1/HPF	(0–2)
Cast	Hyalin	(Neg)

TABLE 8–6. CHEMISTRY

Glucose	90 mg/dL	(65–110)
Creatinine	1.9 mg/dL	(0.7–1.4)
BUN	29 mg/dL	(7–24)
Uric acid	9 mg/dL	(3.0–8.5)
Cholesterol	199 mg/dL	(150–240)
Calcium	12 mg/dL	(8.5–10.5)
Protein	10.9 g/dL	(6–8)
Albumin	3.7 g/dL	(3.7–5.0)
LDH	270 U/L	(100–250)
Alk Phos	210 U/L	(30–120)
AST	50 U/L	(0–55)
GGTP	35 U/L	(0–50)
Bilirubin	0.7 mg/dL	(0.0–1.5)
Bilirubin, direct	0.11 mg/dL	(0.02–0.18)

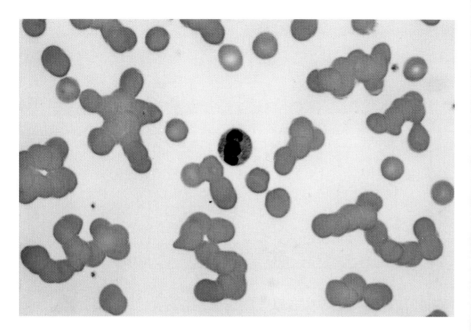

FIGURE 8–3. Peripheral blood smear. Wright/Giemsa stain. Original magnification ×252.

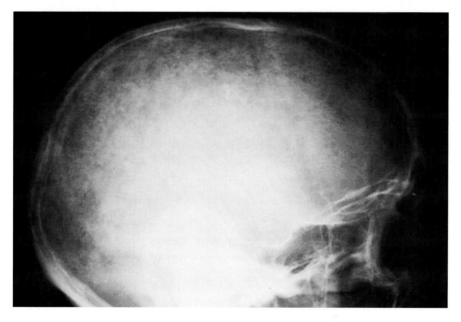

FIGURE 8–4. Skull x-ray.

NOTES

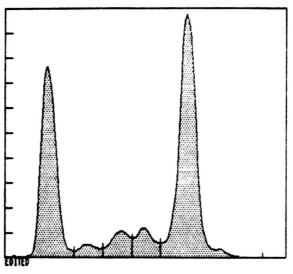

Fraction	%	MG/DL	MG/DL Range	
ALBUMIN	33.8	3.7	3.6	5.4
ALPHA-1	3.0	0.3	0.1	0.3
ALPHA-2	6.1	0.7	0.4	0.9
BETA	6.2	0.7	0.5	1.1
GAMMA	50.9	5.5 hi	0.6	1.6
Total Protein		10.9 hi	6.0	8.2

FIGURE 8–5. Serum protein electrophoresis.

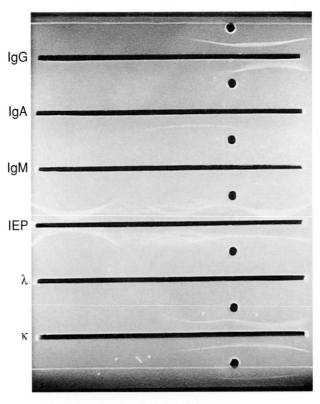

FIGURE 8–6. Serum immunoelectrophoresis.

▶ Questions

5. The morphological findings on the peripheral blood smear (Figure 8–3):
   a. indicate severe dehydration
   b. are characteristic of lead poisoning
   c. are characteristic of hyperglobulinemia
   d. show an air-dried artifact

6. The serum electrophoresis shown in Figure 8–5 indicates the presence of:
   a. agammaglobulinemia
   b. polyclonal gamma globulin elevation
   c. monoclonal gammopathy
   d. elevation of the alpha-2 globulin band

7. Immunofixation electrophoresis is useful for:
   a. demonstration of monoclonal proteins
   b. differentiation between monoclonal and polyclonal proteins
   c. identification of monoclonal proteins
   d. all of the above
   e. none of the above

8. The changes seen in the skull x-ray (Figure 8–4) are associated with:
   a. the occurrence of pathological fractures
   b. the activation of osteoclasts by cytokines
   c. bone resorption
   d. all of the above
   e. none of the above

9. Hypercalcemia in this patient is mainly due to:
   a. primary hyperparathyroidism
   b. bone resorption due to osteoclastic activation
   c. vitamin D toxicity
   d. all of the above
   e. none of the above

10. In patients with this disease, the main cause of renal dysfunction is:
    a. Bence-Jones proteinuria
    b. hypercalcemia
    c. amyloidosis
    d. urinary tract infection
    e. all of the above

11. All of the following statements about this patient's disease are correct EXCEPT:
    a. recurrent infections are common
    b. humoral immunity is intact
    c. hypercalcemia leads to neurological manifestations such as confusion, weakness, and lethargy
    d. development of a hyperviscosity syndrome is common
    e. renal insufficiency is a common cause of death

NOTES

► Figure Descriptions

Figure 8–1. Culture of sputum. Gram stain. Original magnification ×315.

The smear from the culture plate shows Gram positive cocci in pairs and chains. This morphology is consistent with *Streptococcus pneumoniae*, and biochemical testing confirmed the result. No other organisms were identified in the culture.

Figure 8–2. Admission chest x-ray.

A bilateral infiltrate is present, which is consistent with bronchopneumonia.

Figure 8–3. Peripheral blood smear. Wright/Giemsa stain. Original magnification ×252.

The marked feature of this patient's peripheral blood smear is rouleaux formation, or the clumping of red blood cells in groups and stacks. This is due to the presence of a circulating paraprotein. The smear also shows a normocytic, normochromic anemia, which may be difficult to appreciate, due the clumped erythrocytes. The neutrophil and platelets present are unremarkable.

Figure 8–4. Skull.

Multiple "punched out" lesions of the calvaria are evident, and consistent with multiple myeloma.

Figure 8–5. Serum protein electrophoresis.

The serum protein electrophoresis shows a sharp peak in the gamma region, which indicates the presence of a monoclonal protein. This procedure does not identify the protein.

Figure 8–6. Serum immunoelectrophoresis.

The plate consists of a series of round wells and horizontal troughs. The patient's serum is placed in the 2nd, 4th, and 6th wells from the top, while normal human serum is placed in the 1st, 3rd, and 5th wells. Antisera to IgG is placed in trough 1, antisera to IgA in trough 2, antisera to IgM in trough 3, polyvalent antisera in trough 4, antisera to Lambda light chain in trough 5, and antisera to Kappa light chain in trough 6. The results show abnormal precipitin arcs against IgG and Kappa light chains. Thus, this patient had an IgG-Kappa monoclonal protein.

► Answers

1. **(a)** This patient had a normocytic, normochromic anemia. In chronic hemorrhage, a microcytic, hypochromic anemia would be expected. Fever and cough, leukocytosis with increased bands, sputum culture showing Gram positive cocci, and chest x-ray suggest the presence of bronchopneumonia. The patient also had a low serum albumin level, which may have been due to mild malnutrition. The combination of hypercalcemia, increased alkaline phosphatase, normal liver function tests, and persistent bone pain suggest the possibility of a pathological process involving the bone. The limited increase in the BUN and creatinine may be due to a prerenal etiology such as dehydration (due to fever). It is not diagnostic of primary renal disease.

2. (**d**) As mentioned above, the patient had a normocytic, normochromic anemia. A reticulocyte count would provide information about erythropoiesis and the delivery of red blood cells to the circulation. Peripheral blood smears would provide additional information about other abnormalities. In addition, iron studies would provide information about the body's iron stores. In this patient, there was no indication for radiological examination of the gastrointestinal tract. The levels of vitamin B12 and folate are primarily useful in investigating macrocytic anemia, which this patient does not have.

3. (**a**) The Gram stain of the sputum culture clearly depicts the presence of Gram-positive cocci in pairs and chains.

4. (**a**) The chest x-ray is most consistent with bronchopneumonia *(see description of Figure 8–2)*. Sarcoidosis most typically affects the hilar lymph nodes. Congestive heart failure may present with a spectrum of changes ranging from vascular congestion to pulmonary edema.

5. (**c**) Figure 8–3 shows red blood cell aggregates that resemble stacks of coins ("rouleaux"). This is due to clumping of the red blood cells by circulating paraproteins. Dehydration does not lead to rouleaux formation, nor does lead poisoning, which causes basophilic stippling.

6. (**c**) Figure 8–5 shows a serum electrophoresis with a monoclonal spike in the gamma globulin region, characteristic of monoclonal gammopathy. Polyclonal gamma globulin elevation would be seen as an increase over the entire gamma zone, and is not present here. The presence of monoclonal gammopathy excludes the possibility of agammaglobulinemia. There is no evidence of elevated alpha-2 globulin.

7. (**d**) Immunofixation is a modification of immunoelectrophoresis. It can be used (like serum protein electrophoresis) to differentiate monoclonal from polyclonal proteins, and to identify the type of immunoglobulin (IgG, IgM, etc).

8. (**d**) Figure 8–4 depicts multiple lytic lesions (soap-bubble appearance) of the skull, which are consistent with bone resorption. They result from the activation of osteoclasts by cytokines produced by the myeloma cells. Such lesions predispose to pathological fractures.

9. (**b**) In multiple myeloma, hypercalcemia results from bone resorption due to activation of osteoclast-activating factors secreted by the myeloma cells (TNF-B, IL-1, IL-2, IL-6, and M-CSF).

10. (**a**) Bence-Jones (BJ) proteinuria, hypercalcemia, amyloidosis, and urinary tract infection may contribute to renal dysfunction in patients with multiple myeloma. However, Bence-Jones (light chain) proteinuria is a major cause of renal dysfunction. Two mechanisms appear to account for the renal toxicity of BJ protein: some of BJ proteins appear to be directly toxic to the renal epithelial cells, and BJ protein also combines with urinary glycoproteins under acidic conditions to form large, tubular casts that may obstruct the tubular lumina and induce a peritubular inflammatory reaction.

11. (**b**) Patients with multiple myeloma frequently suffer from recurrent infections, primarily with encapsulated bacteria such as pneumococci, due to the excessive production of an abnormal immunoglobulin. The hypercalcemia due to bone resorption may lead to many neurological manifestations, such as confusion and lethargy, and pathological fractures of bone. A hyperviscosity syndrome occurs due to an increased production of abnormal large protein molecules. Renal involvement is common in multiple myeloma, and renal insufficiency is second only to infection as a cause of death.

▶ Final Diagnosis and Synopsis of Case

• Bilateral Bronchopneumonia
• Multiple Myeloma

A 60-year-old woman presented with a pneumococcal bronchopneumonia, which responded to antibiotic therapy, and low back pain, rib pain, and extreme fatigue. Laboratory findings revealed a normocytic, normochromic anemia with rouleaux formation on the peripheral blood smear, hypercalcemia, increased alkaline phosphatase, and abnormal renal function. The x-ray of the skull revealed "punched out" lesions consistent with bone resorption. Similar lesions accounted for the rib pain present in the patient. All these changes are characteristically found in multiple myeloma. The diagnosis was confirmed by the demonstration of a monoclonal serum protein peak, which was identified as an IgG immunoglobulin. The patient also had Bence-Jones proteinuria. Bone marrow biopsy (not shown) showed an infiltration by plasma cells, which constituted approximately 50% of all cells in the bone marrow. The patient was referred to an oncologist for further evaluation and treatment. Multiple myeloma is a malignant process involving plasma cells. In spite of the progress in its treatment, the prognosis remains poor, with median survival of about 3 years.

LAB TIPS

Serum Protein Electrophoresis

Since most biological polymers are electrically charged, we can use their movement through a solvent by an electrical field (ie, electrophoresis), as a means of detection and separation. The electrophoretic separation of these major serum proteins will sometimes produce a distinct pattern, highly specific for a certain disease process. Several of these disease patterns are listed in the table below.

SERUM PROTEIN ELECTROPHORESIS—PATTERNS IN SELECTED CONDITIONS

Albumin Zone	α_1-Globulin Zone	α_2-Globulin Zone	β-Globulin Zone	γ-Globulin Zone
Cirrhosis				
Marked decrease		Decreased	Decreased	Polyclonal increase (β-γ bridging)
Acute Phase Reaction Pattern				
Decreased	Increased	Increased		Increased in prolonged inflammation
Paraprotein				
Decreased				Monoclonal increase
Nephrotic Syndrome				
Marked decrease		Marked increase		Decreased
Hypogammaglobulinemia				
				Marked decrease
Protein–Losing Enteropathy				
Marked decrease		Increased		Decreased
α_1-Antitrypsin Deficiency				
	Marked decrease			
Major Normal Components				
Albumin, pre–albumin	α-lipoproteins, α_1–anti-trypsin	Haptoglobin, α_2–macro-globulin, β–lipopro-teins,	Antithrombin III, transferrin, complement	Immuno-globulins complement, fibrinogen

(Continued)

Lab Tips (continued)

Immunoelectrophoresis

Serum protein electrophoresis can establish the presence of a paraprotein, but can not identify it. However, if we combine immunoprecipitation with electrophoresis, we can produce a precipitin arc for each protein for which an antibody is present in the system. Typically, the protein sample to be separated and identified is placed in a well on a gel plate, and electrophoresis is allowed to occur in order to separate the proteins present. Following electrophoresis, an antibody solution is placed in adjacent trough, and the development of any of the immunoprecipitation arcs, indicative of an antigen-antibody reaction, may be noted. The gel plates are of sufficient size to allow a patient's serum to be tested with several different antibody solutions. Normally, one would test for the presence of IgG, IgM, IgA, kappa, and lambda chains.

▶ **Clinical History and Presentation**

A 79-year-old man with a history of hypertension was brought to the emergency room complaining of severe suprapubic pain associated with hematuria. On rectal examination he was found to have an enlarged prostate. He was admitted, treated for pain, and a work-up for hematuria was pursued. His initial blood pressure was 200/100 mmHg, which decreased to 170/80 mmHg, and subsequently to 150/82 mmHg over a period of 48 hours. The investigation of hematuria included intravenous pyelography, computerized tomography, and a surgical procedure.

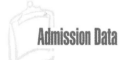

Admission Data

TABLE 9–1. HEMATOLOGY		
WBC	8.1 thousand/µL	(3.6–11.2)
Neut	83%	(44–88)
Band	0%	(0–10)
Lymph	9%	(12–43)
Mono	7%	(2–11)
Eos	1%	(0–5)
Baso	0%	(0–2)
RBC	4.32 million/µL	(4.0–5.6)
Hgb	12.7 g/dL	(12.6–17.0)
HCT	38.2%	(37.2–50.4)
MCV	88.6 fL	(80.5–102.1)
MCH	29.3 pg	(27.0–35.0)
MCHC	33.1 g/dL	(30.7–36.7)
Plts	164 thousand/µL	(130–400)

TABLE 9–2. URINALYSIS		
pH	6	(5.0–7.5)
Protein	3+	(Neg)
Glucose	Neg	(Neg)
Ketone	Trace	(Neg)
Color	Amber	(Yellow)
Clarity	Hazy	Clear
Sp. grav	1.021	(1.010–1.055)
WBC	19/HPF	(0–5)
RBC	49/HPF	(0–2)
Hyaline cast	10/LPF	(Neg)
Bact	2+	(Neg)
Mucus	1+	(Neg)
Urobil	Neg	(Neg)

TABLE 9–3. CHEMISTRY

Glucose	110 mg/dL	(65–110)
Creatinine	1.2 mg/dL	(0.7–1.4)
BUN	17 mg/dL	(7–24)
Uric acid	6.2 mg/dL	(3.0–8.5)
Cholesterol	257 mg/dL	(150–240)
Calcium	9.4 mg/dL	(8.5–10.5)
Protein	7.1 g/dL	(6–8)
Albumin	4.1 g/dL	(3.7–5.0)
LDH	242 U/L	(100–225)
Alk Phos	103 U/L	(30–120)
AST	15 U/L	(0–55)
GGTP	12 U/L	(0–50)
Bilirubin	0.8 mg/dL	(0.0–1.5)
Bilirubin, direct	0.18 mg/dL	(0.02–0.18)

TABLE 9–4. ELECTROLYTES

Na	133 mEq/L	(134–143)
K	5.0 mEq/L	(3.5–4.9)
Cl	98 mEq/L	(95–108)
CO_2	24 mEq/L	(21–32)

TABLE 9–5. TUMOR MARKERS

Prostate specific antigen	2.95 ng/mL	(0–4)

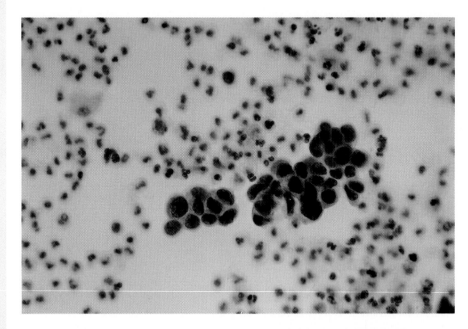

FIGURE 9–1. Patient's urine cytology. Papanicolaou stain. Original magnification ×125.

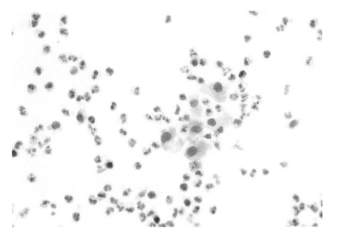

FIGURE 9–2. Urine cytology from another patient. Papanicolaou stain. Original magnification ×125.

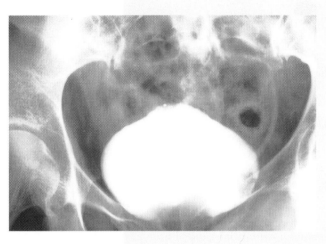

FIGURE 9–3. Intravenous pyelogram.

▶ Questions

On the basis of the preceding information, you can best conclude the following:

1. Based on the patient's urinalysis, the LEAST likely cause of his hematuria is:
   a. acute glomerulonephritis
   b. cystitis
   c. bladder carcinoma
   d. urethral infection

2. The presence of hyaline casts is best related to the patient's:
   a. hematuria
   b. proteinuria
   c. pyuria
   d. bacteriuria

3. Urine cytology in this case (Figure 9–1) is strongly suggestive of which of the following?
   a. pyelonephritis
   b. glomerulonephritis
   c. cystitis
   d. neoplasia

4. The radiographic appearance in Figure 9–3 suggests the presence of which of the following?
   a. a filling defect in the bladder
   b. a possible blood clot in the bladder
   c. a possible neoplasm
   d. all of the above

▶ Clinical Course

The surgical procedure was a transurethral resection, performed under general anesthesia, of the prostate and of a solid mass in the bladder wall. The patient tolerated surgery well, and was soon temporarily discharged to attend to some personal affairs. It was explained to him that he would need re-admission for additional work-up.

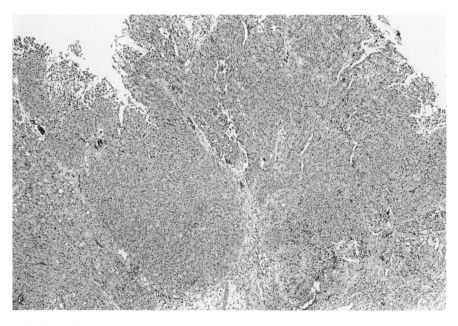

FIGURE 9–4. Endoscopic bladder biopsy (patient). Hematoxylin–eosin stain. Original magnification ×12.

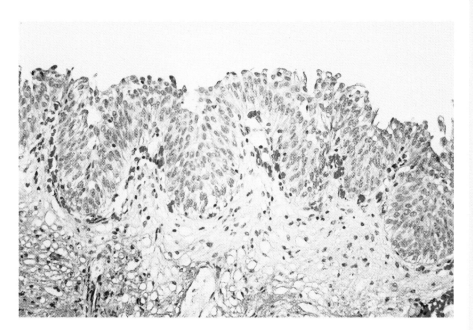

FIGURE 9–5. Normal bladder mucosa. Hematoxylin–eosin stain. Original magnification ×50.

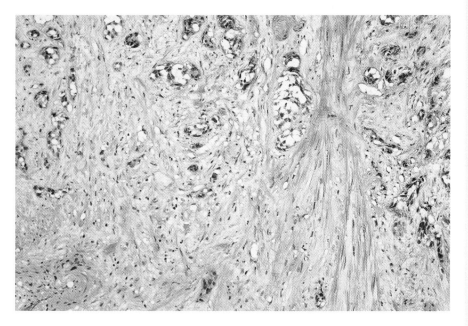

FIGURE 9–6. Portion of muscular wall of bladder (patient). Hematoxylin–eosin stain. Original magnification ×31.

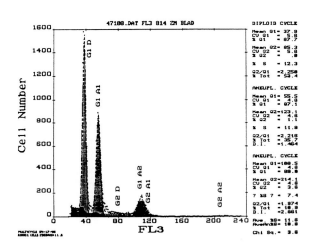

FIGURE 9–7. DNA histogram of the bladder mass.

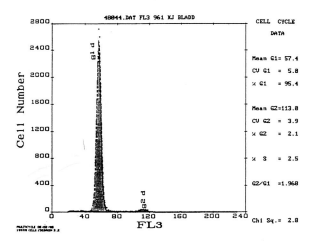

FIGURE 9–8. DNA histogram of normal bladder (control).

▶ Questions

5. The bladder biopsy (Figures 9–4 and 9–6) shows:
   a. normal bladder mucosa
   b. bladder mucosa and a granulomatous process
   c. a neoplastic process
   d. malakoplakia of the bladder

6. All of the following statements concerning the lesion depicted in Figures 9–4 and 9–6 are correct EXCEPT:
   a. it is often recurrent
   b. it has been associated with p53 gene mutations
   c. it is often multicentric
   d. it arises only in the bladder
   e. it is thought to be clonal in nature

7. All of the following statements about the type of lesions depicted in Figures 9–4 and 9–6 are correct EXCEPT:
   a. they have been etiologically associated with the therapeutic use of the anti-tumor agent cyclophosphamide
   b. they have been etiologically associated with nephropathy due to the prolonged use of phenacetin
   c. they have been etiologically associated with cigarette smoking
   d. they more often affect inhabitants of rural rather than those of urban areas
   e. they affect males predominantly

8. All of the following statements about the DNA histogram in Figure 9–7 are correct EXCEPT:
   a. it depicts a diploid DNA peak
   b. it depicts an aneuploid DNA content
   c. with respect to DNA content, it depicts more than one abnormal cell population
   d. the abnormal cell population has a smaller amount of DNA per one cell than the normal cell population
   e. the estimation of the "S phase" fraction of the diploid cell population is complicated by the presence of the aneuploid DNA peaks

9. All of the following statements about this patient's disease are correct EXCEPT:
   a. hematuria is the most common clinical manifestation
   b. it may lead to pyelonephritis
   c. it may lead to hydronephrosis
   d. when first discovered, it is usually multifocal and localized outside the bladder in the majority of patients

NOTES

▶ Figure Descriptions

Figure 9–1. Patient's urine cytology. Papanicolaou stain. Original magnification ×125.

Two groups of hyperchromatic, pleomorphic cells are present near the center of the photomicrograph. The nuclear/cytoplasmic ratio is high, nuclear chromatin distribution is irregular, and the nuclear membrane is uneven. These findings are consistent with a high-grade transitional cell carcinoma. A number of inflammatory cells are also present.

Figure 9–2. Urine cytology from another patient. Papanicolaou stain. Original magnification ×125.

Here the transitional cells have abundant, delicate cytoplasm. The nuclear chromatin is fine and evenly dispersed throughout the nucleus. Inflammatory cells are also present in this specimen.

Figure 9–3. Intravenous pyelogram (patient).

The pyelogram reveals an irregular, 2 cm filling defect in the left bladder consistent with a tumor or blood clot.

Figure 9–4. Endoscopic bladder biopsy (patient). Hematoxylin–eosin stain. Original magnification ×12.

The bladder mucosa is markedly thickened by a papillary and solid transitional cell carcinoma. In this part of the tumor, the transitional nature of the cells is still evident, but mitotic figures, loss of polarity, and glandular metaplasia are apparent.

Figure 9–5. Normal bladder mucosa. Hematoxylin–eosin stain. Original magnification ×50.

At a much higher magnification, the thinness of the bladder mucosa may be noted and compared to that in Figure 9–4. Here, it is 3 to 4 cells deep, and the nuclei are regular in appearance and maintain polarity with the basement membrane.

Figure 9–6. Portion of muscular wall of bladder (patient). Hematoxylin–eosin stain. Original magnification ×31.

One of the pieces of tissue obtained by endoscopy contained bladder musculature and shows separation of muscle fibers by infiltrating tumor. Here, the cells are not easily recognizable as transitional cells, and glandular metaplasia (vacuolization) is more prominent. When glandular or squamous metaplasia occurs in an otherwise transitional cell carcinoma, the convention is to classify it as a transitional cell carcinoma with metaplasia (glandular or squamous). True adenocarcinomas and squamous carcinomas of the bladder do occur, but are much less common.

Figure 9–7. DNA histogram (patient).

This is a DNA histogram obtained by flow cytometric analysis of a tumor cell population. The DNA content (intensity of DNA staining) is plotted on the X-axis, and the number of cells of any given staining intensity is plotted on the Y-axis. The pattern seen shows three DNA peaks, reflecting the G_0/G_1 phases of the diploid and of the two aneuploid cell populations. The presence of aneuploid DNA peaks is a distinctively abnormal finding. The area between the G_0/G_1 and G_2/M peaks under the curve defines the "S-phase" fraction, {ie, the proportion of cells in the synthetic phase with an intermediate amount of DNA). Both DNA ploidy and "S-phase" values are important in the interpretation of histograms.

Figure 9–8. DNA histogram (control).

A normal diploid DNA histogram with one DNA peak, a low "S-phase" fraction and a small G_2/M population.

▷ **Answers**

1. (**a**) This patient has hematuria, pyuria, and bacteriuria without any cellular casts. These findings indicate that the diagnosis of acute glomerulonephritis is least likely. Cystitis, bladder carcinoma and urethral infection are postrenal disorders and therefore do not lead to cast formation.

2. (**b**) Hyaline casts are composed of protein alone and pass through the urinary tract virtually unchanged. Since the cast formation occurs principally in the distal and collecting tubules, hyalin casts reflect the presence of a renal proteinuria. Postrenal proteinuria is not associated with hyalin cast formation.

3. (**d**) Urine cytology (Figure 9–1) shows hyperchromatic neoplastic epithelial cells consistent with transitional cell carcinoma. These cells would not be seen in cystitis or in pyelonephritis where acute inflammatory cells would be prominent. Acute inflammatory cells can also be seen in the urine cytology of patients with carcinoma, as in this case. In glomerulonephritis, abundant red blood cells might be encountered, but neoplastic cells are not a feature of that disease.

4. (**d**) The intravenous pyelogram shows a filling defect in the left portion of the urinary bladder. This could represent a blood clot or a neoplasm.

5. (**c**) The tissue depicted in Figures 9–4 and 9–6 is a grade III transitional cell carcinoma of the bladder, and shows invasion of the muscular bladder wall. While it is bladder tissue, it is neither normal nor granulomatous.

6. (**d**) The lesion shown in Figures 9–4 and 9–6 is a transitional cell carcinoma. Tumors of this type can arise in the renal pelvis, ureter, bladder, or prostatic urethra. They are often recurrent and/or multicentric, but nevertheless are regarded as clonal in origin (ie, arising from a single cell). Their clonal character has been deduced on the basis of studies of p53 gene mutations and other molecular genetic studies.

7. (**d**) Epidemiologically the male to female ratio of the incidence of transitional cell carcinoma is about 3 to 1, and the disease is more common in those who live in urban rather than rural areas. Transitional cell carcinoma has been associated with cigarette smoking, and with both phenacetin overuse and analgesic nephropathy in general. Treatment with cyclophosphamide, an antitumor and immunosuppressive agent, may cause severe cystitis and increase the risk of bladder cancer.

8. (**d**) The histogram in Figure 9–7 shows both diploid and aneuploid DNA peaks. There are two aneuploid peaks, reflecting the presence of two aneuploid cell populations. The DNA content of the aneuploid populations is higher (a higher staining intensity points to a higher content of DNA) than that of a diploid population. The DNA Index (DI) is a value given to express the aneuploid DNA content relative to the normal cell complement of DNA. The estimation of an "S phase" fraction, which is a measure of the proliferative activity of a given cell population, is complicated when two or more cell populations are present. Several studies have indicated that tumor recurrence and progression are more frequently seen in aneuploid bladder tumors.

9. (**d**) When first diagnosed, the majority of bladder cancers present as a single lesion, which is localized in the bladder. Hematuria is the most common and sometimes the only manifestation of bladder cancer. The cancer can cause urinary outflow obstruction, which would predispose the patient to pyelonephritis or hydronephrosis.

▷ Final Diagnosis and Synopsis of Case

- Transitional Cell Carcinoma of the Bladder
- Glandular Metaplasia
- Right Hydronephrosis and Hydroureter

The patient, a 79-year-old man with a history of hypertension, was admitted for treatment of hematuria and severe abdominal pain. Intravenous pyelography and computer tomography revealed a space occupying lesion in the bladder. The pathological diagnosis on resected tissue was one of grade III transitional cell carcinoma of the bladder with glandular metaplasia. The carcinoma proved to be aneuploid, and extensively invaded the attached muscular wall. The patient was to be followed up for the evaluation of possible metastasis of his tumor.

LAB TIPS

Urine Cytology

The light microscopic examination of the unstained urine sediment is usually a part of the routine urinalysis. It is a useful technique for the diagnosis of a number of different genitourinary tract diseases. Many different formed elements (eg, white blood cells, red blood cells, epithelial cells, casts, crystals, and organisms) can be identified by this method. However, this method is not sufficiently sensitive for the diagnosis of genitourinary tract neoplasms. When malignancy is suspected, the urine is sent for "urine cytology," which usually includes cytocentrifugation and Papanicolaou staining. Besides urine, urinary tract specimens for cytology may also be obtained from urinary tract washings and brushings, and also from fine needle aspiration of a suspected lesion. In order for the cytopathologist to make an accurate diagnosis of malignancy, the specimen should have been optimally obtained and prepared, and also be representative of the lesion in question. As there is no single cytologic feature conclusive for malignancy, the diagnosis rests on the nuclear criteria listed in the table below.

GENERAL CYTOLOGIC CRITERIA OF MALIGNANCY (SITE INDEPENDENT)	
Nuclear Feature	**Comment**
Nuclear size	Nuclei vary in size, but are generally larger than the benign equivalent
Nuclear shape	Nuclei vary in shape
Nuclear–cytoplasmic ratio	Increased
Nuclear membrane	Unevenly thickened, often indented and angulated
Chromatin	Chromatin distribution irregular; chromatin varies in size and shape; may be coarse or clumped
Number of nuclei	May be multinucleated but unreliable as a criterion of malignancy
Mitoses	Abnormal mitoses, aneuploidy are reliable; increased number of mitoses is not a reliable criterion

URINARY TRACT CYTOLOGY	
Site	**Source of Cells**
Kidney	Renal parenchymal cells—renal parenchymal tumors are rarely diagnosed by cytology
Lower urinary tract (bladder and urethra)	Transitional cells—major epithelium of bladder and urethra
	Glandular cells—trigone and dome of bladder; prostate gland; paraurethral glands; cells from Brunn's nests
	Squamous epithelium—vaginal contamination in women; from distal penile urethra; trigone of women; squamous metaplasia
Upper urinary tract (calyces, renal pelvis, and ureters)	Transitional cells—major epithelium of all three sites
	Squamous epithelium—squamous metaplasia

An 80-Year-Old Man With Abdominal Pain and Weight Loss

▶ **Clinical History and Presentation**

An 80-year old man was admitted to the hospital because of complaints of lower abdominal pain. He had lost 16 lbs in recent months. There was no other significant medical or surgical history, and the patient was on no medication. On physical examination, he looked comfortable and alert. He answered simple questions appropriately, but his memory was very poor. Blood pressure was 130/80 mmHg, heart rate was 70 per minute. He was afebrile. Examination of the chest did not reveal any abnormalities. The abdomen was soft; bowel sounds were present. There was tenderness to palpation in the left lower quadrant. The rectal examination revealed an enlarged, hard prostate. The stool was negative for occult blood. A CT scan of the abdomen (Figure 10–3) was performed.

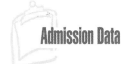

Admission Data

TABLE 10–1. HEMATOLOGY		
WBC	12.4 thousand/μL	(3.6–11.2)
Neut	91%	(44–88)
Band	0%	(0–10)
Lymph	5%	(12–43)
Mono	2%	(2–11)
Eos	1%	(0–5)
Baso	1%	(0–2)
RBC	2.84 million/μL	(4.0–5.6)
Hgb	8.7 g/dL	(12.6–17.0)
HCT	28.5%	(37.2–50.4)
MCV	100.5 fL	(80.5–102.1)
MCH	30.5 pg	(27.0–35.0)
MCHC	30.4 g/dL	(30.7–36.7)
Plts	412 thousand/μL	(130–400)

TABLE 10–2. CHEMISTRY		
Glucose	122 mg/dL	(65–110)
Creatinine	1.3 mg/dL	(0.7–1.4)
BUN	24 mg/dL	(7–24)
Uric acid	6.6 mg/dL	(3.0–8.5)
Cholesterol	240 mg/dL	(150–240)
Calcium	9.1 mg/dL	(8.5–10.5)
Protein	6.6 g/dL	(6–8)
Albumin	3.6 g/dL	(3.7–5.0)
LDH	282 U/L	(100–250)
Alk Phos	63 U/L	(30–120)
AST	12 U/L	(0–55)
Bilirubin	0.3 mg/dL	(0.0–1.5)
Bilirubin, direct	0.05 mg/dL	(0.02–0.18)
Amylase	71 U/L	(23–85)

TABLE 10–3. URINALYSIS

Sp. grav	1.010	(1.010–1.055)
pH	7	(5.0–7.5)
Protein	Neg	(Neg)
Glucose	Neg	(Neg)
Ketone	Neg	(Neg)
Occult blood	3+	(Neg)
Color	Yellow	(yellow)
Clarity	Clear	(Clear)
WBC	1/HPF	(0–5)
RBC	29/HPF	(0–2)

TABLE 10–4. COAGULATION

PT	10.5 sec	(11–14)
aPTT	20 sec	(19–28)

TABLE 10–5. ELECTROLYTES

Na	143 mEq/L	(134–143)
K	4.7 mEq/L	(3.5–4.9)
Cl	109 mEq/L	(95–108)
CO_2	17 mEq/L	(21–32)

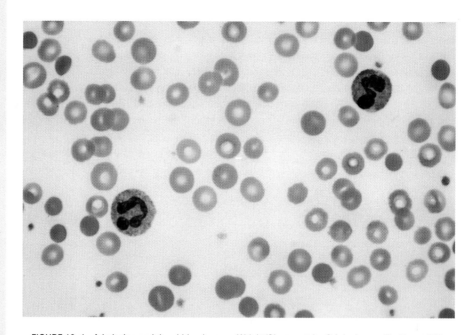

FIGURE 10–1. Admission peripheral blood smear. Wright/Giemsa stain. Original magnification ×252.

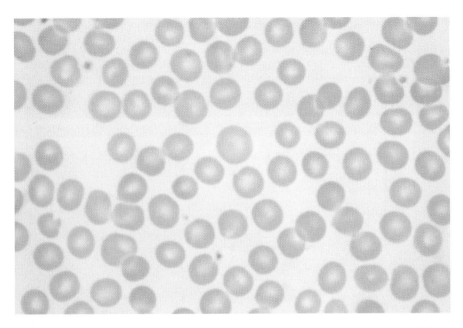

FIGURE 10–2. Normal peripheral blood smear. Wright/Giemsa stain. Original magnification ×315.

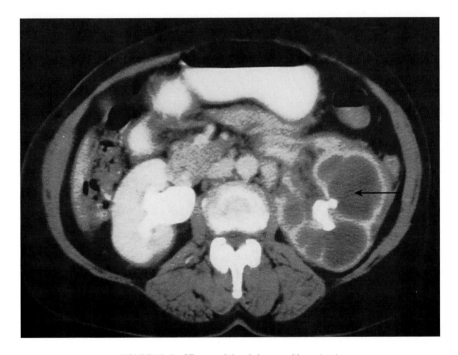

FIGURE 10–3. CT scan of the abdomen with contrast.

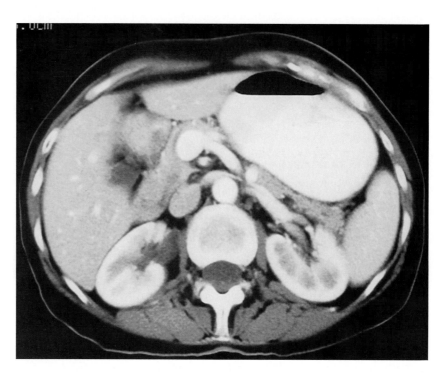

FIGURE 10–4. Normal CT scan.

► Questions

On the basis of the preceding information, you can best conclude the following:

1. The hematology values and the appearance of the peripheral blood smear depicted in Figure 10–1 are most consistent with:
   a. megaloblastic anemia
   b. spherocytosis
   c. iron deficiency anemia
   d. anemia of chronic disease

2. The LEAST likely diagnosis of the patient's prostatic problem would be:
   a. acute bacterial prostatitis
   b. cancer of the prostate
   c. benign prostatic hyperplasia
   d. cancer of the prostate and prostatic intraepithelial neoplasm

3. The LEAST helpful test for the diagnosis of this patient's prostatic problem is:
   a. rectal examination
   b. serum prostatic acid phosphatase
   c. serum prostate specific antigen
   d. examination of expressed prostatic secretion (EPS)
   e. biopsy of the prostate

4. All of the following statements about the appearance of the patient's left kidney (Figure 10–3) or the process leading to this appearance are correct EXCEPT:
   a. the kidney shows parenchymal thinning
   b. such thinning may develop over a prolonged period of time
   c. the process may occur virtually asymptomatically
   d. this process is by itself sufficient to cause an acute renal failure in this patient

5. The underlying cause of the abnormal appearance of the left kidney seen in the abdominal CT scan shown in Figure 10–3 is known to be associated with all of the following EXCEPT:
   a. hematuria
   b. remaining asymptomatic for a long period of time
   c. infection by urea splitting organisms
   d. acute renal failure

▶ Clinical Course

Additional work-up consisted of a needle biopsy of the prostate (Figure 10–5) followed by a bone scan (Figure 10–9). The treatment options were discussed with the patient and his family.

TABLE 10–6. TUMOR MARKERS

Prostate specific antigen (PSA)	51.6 ng/mL	(0–4)
Prostatic acid phosphatase (PAP)	23.8 ng/mL	(<3.7)

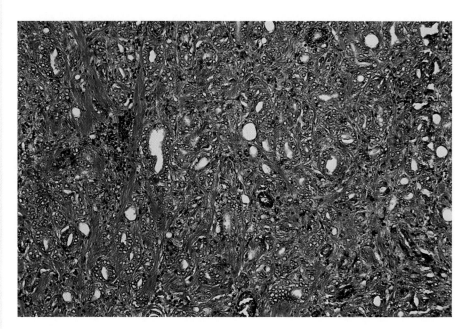

FIGURE 10–5. Prostate gland biopsy. Hematoxylin–eosin stain. Original magnification ×31.

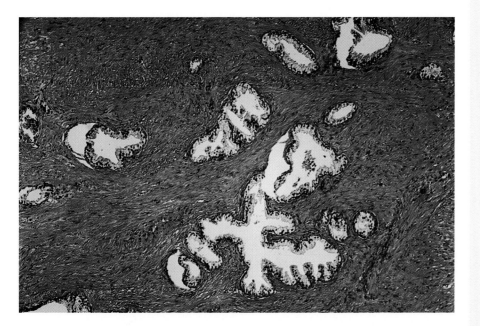

FIGURE 10–6. Normal prostate gland. Hematoxylin–eosin stain. Original magnification ×12.

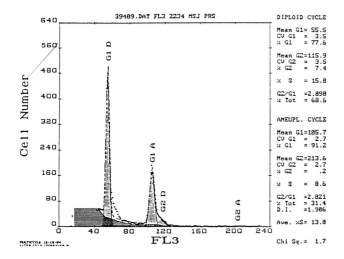

FIGURE 10–7. DNA ploidy/cell cycle analysis of prostate (patient).

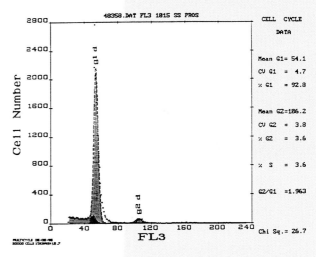

FIGURE 10–8. DNA ploidy/cell cycle analysis of normal prostatic tissue.

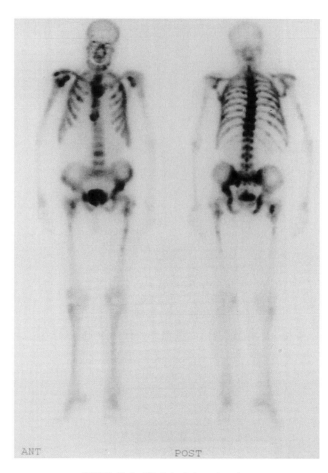

FIGURE 10–9. Whole body bone imaging.

▶ Questions

6. Elevated prostate specific antigen level:
   a. may be seen in benign prostatic hyperplasia
   b. may be seen in prostatic inflammation or infarction
   c. may be seen in prostatic neoplasia without metastases
   d. is the most sensitive test for the early detection of prostatic cancer
   e. all of the above statements are correct

7. The biopsy of the prostate depicted in Figure 10–5 is consistent with:
   a. normal prostatic tissue
   b. benign prostatic hyperplasia
   c. adenocarcinoma of the prostate
   d. chronic prostatitis
   e. none of the above

8. A "hot spot" in a ^{99m}Tc (technetium) diphosphonate bone scan such as the one shown in Figure 10–9 may indicate:
   a. an increased blood flow
   b. reactive bone formation
   c. destructive lesions
   d. inflammatory lesions
   e. all of the above

NOTES

▶ Figure Descriptions

Figure 10–1. Admission peripheral blood smear. Wright/Giemsa stain. Original magnification ×252.

This photomicrograph illustrates the patient's normocytic, normochromic anemia. The red cell population is decreased in numbers but most of the cells are normal in size and shape. The platelets and two neutrophils present are unremarkable.

Figure 10–2. Normal peripheral blood smear. Wright/Giemsa stain. Original magnification ×315.

These red blood cells do not appear dissimilar in terms of shape and size from those in Figure 10–1, however, there appears to be more of them.

Figure 10–3. CT scan of abdomen with contrast.

The left kidney (arrow) is enlarged, hydronephrotic, and contains a staghorn calculus. The left renal cortex is markedly thinned. The right kidney appears to be normal.

Figure 10–4. Normal CT scan.

Both kidneys are normal in shape and size with well-defined renal cortices. This image is at a higher level than that in Figure 10–3 and we can see portions of the liver and spleen, which appear normal.

Figure 10–5. Prostate gland biopsy. Hematoxylin–eosin stain. Original magnification ×31.

Almost all of the tissue obtained showed infiltration of the gland by numerous, small, tightly-packed acini that have lost their normal convolutions. The cells appear cuboid, the nuclei are enlarged, irregular, and contain prominent nucleoli. These histologic findings are diagnostic of prostatic adenocarcinoma. It should be remembered that this is only one of several patterns of adenocarcinoma of the prostate gland, though it is probably the most common one.

Figure 10–6. Normal prostate gland. Hematoxylin–eosin stain. Original magnification ×12.

Note the irregularly-shaped alveoli scattered throughout the fibromuscular stroma. These glands are lined by columnar epithelium with round or oval nuclei having inconspicuous nucleoli.

Figure 10–7. DNA/Cell cycle analysis of prostate (patient).

This DNA histogram was obtained by flow cytometric analysis of the patient's prostatic tissue. The DNA content (reflected by the intensity of DNA staining) is plotted on the X-axis, and the number of cells of any given staining intensity is plotted on the Y-axis. The first DNA peak (G_1D) represents G_0/G_1 phase of the diploid cell population. The second peak represents G_0/G_1 phase of the aneuploid cell population, which is an abnormal finding. The area between the G_0/G_1 and G_2M phases of each (diploid and aneuploid) cycle defines the "S-phase" fraction, (ie, the proportions of cells in the synthetic phase with an intermediate amount of DNA). Both DNA ploidy and "S-phase" values are important in the interpretation of histograms. About 31% of cells in this specimen have an aneuploid DNA content. The DNA index (DI) is 1.9. DNA index defines the amount of abnormal DNA relative to a normal DNA control, (ie, DNA index = peak channel number of aneuploid G_0/G_1 peak/peak channel number of diploid G_0/G_1 peak).

Figure 10–8. DNA/Cell cycle analysis of normal prostatic tissue.

This DNA histogram shows a diploid DNA peak (G_1D) containing 92.8% of a total cell population and a small G_2D phase with a total proportion of 3.6% of cells, which is within the normal range (<6.0%).

Figure 10–9. Whole body bone imaging.

The imaging agent was a technetium-labeled phosphate (^{99m}Tc-diphosphate) that was administered intravenously. Anterior and posterior images were obtained. They showed numerous abnormal foci of accumulation of the imaging agent. While the "hot spots" are more numerous in the axial skeleton, involvement of the appendicular skeleton is also present.

▶ Answers

1. (**d**) The laboratory values and the blood smear are consistent with anemia of chronic disease. The macrocytosis characteristic of the megaloblastic anemias of vitamin B_{12} and folate deficiency and some forms of chronic liver disease is not evident. Microcytosis and hypochromia of iron deficiency anemia and spherocytes are not apparent.

2. (**a**) Acute bacterial prostatitis is a suppurative inflammation of the prostate. Patients have systemic symptoms, such as fever and chills, and they experience dysuria. The prostate is very tender to palpation. Our patient has none of these symptoms. The diagnosis of prostatic carcinoma should be considered because of the finding on rectal examination of a hard, enlarged prostate and because of the patient's age, anemia, and weight loss. Cancer of the prostate is often combined with prostatic intraepithelial neoplasia. Benign prostatic hyperplasia is extremely common in this age group and should be considered in the differential diagnosis.

3. (**d**) The rectal examination revealed a hard, enlarged prostate. This should raise the suspicion of a prostatic carcinoma. Serum prostatic acid phosphatase (PAP) and serum prostate specific antigen (PSA) are two biochemical markers produced by both normal and neoplastic prostatic epithelium. Serum levels of prostatic acid phosphatase are elevated in locally invasive or widely metastatic prostatic carcinoma. Serum levels of prostate specific antigen (PSA) are proportional to the volume of the tumor. These blood tests in themselves do not provide a direct diagnosis, but are helpful in combination with other diagnostic modalities and in the management of prostatic cancer. Biopsy of the prostate provides the ultimate histological diagnosis. Examination of expressed prostatic secretions (EPS) is helpful as a part of the work-up of an enlarged, painful prostate (prostatitis) to identify a suspected microbial agent. However, examination of EPS is not useful in investigating hard, non-tender prostatic enlargement in older men.

4. (**d**) Figure 10–3 shows hydronephrosis of the left kidney, and the presence of a "staghorn" stone in the renal pelvis. Dilatation of the kidney pelvis and calyces (hydronephrosis) is caused by obstruction to the outflow of the urine. In this case, the obstruction was caused by a stone. It may occur slowly and asymptomatically; the function of the affected kidney diminishes with time, but the contralateral, unaffected, kidney can maintain adequate renal function, and therefore the syndrome of acute renal failure does not occur.

5. (**d**) The larger renal stones develop over a long period of time. They usually manifest themselves by hematuria and are often associated with infections, mostly by urea splitting bacteria. The majority of renal stones are unilateral. The "staghorn" calculus, seen in this patient, led to the left hydronephrosis. The patient was not in renal failure, since the uninvolved contralateral kidney was capable of maintaining normal renal function.

NOTES

6. (**e**) Serum prostate specific antigen (PSA) may be elevated in any of the conditions listed (normal prostatic tissue, benign prostatic hyperplasia, cancer of the prostate, and chronic prostatitis), and hence it is not a specific test. However, it is the most sensitive test for the early detection of prostatic carcinoma, and unlike the acid phosphatase level, it can detect localized disease. In contrast, serum acid phosphatase is usually elevated only when the tumor has spread outside the prostate or metastasized. Serial PSA determinations provide the best means of monitoring the response to treatment.

7. (**c**) The needle biopsy shows numerous small glands of irregular shape with large vacuolated nuclei and often prominent nucleoli, often lying back to back, infiltrating the prostatic stroma. These structures are smaller than normal prostatic glands, and even more so than the dilated glands of prostatic hypertrophy. There is no evidence of aggregates of lymphocytes, plasma cells, macrophages and neutrophils, typical of chronic prostatitis.

8. (**e**) The radionuclide technetium (^{99m}Tc) diphosphonate detects "hot spots," or areas of increased blood flow or reactive bone formation associated with destructive, inflammatory, or arthritic lesions. Since cancer metastases are often lytic or associated with bone formation, they can produce any of the reactions listed. However, some metastatic tumors, such as multiple myeloma, may escape detection by ^{99m}Tc scans. Thus ^{99m}Tc may be used for bone scans to demonstrate any of the reactions or lesions listed. It is a sensitive, though not specific, test for metastases to bone.

▶ Final Diagnosis and Synopsis of Case

- Adenocarcinoma of the Prostate Gland With Widespread Bony Metastatic Disease
- Staghorn Calculus
- Left Hydronephrosis
- Anemia of Chronic Disease

The patient, an 80-year-old man, was admitted for evaluation of his abdominal pain and weight loss. He was found to be severely anemic. Computed tomography showed hydronephrosis of the left kidney and a "staghorn" stone. Rectal examination revealed a hard, enlarged prostate, which on biopsy showed poorly differentiated adenocarcinoma. A bone scan showed multiple foci of increased activity, which were interpreted as evidence of metastatic disease. This classified the patient as having stage D disease. The patient will undergo transurethral resection of the prostate and hormonal therapy.

LAB TIPS

Carcinoma of the Prostate Gland: Gleason Grading System

Several different grading systems exist for adenocarcinoma of the prostate gland. The Glisson system is not based on the cytologic features of the malignant cells, but on the glandular pattern of the tumor as observed by the microscope under low magnification. Five grades are identified, from grade 1, the most differentiated, composed of closely packed, uniformly-shaped single glands, to grade 5 (undifferentiated) which shows no glandular differentiation. In any particular case, the two most prevalent patterns are identified, each is assigned a grade from 1 to 5, and the total grade is their sum. The other commonly used grading system, the three grade system, relies on both the pattern of the tumor and its cytology. This system contains three categories: grade 1, well differentiated; grade 2, moderately differentiated; and grade 3, poorly differentiated. In many institutions, the surgical pathology report will show the grades from both systems. The table below illustrates the relatively good correlation between these two systems.

PROSTATE CARCINOMA: GRADE VERSUS PROGNOSIS

Three Grade System	Combined Gleason Grade[a]	Clinical Stage[b]	Average Incidence of Lymph Node Metastasis
Well differentiated	Usually grades 2 to 4	Usually A or B1	12%
Moderately differentiated	Usually grades 5 to 7		35%
Poorly differentiated	Usually grades 8 to 10	Usually B2 or higher	61%

[a]Discrepancies may occur between the two grading systems when there is a marked difference in the primary and secondary patterns of the Gleason system.
[b]Clinical Staging of prostate carcinoma (abbreviated):
    Stage A—Clinically unsuspected tumor, found incidently in specimens removed presumably for benign nodular hyperplasia.
    Stage B1—Tumor localized to one lobe of gland (usually <2.0 cm).
    Stage B2—Larger tumors still confined to the prostate gland.
    Stage C—Tumor has extended out of the prostate gland and may or may not involve the seminal vesicles.
    Stage D1—Tumor has metastasized to regional lymph nodes.
    Stage D2—Tumor has metastasized to distant sites.

Immunoperoxidase Staining in Prostate Carcinoma

Antisera to prostate-specific acid phosphatase (PSAP) and prostate-specific antigen (PSA) show immunoreactivity to most adenocarcinomas of the prostate and have been used to help identify poorly-differentiated tumors in the prostate gland and establish the prostatic origin of metastases. One should stain for both PSAP and PSA, since not all prostate carcinomas, especially poorly differentiated tumors, stain for both substances. While there are some non-prostatic tumors (eg, breast, carcinoid, and renal) that will stain with PSAP, no non-prostatic tumors have stained with PSA.

A 33-Year-Old Woman With a Sudden Loss of Vision

► **Clinical History and Presentation**

A 33-year-old woman was admitted to the hospital for sudden bilateral loss of vision. About a year ago, the patient also noticed some difficulty in walking, which improved two weeks later. She also reported an occasional tingling and an "electrical" sensation down her back when she flexed her neck. She occasionally had difficulty in expressing herself verbally. Physical examination revealed an alert and oriented woman in mild distress. Her speech was normal. There was no light perception in either eye. Ocular movements were intact. There was no nystagmus and the pupils were sluggishly reactive to light. The patient had paraparesis with spasticity and dissociated sensory loss in the lower extremities. Her sensory level was at T7. Also, there were brisk deep tendon reflexes of the knees and a bilaterally positive Babinski's sign. The rest of the physical examination was unremarkable. A lumbar puncture was performed on admission.

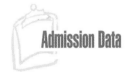

Admission Data

TABLE 11–1. HEMATOLOGY

WBC	7.4 thousand/μL	(4.5–11.0)
Neut	52%	(44–88)
Band	0%	(0–10)
Lymph	40%	(12–43)
Mono	6%	(2–11)
Eos	1%	(2–5)
Baso	1%	(0–2)
RBC	4.53 million/μL	(3.9–5.0)
Hgb	13.1 g/dL	(12.0–15.0)
HCT	39.1%	(36.0–44.0)
MCV	86.5 fL	(79.0–96.0)
MCH	29.0 pg	(26.0–32.0)
MCHC	33.5 g/dL	(32.5–36.0)
Plts	217 thousand/μL	(150–400)

TABLE 11–2. CEREBROSPINAL FLUID

Color	Colorless	(Colorless)
Clarity	Clear	(Clear)
WBC, total	12/μL	(0–5)
Neut	0%	(0)
Lymph	12%	(0)
RBC	Neg	(Neg)
GLUC	70 mg/dL	(40–80)
Protein, total	56 mg/dL	(15–45)
Albumin	21.1 mg/dL	(9–30)
IgG	6 mg/dL	(0.7–3.5)
IgG INDEX	1.1	(0.3–0.7)
VDRL	Neg	(Neg)
Myelin basic protein	6 ng/mL	(0–4)

NOTES

TABLE 11–3. CHEMISTRY

Glucose	87 mg/dL	(65–110)
Creatinine	1.0 mg/dL	(0.7–1.4)
BUN	12 mg/dL	(7–24)
Uric acid	3.1 mg/dL	(3.0–7.5)
Cholesterol	157 mg/dL	(150–240)
Calcium	9.5 mg/dL	(8.5–10.5)
Protein	6.9 g/dL	(6–8)
Albumin	4.0 g/dL	(3.7–5.0)
LDH	130 U/L	(100–250)
Alk Phos	46 U/L	(30–120)
AST	22 U/L	(0–55)
GGTP	20 U/L	(0–50)
Bilirubin	0.5 mg/dL	(0.0–1.5)
Bilirubin, direct	0.14 mg/dL	(0.02–0.18)
Serum IgG	1020 mg/dL	(564–1765)

TABLE 11–4. IMMUNOLOGY

Lyme disease	Negative
RA factor	Negative
Syphilis	Negative
Crypto	Negative
ANA	Negative

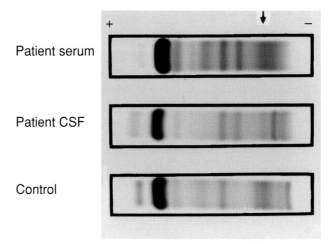

FIGURE 11–1. Cerebrospinal fluid electrophoresis.

▶ Questions

On the basis of the preceding information, you can best conclude the following:

1. The cerebrospinal fluid (CSF) myelin basic protein (MBP) level is elevated in all of the following conditions EXCEPT:
   a. head trauma
   b. primary syphilis
   c. leukodystrophies
   d. Guillain-Barré syndrome
   e. multiple sclerosis

2. Elevated CSF protein levels may be seen in all of the following conditions EXCEPT:
   a. bacterial meningitis
   b. aseptic meningitis
   c. central nervous system (CNS) lymphoma
   d. traumatic dural tear with CSF rhinorrhea
   e. traumatic tap

3. An increased CSF IgG index indicates:
   a. traumatic tap
   b. increased serum IgG transudation to CSF
   c. increased IgG production within the central nervous system (CNS)
   d. a dural tear

4. All of the following statements about the IgG and albumin in the CSF are correct EXCEPT:
   a. the IgG/albumin ratio in the CSF can be different from that in the serum
   b. CSF IgG and albumin can both be secreted into the CNS
   c. IgG and albumin found in the CSF could have diffused into the CSF from the blood
   d. the CSF IgG may be increased without a concurrent increase in the CSF albumin level

5. The CSF electrophoretic pattern seen in Figure 11–1 shows:
   a. CSF monoclonal gammopathy
   b. CSF oligoclonal bands
   c. hypogammaglobulinemia
   d. none of the above

Clinical Course

MRI of the brain, sella, thoracic spine, and orbit were performed. The patient was treated with steroid hormones and discharged several days later.

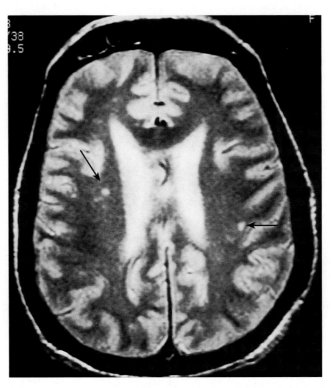

FIGURE 11–2. MRI of the brain.

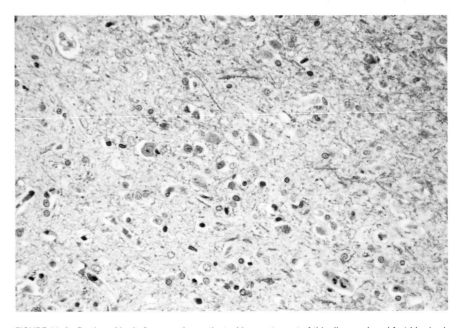

FIGURE 11–3. Portion of brain from another patient with recent onset of this disease. Luxol fast blue/periodic acid-Schiff stain. Original magnification ×78.

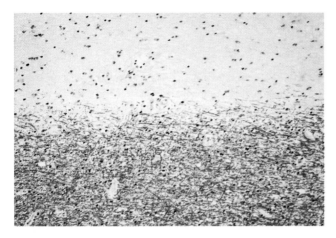

FIGURE 11–4. Portion of brain from another patient with longstanding disease. Luxol fast blue/periodic acid-Schiff stain. Original magnification ×31.

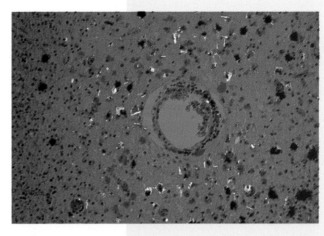

FIGURE 11–5. Portion of brain from another patient with recent onset of this disease. Oil red O stain. Polarized light. Original magnification ×50.

▶ Questions

6. All of the following mechanisms have been suggested to play a role in the pathogenesis of this patient's disorder EXCEPT:
   a. genetic influences
   b. environmental factors
   c. an aberrant immune response
   d. neoplastic proliferation

7. All of the following statements about this disease process are correct EXCEPT:
   a. The abnormal finding in the CSF electrophoresis (Figure 11–1) is due to an increased production of IgG within the central nervous system (CNS)
   b. the early lesions of this disorder are characterized by severe axonal loss
   c. there is a depletion of oligodendrocytes in active plaques
   d. neurological findings are characteristic of upper motor neuron lesions
   e. there is no effective treatment for this disorder

▶ Figure Descriptions

Figure 11–1. Cerebrospinal fluid electrophoresis.

This photomicrograph shows three electrophoretic patterns. The top pattern is that of the patient's serum and shows one broad band in the gamma region (arrow). The middle pattern is that of the patient's cerebrospinal fluid and shows several distinct bands, indicative of oligoclonal bands, in the same region. The bottom is a manufacturer's control that is positive for oligoclonal bands.

Figure 11–2. MRI of brain.

Several areas of increased signal density are present in the deep white matter of the brain (arrows) and represent the demyelinated plaques of multiple sclerosis.

Figure 11–3. Portion of brain from another patient with acute onset of this disease. Luxol fast blue/periodic acid-Schiff stain. Original magnification ×78.

This is an evolving plaque of multiple sclerosis and shows several macrophages containing blue fragments of myelin. PAS-positive material, which is difficult to see in the photomicrograph, represents the breakdown products of myelin.

Figure 11–4. Portion of brain from another patient with longstanding disease. Luxol fast blue/periodic acid-Schiff stain. Original magnification ×31.

This is the edge of an old plaque of multiple sclerosis. The plaque in the upper portion of the image shows almost complete demyelination. Normal myelinated white matter is present in the bottom half of the field.

Figure 11–5. Portion of brain from another patient with acute onset of this disease. Oil red O stain. Polarized light. Original magnification ×50.

This is a frozen section preparation of a portion of an active plaque from a patient with multiple sclerosis. With the oil red O stain, intact myelin stains red and is not birefringent. The breakdown products of myelin, however, are birefringent and under polarized light appear as yellow and blue crystals within the macrophages.

▶ Answers

1. **(b)** Myelin basic protein (MBP) in the cerebrospinal fluid (CSF) is elevated in about 90% of multiple sclerosis (MS) patients during the acute exacerbation stage. An elevated MBP level in the CSF, however, is not specific for MS. It may be also elevated in other conditions, such as neurosyphilis (the tertiary, not the primary, stage of syphilis), head trauma, leukodystrophies, leukemia, hypoxia, cerebrovascular accidents, intrathecal chemotherapy, post irradiation status, Guillain-Barré syndrome, leukoencephalopathy, etc.

2. **(d)** An elevated level of CSF protein is seen with traumatic tap (due to plasma contamination), increased permeability of the blood-CSF barrier, decreased removal of protein (eg, meningitis), obstruction to CSF circulation by tumor, herniation, or adhesions (which would lead to increased water resorption), and increased synthesis of immunoglobulin within the central nervous system (eg, CNS lymphoma). Decreased levels of CSF protein are seen with CSF leakage (trauma), upon removal of a large amount of the CSF during a spinal tap, and in hypothyroidism.

3. (**c**) The cerebrospinal fluid (CSF) IgG index is calculated according to the formula:

$$\frac{\text{CSF IgG}}{\text{serum IgG}} \times \frac{\text{serum albumin}}{\text{CSF albumin}}$$

When the CSF IgG is increased, the IgG index will help to differentiate between an increase in CNS production of IgG and an increase due to serum IgG transudation into the CSF. The normal range for the CSF IgG index is 0–0.77. The presence of an increased CSF IgG and an increased CSF IgG index indicate an increased IgG production within the CNS. In traumatic taps and dural tears, the increase in the CSF IgG level is mainly due to the increased transudation of serum IgG into the CSF.

4. (**b**) IgG can be produced locally in the CNS by B cells, while albumin is produced by the liver. In multiple sclerosis proliferation of B lymphocytes in the CNS will increase the IgG level, but not the albumin level. Both IgG and albumin can, however, diffuse from the blood into the CSF.

5. (**b**) The electrophoretic pattern depicted in Figure 11–1 shows an increased proportion of IgG and oligoclonal bands. There is no monoclonal band in the CSF. The increased level of IgG in the CSF is mainly due to increased proliferation of B lymphocytes in the CNS.

6. (**d**) Multiple sclerosis is the most common of demyelinating disorders. The etiology and pathogenesis of MS are still unknown. MS is clearly not characterized by neoplastic growth. Present evidence suggests that MS is the result of an interaction of genetic, environmental and immune mechanisms that may operate at different stages of the disease.

7. (**b**) The characteristic features of multiple sclerosis include an elevated level of CSF IgG, an increased CSF IgG index, and the presence of oligoclonal bands due to the increased production of IgG by activated B lymphocytes within the CNS. An active plaque of MS is characterized by active demyelination, increased numbers of lipid-laden macrophages, perivascular mononuclear inflammatory cell infiltrates, oligodendrocyte loss, and by astrocytes with reactive changes. The axons, however, are relatively preserved within the active plaque. MS affects the central nervous system (brain and spinal cord) and accordingly, its neurological effects are those characteristic of upper motor neuron lesions. There is no specific or effective therapy for MS. The treatment is usually supportive. Corticosteroids may be helpful in the acute attack.

▶ Final Diagnosis and Synopsis of the Case

• Multiple Sclerosis

A 33-year-old woman presented with an acute onset of vision loss and with multiple sensory and motor problems which had begun approximately a year before. Immunological studies revealed an elevated level of cerebrospinal fluid (CSF) IgG and an increased cerebrospinal fluid IgG index, suggesting a local IgG production. Examination of the cerebrospinal fluid revealed the presence of oligoclonal IgG bands, a slight increase in mononuclear cells, and an increased level of myelin basic protein. The MRI of the brain showed the presence of several deep white matter lesions. The clinical presentation, laboratory findings, and the exclusion of some other possible diagnostic options led to the diagnosis of multiple sclerosis. The patient was treated with steroid hormones, which are known to lessen the severity of the symptoms. However, they do not provide a cure for the disease. The clinical course of this disease is unpredictable, ranging from rare fulminant cases to cases characterized by exacerbations and remissions over the period of many years.

LAB TIPS

Cerebrospinal Fluid Electrophoresis

The electrophoretic pattern of normal cerebrospinal fluid differs in the relative concentrations of various proteins from that of serum. CSF electrophoresis is mainly used to identify oligoclonal IgG bands which are present in 70% to 90% of patients with multiple sclerosis. A serum electrophoresis must be performed simultaneously to ensure that any CSF bands that are present were not derived from serum proteins. Oligoclonal IgG bands can also be found in subacute sclerosing panencephalitis, mumps encephalitis, HIV infection, neurosyphilis (60% of patients), bacterial and viral meningoencephalitis (40% of patients), meningeal carcinomatosis, herpes simplex encephalitis, and so on.

CEREBROSPINAL FLUID ELECTROPHORESIS

Component	Normal Range	Comments
Total protein	20–50 mg/dL	Elevated with CSF leukocytosis (infections), CSF blood (hemorrhage, traumatic tap), tumors, collagen diseases, multiple sclerosis, toxic encephalopathies, etc
Pre–albumin (transthyretin)	2–7%	Increased in cerebral atrophy
Albumin	56–76%	Reflects, as does total protein, the permeability of the blood–brain barrier
α_1–Globulin	2–7%	Increased in tumors, and extensive cerebrovascular damage
α_2–Globulin	4–12%	Increased in infections, inflammations
β–Globulin	8–18%	Increased in meningeal hemorrhage, some degenerative disorders
γ–Globulin	3–12%	Mainly IgG; elevated: (1) with increased permeability of blood–brain barrier, (2) when there is an increased serum immunoglobulin (eg, chronic infections and inflammations), and (3) CSF production of immunoglobulins (multiple sclerosis, etc)

▶ Clinical History and Presentation

A 64-year-old man was found to have a significantly elevated serum ferritin. Other than excessive fatigue, the patient had minimal general complaints and no known medical problems. He admitted to moderate consumption of alcohol, and did not take any medication or vitamin supplements. Physical examination revealed a well-nourished man in no acute distress. Pertinent physical findings included a somewhat grayish color of the skin, an enlarged liver palpable 8 cm below the right costal margin, and a symmetrically enlarged and soft prostate on rectal examination.

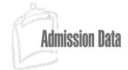

Admission Data

TABLE 12–1. HEMATOLOGY		
WBC	4.9 thousand/μL	(3.6–11.2)
Neut	57%	(44–88)
Band	0%	(0–10)
Lymph	31%	(12–43)
Mono	9%	(2–11)
Eos	2%	(0–5)
Baso	1%	(0–2)
RBC	4.87 million/μL	(4.0–5.8)
Hgb	15.3 g/dL	(12.6–17.0)
HCT	44.8%	(42.0–52.0)
MCV	91.9 fL	(80.0–102.0)
MCH	31.4 pg	(27.0–35.0)
MCHC	34.2 g/dL	(30.7–36.7)
Plts	162 thousand/μL	(130–400)

TABLE 12–2. URINALYSIS		
pH	6	(5.0–7.5)
Protein	Neg	(Neg)
Glucose	Neg	(Neg)
Ketone	Neg	(Neg)
Occult blood	Neg	(Neg)
Color	Yellow	(Yellow)
Sp. grav	1.020	(1.010–1.055)
WBC	1/HPF	(0–5)
RBC	0/HPF	(0–2)
Bacteria	Neg	(Neg)

TABLE 12–3. CHEMISTRY

Glucose	160 mg/dL	(65–110)
Creatinine	1.2 mg/dL	(0.7–1.4)
BUN	22 mg/dL	(7–24)
Uric acid	8.5 mg/dL	(3.0–8.5)
Cholesterol	240 mg/dL	(150–240)
Calcium	9.3 mg/dL	(8.5–10.5)
Protein	7.0 g/dL	(6–8)
Albumin	4.7 g/dL	(3.7–5.0)
LDH	165 U/L	(100–250)
Alk Phos	84 U/L	(0–120)
AST	17 U/L	(0–55)
GGTP	12 U/L	(0–50)
Bilirubin	0.5 mg/dL	(0.0–1.5)
Biluribin, direct	0.09 mg/dL	(0.02–0.18)

TABLE 12–4. COAGULATION

PT	12 sec	(11–14)
aPTT	24 sec	(19–28)

TABLE 12–5. ELECTROLYTES

Na	139 mEq/L	(134–143)
K	3.7 mEq/L	(3.5–4.9)
Cl	96 mEq/L	(95–108)
CO_2	26 mEq/L	(21–32)

TABLE 12–6. SERUM IRON STUDIES

Iron	275 μg	(80–160)
Ferritin	465 ng/mL	(20–300)
Total iron binding capacity (TIBC)	200 μg/dL	(250–410)
Transf. saturation	85%	(20–55)

TABLE 12–7. SPECIAL STUDIES

Prostate specific antigen (PSA):	2.7 ng/mL	(<4.0)

▶ **Questions**

On the basis of the preceding information, you can best conclude the following:

1. All of the following statements about ferritin are correct EXCEPT:
   a. it represents the storage form of iron
   b. it is a protein-iron complex
   c. most of the body ferritin circulates in plasma
   d. an increased plasma level of ferritin does not always represent increased body iron
   e. ferritin can be stored in both parenchymal and mononuclear phagocytic cells

2. All of the following statements about transferrin are correct EXCEPT that:
   a. it is an iron binding glycoprotein
   b. it is a product of hemoglobin catabolism
   c. it delivers iron to the cells
   d. it is produced in the liver
   e. almost all of the plasma iron is bound to transferrin

3. An increased serum level of ferritin is seen in all of the following conditions EXCEPT:
   a. iron deficiency anemia
   b. idiopathic hemochromatosis
   c. chronic inflammatory conditions
   d. hemolytic anemia
   e. liver damage

4. The patient's CBC and iron studies are suggestive of:
   a. acute blood loss
   b. a chronic iron deficiency state
   c. hemochromatosis
   d. polycythemia vera
   e. anemia of chronic disease

5. Considering all the abnormal findings in this patient, all of the following statements are correct EXCEPT:
   a. the increase in blood glucose is most likely etiologically related to the underlying disease process
   b. the liver enlargement is due to the underlying disease process
   c. the color of the patient's skin is due to the underlying disease process
   d. the enlarged prostate is most likely due to the underlying disease process
   e. a liver biopsy would confirm the diagnosis

NOTES

▶ Clinical Course

All abnormal laboratory tests were repeated and confirmed. The patient was admitted for a liver biopsy (Figures 12–1 and 12–2).

TABLE 12–8. LIVER IRON CONTENT	
Patient	Normal
2050 mg/100 mg of dry liver	(<200 mg/100 mg of dry liver)

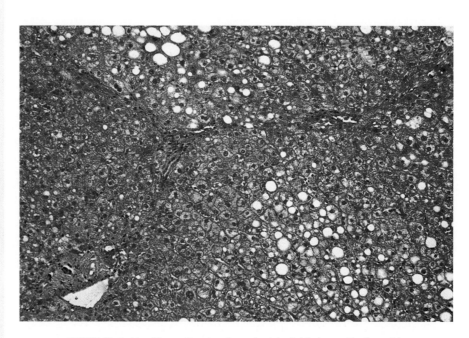

FIGURE 12–1. Liver biopsy. Hematoxylin–eosin stain. Original magnification ×31.

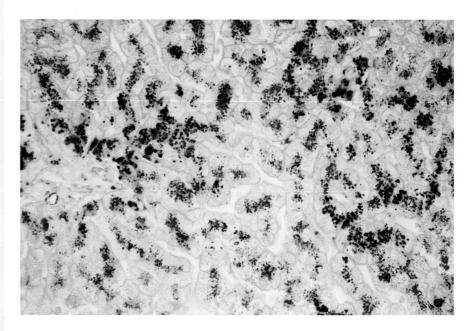

FIGURE 12–2. Liver biopsy. Iron stain. Original magnification ×78.

▶ **Questions**

6. The microscopic appearance of the liver (Figure 12–1):
   a. depicts a granulomatous lesion
   b. suggests the presence of metastatic carcinoma
   c. depicts a liver abscess
   d. shows changes characteristic of right-sided heart failure
   e. shows fatty change and increased portal fibrosis

7. Identify the INCORRECT statement about the accumulation of iron as detected by a Prussian blue stain in Figure 12–2:
   a. it may occur in the parenchymal cells of the liver
   b. it may occur in the Kupffer cells
   c. it may occur in the epithelial cells of the bile duct
   d. it may lead to organ injury
   e. it is irreversible

8. An iron overload disorder may be due to:
   a. multiple blood transfusions
   b. high iron intake
   c. ineffective erythropoiesis
   d. genetic abnormality
   e. all of the above

9. All of the following statements regarding this patient's primary disorder are true EXCEPT that:
   a. it is known to be associated with the HLA-A3 allele
   b. family studies suggest an autosomal recessive inheritance of the susceptibility gene
   c. there is a strong male predominance of the fully developed disease
   d. the excess iron predominantly accumulates in the cytoplasm of the parenchymal cells
   e. carcinoma of the liver in patients with this disease is an extremely rare finding

10. All of the following statements concerning this patient's condition are correct EXCEPT:
   a. phlebotomy is an appropriate treatment
   b. the HLA typing of family members and close relatives is justified
   c. the prostatic enlargement is most likely of benign character
   d. the patient is at increased risk of developing squamous cell carcinoma of the skin
   e. the patient could develop arrhythmias or congestive heart failure as a consequence of his disease

Figure Descriptions

Figure 12–1. Liver biopsy. Hematoxylin–eosin stain. Original magnification ×31.

The junction of several lobules are visible here. There is a slight increase in portal fibrosis with some extension between adjacent portal areas, but true cirrhosis is not present. Moderate fatty change is evident.

Figure 12–2. Liver biopsy. Prussian blue stain. Original magnification ×78.

The Prussian blue stain for iron clearly shows a marked increase in iron content, primarily in hepatocytes, but also in sinusoidal macrophages.

Answers

1. (**c**) Ferritin is a water soluble protein-iron complex which represents, together with hemosiderin, a storage form of iron. Most of ferritin is stored within the parenchymal and the mononuclear phagocytic cells. Only a very small amount of ferritin circulates in the plasma. The plasma level of ferritin is generally a good indicator of iron stores in the body. In fact, serum ferritin is (except for bone marrow iron stains) the most sensitive test for detection of iron deficiency. However, in certain conditions, an elevated serum ferritin does not necessarily indicate excessive body iron stores; such conditions include inflammatory processes, neoplasia, or liver disease. In these conditions, an increased ferritin level represents an acute phase response which may persist for several weeks.

2. (**b**) Transferrin is an iron-binding glycoprotein which is synthesized primarily by the liver. Almost all plasma iron is bound to transferrin, which transports iron from its absorption site, the intestine, or from the reticuloendothelial system (RBC catabolism), to other cells. Transferrin is not a product of hemoglobin catabolism.

3. (**a**) Iron deficiency anemia leads to a decreased, not an increased, serum ferritin level. All other conditions listed (idiopathic hemochromatosis, chronic inflammatory conditions, hemolytic anemia, and liver damage) present with an increased ferritin level.

4. (**c**) The patient's iron studies show increased serum levels of iron and ferritin and an increase in transferrin saturation. The total iron binding capacity (TIBC) is decreased. These findings indicate an iron overload condition, typically seen in hemochromatosis. The patient's CBC is normal, which is also compatible with hemochromatosis. A chronic iron deficiency state and anemia of chronic disease show abnormalities of CBC and an iron deficiency; polycythemia vera is a myeloproliferative disorder which is associated with an increased RBC count and hematocrit, not present in this patient. Acute blood loss does not present with a picture of an iron overload.

5. (**d**) If the diagnosis of hemochromatosis is suspected, the only abnormality that is not a feature of this disease is the enlarged prostate. Diabetes mellitus, hepatomegaly and metallic discoloration of the skin are the classic presenting features, and liver biopsy would confirm the diagnosis.

6. (**e**) The microscopic appearance of the liver shows fatty change and a slight increase in portal fibrosis. There are no features of right-sided heart failure, liver abscess, granuloma formation, or metastatic carcinoma.

7. (**e**) The accumulation of iron in the hepatocytes is reversible. It may occur in the parenchymal cells of the liver, the Kupffer cells, or the epithelial cells of the bile duct and may lead to liver injury.

8. (e) Iron overload with excessive iron deposits can be observed in anemias with ineffective erythropoiesis, when iron absorption by the body continues despite the inability of the erythrocytes to properly utilize iron in heme synthesis. Multiple blood transfusions can produce a clear iron overload. High iron intake leading to iron overload has been described in South African blacks following the drinking of iron-contaminated alcoholic beverages. A genetic role in iron overload disorders is best documented in hemochromatosis.

9. (e) The patient had primary hemochromatosis. It is a genetically determined disease. The gene for hemochromatosis is located on the sixth chromosome close to the HLA-A locus. The strongest association is with the HLA-A3 allele. The mode of inheritance is autosomal recessive and men are affected 10 times more often than women. Parenchymal cells are preferentially affected by iron deposition. Hepatocellular carcinoma is a relatively frequent complication, especially in patients with cirrhosis.

10. (d) Phlebotomy therapy is the preferred treatment for the removal of excess iron. The removal of one unit of blood depletes the body of 200-250 mg of iron. It is done weekly or twice a week, and is closely monitored by plasma iron and ferritin levels. All family members should have an HLA typing performed and be tested for iron overload to detect possible disease as early as possible. Cardiac involvement in hemochromatosis is frequent. The symmetrical prostatic enlargement with normal PSA is most likely benign, but should be followed up. Squamous cell carcinoma of the skin is not seen with increased frequency in patients with idiopathic hemochromatosis.

Final Diagnosis and Synopsis of the Case

- Hemochromatosis
- Diabetes Mellitus
- Benign Prostatic Hyperplasia

A 64-year-old man without any significant medical or surgical history was found, on routine examination, to have a significantly increased serum level of ferritin and glucose. The patient's physician also noted an abnormal metallic color of the skin and an enlarged liver. Complete iron studies showed an increased serum iron, a high transferrin saturation, and a decreased total iron binding capacity (TIBC). The physical and laboratory data suggested the diagnosis of an iron overload disorder. In the absence of anemia, or a history of multiple blood transfusion or other source of high iron intake, idiopathic hemochromatosis was considered the most likely diagnosis. Liver biopsy showing an increased iron concentration confirmed the diagnosis. The increased glucose level reflected pancreatic involvement due to ferritin and hemosiderin deposition. The skin discoloration was also due to the accumulation of hemosiderin in the dermal macrophages and fibroblasts, combined with an increased amount of melanin. The symmetrically enlarged soft prostate in the presence of a normal prostate specific antigen (PSA) level was most likely due to a benign prostatic hypertrophy, which is extremely common in this age category. Hemochromatosis affects predominantly liver, pancreas, heart, synovium, skin, and endocrine glands owing to the accumulation of ferritin and hemosiderin. Therapy involves the removal of 500 mL of blood by phlebotomies once or twice weekly until a desirable plasma iron concentration is reached. The life expectancy of symptomatic patients is extended by the treatment and is virtually normal in treated asymptomatic patients.

LAB TIPS

Acute Phase Reactants

One of the most common findings on the serum protein electrophoresis of hospitalized patients is the acute phase reaction pattern (showing decreased albumin level and elevated alpha 2-globulin level) that occurs with infection, trauma (including surgery), injury, or other conditions in which there is tissue necrosis. Other determinations that can be used to monitor an inflammatory state include elevations in the patient's temperature, white blood cell count, and sedimentation rate. The measurement of serum acute phase reactants is useful in several situations, including patients with an occult infection or autoimmune disorders.

THE ACUTE PHASE REACTANTS

Protein	Reference Range	Function	Level in Acute Phase
Prealbumin	20–40 mg/dL	Transport protein	Decreased
Albumin	3.5–5.0 g/dL	Transport protein; maintains colloid osmotic pressure in vessels	Decreased
α_1–Acid glycoprotein (orosomucoid)	50–150 mg/dL	Unknown	Increased
α_1–Antitrypsin	80–200 mg/dL	Neutralizes trypsin from leukocytes	Increased
Haptoglobin	30–220 mg/dL	Binds hemoglobin (preserves iron stores)	Increased
Fibrinogen	100–400 mg/dL	Clot formation (healing of wounds uses a large amount of fibrinogen)	Increased
C–reactive protein	500–1300 ng/mL	Scavenger protein; aids in opsonization; activates classic complement pathway (lyses foreign cells); detoxification	Increased (markedly)
Serum Ferritin	15–200 ng/mL (Male) 12–150 ng/mL (Female)	Regulates iron transport	Increased

Lab Tips (continued)

THE IRON PANEL IN VARIOUS CONDITIONS

Condition	Serum Iron	TIBC[a]	Serum Ferritin	Transferrin Saturation
Normal range	60–150 µg/dL	250–400 µg/dL	15–200 ng/mL (male) 12–150 ng/mL (female)	20–55%
Iron deficiency	Decreased	Increased	Decreased	Decreased
Hemochromatosis	Increased	Normal or decreased	Increased	Increased
Thalassemia	Increased	Decreased	Increased	Increased
Chronic infection	Decreased	Decreased	Increased	Decreased
Acute liver disease	Increased	Increased	Increased	Normal or increased
Chronic liver disease	Normal or decreased	Decreased	Increased	Normal or increased
Malignancy	Decreased	Decreased	Increased	Decreased

[a]TIBC—Total iron–binding capacity

► **Clinical History and Presentation**

A 30-year-old man was admitted to the hospital with a chief complaint of severe squeezing chest pain of ten minutes' duration which had begun after dinner while he was watching television. The pain radiated to the left shoulder and jaw and was associated with palpitations and shortness of breath. The patient also recalled a similar episode the previous month that had lasted only about two minutes. The patient was a heavy cigarette smoker. His family history showed that his grandfather, father, and sister had died from heart attacks at an early age. The patient's older brother, and his father's brother and sister were alive and well. Physical examination revealed a pale and restless young man in severe distress due to his chest pain. The pain subsided after he was given a vasodilator. Blood pressure was 120/80 mmHg, heart rate was 60 per minute and regular, and temperature was 98° F. Chest and abdominal examinations were unremarkable. White deposits were noted on the lateral side of both corneas. There were nodular swellings of the Achilles tendons and of the tendons of both knees. EKG showed elevated ST segments in the precordial leads. A coronary arteriogram was performed and showed a fixed 80% stenosis of the left anterior descending artery and 60% stenosis of the right coronary artery. A repeated EKG was normal.

Admission Data

TABLE 13–1. HEMATOLOGY

WBC	6.3 thousand/μL	(3.3–11.0)
Neut	75%	(44–88)
Band	0%	(0–10)
Lymph	21%	(12–43)
Mono	3%	(2–11)
Eos	1%	(0–5)
Baso	0%	(0–2)
RBC	4.44 million/μL	(3.9–5.0)
Hgb	13.5 g/dL	(11.6–15.6)
HCT	41%	(37.0–47.0)
MCV	92.4 fL	(79.0–99.0)
MCH	30.3 pg	(26.0–32.6)
MCHC	32.8 g/dL	(31.0–36.0)
Plts	236 thousand/μL	(130–400)

TABLE 13–2. CHEMISTRY

Glucose	92 mg/dL	(65–110)
Creatinine	1.0 mg/dL	(0.7–1.4)
BUN	18 mg/dL	(7–24)
Uric acid	4 mg/dL	(3.0–8.5)
Cholesterol	400 mg/dL	(150–240)
Calcium	9 mg/dL	(8.5–10.5)
Protein	7.5 g/dL	(6–8)
Albumin	4.4 g/dL	(3.7–5.0)
LDH	200 U/L	(100–250)
Alk Phos	50 U/L	(0–120)
AST	55 U/L	(0–55)
GGTP	27 U/L	(0–50)
Bilirubin	0.7 mg/dL	(0.0–1.5)
Bilirubin, direct	0.18 mg/dL	(0.02–0.18)

TABLE 13–3. CARDIAC ENZYMES

CK	216 U/L	(55–215)
CK–MB	3%	(<5%)
LDH	200 U/L	(100–250)
LDH_1	20%	(17–28)
LDH_2	40%	(30–36)
LDH_3	20%	(19–25)
LDH_4	13%	(10–16)
LDH_5	7%	(6–13)

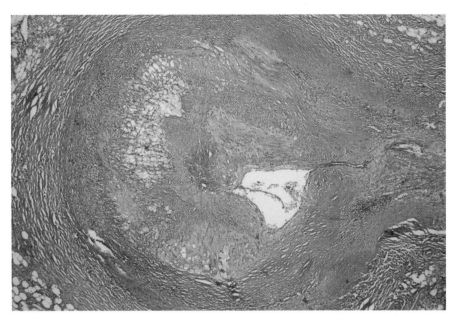

FIGURE 13–1. Coronary artery from another patient with this disease. Hematoxylin–eosin stain. Original magnification ×8.

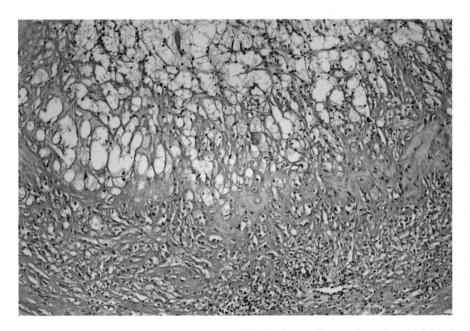

FIGURE 13–2. Coronary artery from another patient with this disease. Hematoxylin–eosin stain. Original magnification ×31.

NOTES

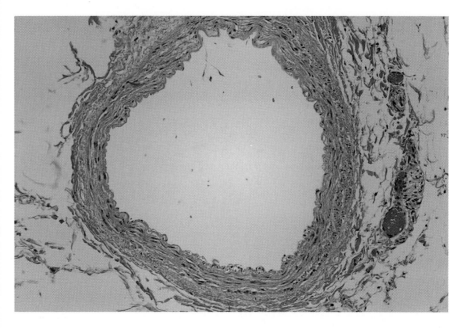

FIGURE 13–3. Normal coronary artery. Hematoxylin–eosin stain. Original magnification ×31.

▶ **Questions**

On the basis of the preceding information, you can best conclude the following:

1. The clinical presentation of the acute problem and related laboratory values are most strongly indicative of:
   a. myocardial infarction
   b. an asthmatic attack
   c. congestive heart failure
   d. variant (Prinzmetal's) angina

2. The patient's clinical presentation may be caused by:
   a. fixed stenosing coronary arteries
   b. vasospasm
   c. platelet aggregation
   d. increased myocardial demand
   e. all of the above

3. All of the following changes would be expected in patients with acute myocardial infarction EXCEPT:
   a. a polymorphonuclear leukocytosis that begins about 24 hours after the onset of acute symptoms
   b. an increased erythrocyte sedimentation rate (ESR) 24 hours after the onset of symptoms
   c. an increased serum LDH level about 48 hours after the onset of the symptoms
   d. an increased serum level of the CK-MB fraction of creatinine kinase (CK) at the end of the first week
   e. changes in the electrocardiogram (EKG)

4. Identify the INCORRECT statement about the lesion depicted in Figures 13–1 and 13–2 that was obtained from the autopsy of another patient with the same underlying disease:
   a. it can undergo calcification
   b. it can lead to cholesterol emboli
   c. it can hemorrhage
   d. it can undergo aneurysmal dilatation
   e. it is often complicated by granuloma formation

▶ Clinical Course

Cardiac enzymes were repeated serially and the results were similar to those obtained on admission. The cholesterol level was repeated in duplicate and it was again elevated (350 mg/dL). The patient was discharged and referred to a lipid consultant for further evaluation. A complete lipid profile *(see below)* and a biopsy of a nodule in one of the Achilles tendons (Figures 13–4 through 13–7) were performed. Dietary therapy alone failed to lower his cholesterol level and he was started on specific therapy. The patient was later advised to bring his 7-month-old son for evaluation.

TABLE 13–4. LIPID PROFILE		
Cholesterol	399 mg/dL	(150–250)
Triglycerides	120 mg/dL	(43–171)
HDL	40 mg/dL	(30–70)
LDL	335 mg/dL	(70–190)
Apoprotein A–1	1.08 g/L	(1.15–1.9)
Apoprotein B100	2.53 g/L	(0.17–1.6)

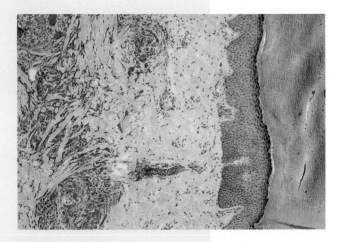

FIGURE 13–4. Biopsy of skin nodule. Oil red O stain. Original magnification ×20.

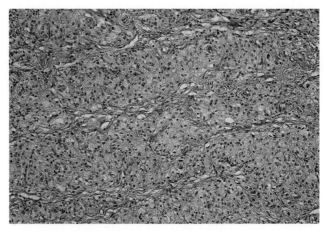

FIGURE 13–5. Biopsy of skin nodule. Hematoxylin–eosin stain. Original magnification ×31.

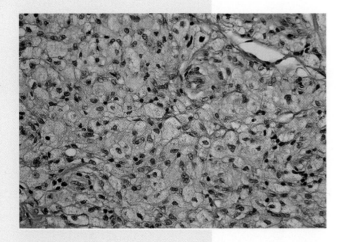

FIGURE 13–6. Biopsy of skin nodule. Hematoxylin–eosin stain. Original magnification ×78.

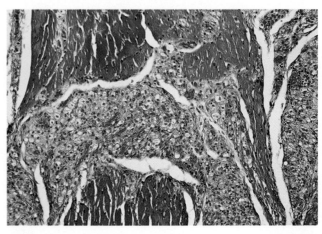

FIGURE 13–7. Biopsy of skin nodule. Trichrome stain. Original magnification ×31.

> ▶ **Questions**

5. The lesion depicted in Figures 13–4 through 13–7 most likely represents:
   a. clear cell sarcoma
   b. xanthoma
   c. chronic granuloma
   d. erythema nodosum

6. The main pathogenetic mechanism underlying this patient's condition is:
   a. deficiency in lipoprotein lipase
   b. increased synthesis of endogenous cholesterol
   c. defective removal of plasma LDL
   d. all of the above
   e. none of the above

7. The probability that this patient's son has the same metabolic problem is at least:
   a. 10%
   b. 25%
   c. 50%
   d. 100%

8. This metabolic problem is known to be associated with:
   a. arcus corneae
   b. hypercholesterolemia
   c. xanthoma
   d. accelerated coronary disease
   e. all of the above

9. All of the following conditions may increase HDL cholesterol levels EXCEPT:
   a. exercise
   b. moderate alcohol consumption
   c. insulin treatment
   d. estrogen
   e. starvation

▶ **Figure Descriptions**

Figure 13–1. Coronary artery from another patient with this disease. Hematoxylin–eosin stain. Original magnification ×8.

The lumen of the artery is greatly reduced in size due to a large atheromatous plaque composed of a fibrous cap and a central necrotic core containing slit-like cholesterol clefts and lipid-laden foam cells. Smooth muscle hypertrophy is evident near the sides of the plaque and the medial wall under the plaque shows marked thinning.

Figure 13–2. Coronary artery from another patient with this disease. Hematoxylin–eosin stain. Original magnification ×31.

Numerous lipid-laden foam cells and debris are present in the central necrotic core. Fibrous tissue and chronic inflammatory cells are also present. The media has been greatly thinned in this area.

Figure 13–3. Normal coronary artery. Hematoxylin–eosin stain. Original magnification ×31.

This is a cross-section of a coronary artery from a teenager and shows an intact intima and no evidence of plaque formation.

Figure 13–4. Biopsy of skin nodule. Oil red O stain. Original magnification ×20.

This is a frozen section of the Achilles tendon nodule and shows the presence of fat within the dermis. Since lipids are dissolved out during routine histological processing, their demonstration in tissue sections requires a frozen section.

Figure 13–5. Biopsy of skin nodule. Hematoxylin–eosin stain. Original magnification ×31.

The nodule is composed of collections of pale-staining cells with abundant cytoplasm and delicate-appearing nuclei.

Figure 13–6. Biopsy of skin nodule. Hematoxylin–eosin stain. Original magnification ×78.

The cells are histiocytes with clear or reticulated cytoplasm that would have contained lipids before histological processing. Since the patient had hyperlipemia, this nodule is an example of a hyperlipemic xanthoma.

Figure 13–7. Biopsy of skin nodule. Masson trichrome stain. Original magnification ×31.

This photomicrograph demonstrates the infiltrative nature of the masses of histiocytes as they separate bands of fibrous tissue overlying the tendon. However, this lesion is technically not a neoplasm and many people would refer to it as an xanthosis rather than an xanthoma.

▶ Answers

1. (**d**) Squeezing chest pain that radiates to the left shoulder and jaw is the classical presentation of myocardial ischemia. In this patient, the duration of pain (10 minutes), the absence of prominent EKG changes, the low MB fraction of CK, and the normal LDH_1 to LDH_2 (1 to 2) ratio favor the diagnosis of variant (Prinzmetal) angina over that of myocardial infarction. There are no signs and symptoms of congestive heart failure or of an asthmatic attack (the lung was clear to auscultation and percussion).

2. (**e**) Fixed stenosis of coronary arteries, vasospasm, platelet aggregation, and increased myocardial demand play an important etiological role in the pathogenesis of all three variants of angina pectoris (typical, variant (Prinzmetal's) and unstable angina).

3. (**d**) In acute myocardial infarction, the CK-MB serum level begins to rise 3–6 hours after the onset of symptoms, reaches its peak in 12–24 hours, and returns to its normal level in 24–48 hours. All other statements are correct (polymorphonuclear leukocytosis and increased erythrocyte sedimentation rate (ESR) begin about 24 hours after the onset of acute symptoms, increased serum LDH level begins about 48 hours after the onset of the symptoms, and specific electrocardiogram changes occur).

4. (**e**) Figures 13–1 and 13–2 depict the typical histological features of coronary atherosclerosis (atheromatous plaque), such as intimal and smooth muscle proliferation, cholesterol clefts, and foamy macrophages. Calcification, cholesterol emboli, hemorrhage, and aneurysmal dilatation are all known complications of atheromas. Granuloma formation is seen with chronic granulomatous inflammation and certain types of vasculitis, but not with coronary atherosclerosis.

5. (**b**) Figures 13–4 through 13–7 represent a skin lesion with the accumulation of lipid-laden macrophages in the dermis typically seen with xanthomas. There are no malignant changes, granuloma formation, or the septal inflammatory cell infiltrate of the subcutaneous adipose tissue characteristic of erythema nodosum.

6. (**c**) The patient had a genetically determined disorder of LDL metabolism known as familial hypercholesterolemia (type IV hyperlipidemia). High levels of serum cholesterol are due to defective removal of plasma LDL and also due to an increased synthesis of LDL. Both metabolic abnormalities result from a mutation in the gene encoding the LDL-receptor. There is no deficiency in lipoprotein lipase, nor an increase in the synthesis of endogenous cholesterol.

7. (**c**) Familial hypercholesterolemia has an autosomal dominant inheritance pattern. Children of heterozygous patients will have a 50% probability of inheriting the disease.

8. (**e**) Familial hypercholesterolemia is associated with LDL-receptor deficiency, an increased LDL level, xanthomas of tendons, xanthelasma, premature ischemic heart disease, hypercholesterolemia, and arcus corneae (faint white deposits on the peripheral aspect of the cornea).

9. (**e**) Starvation leads to a decrease in HDL cholesterol levels, not an increase. The other options, which are exercise, moderate alcohol consumption, insulin treatment, and estrogens all increase the HDL cholesterol levels.

▶ Final Diagnosis and Synopsis of the Case

- Coronary Artery Atherosclerosis
- Variant (Prinzmetal's) Angina
- Familial Hypercholesterolemia With Hyperlipemic Xanthosis

A 30-year-old man presented with chest pain which subsided after vasodilator treatment. Acute myocardial infarction was ruled out, but a coronary arteriogram revealed 80% stenosis of the left anterior descending artery and the diagnosis of variant (Prinzmetal's) angina was made. The patient had a strong family history of ischemic heart disease and his lipid profile showed elevated cholesterol, LDL cholesterol and apoprotein B100 levels, and normal triglycerides and HDL cholesterol levels. The patient's family history and lipid profile in the presence of arcus corneae (faint white deposits on the peripheral aspect of the cornea) and tendon xanthoma (Achilles tendon and tendon of both knees) confirmed the diagnosis of familial hypercholesterolemia. Familial hypercholesterolemia is an autosomal dominant genetic disorder (perhaps the most common metabolic disorder), which is most likely due to the deficiency of the LDL-receptor. The family history of the patient suggested that he was heterozygous for the disease. This patient's son will have a 50% chance of inheriting the mutant gene. Familial hypercholesterolemia can be diagnosed at birth (umbilical blood would show a 2–3 fold increase in LDL concentration).

LAB TIPS

The Lipid Panel

There is considerable variation among different institutions as to the makeup of the laboratory tests in the lipid profile. Listed below are a number of tests that are currently being used to assess the risk of coronary heart disease (CHD).

TESTS USED TO ASSESS THE RISK OF CORONARY HEART DISEASE

Test	Reference Ranges (Adult)	Comments
Serum cholesterol, total	Desirable level <200 mg/dL Borderline risk 200–239 mg/dL High risk level >240 mg/dL	Biologic, diurnal, and seasonal variations are known to occur; varies with diet, age, sex, alcohol intake, and exercise
Serum triglycerides	10–190 mg/dL	Used in differential diagnosis of primary or secondary hyperlipidemia; determines risk factor for acute pancreatitis, not an independent risk factor for CHD *Increased* in alcoholism, diabetes, hypertension, hyperuricemia, pregnancy, etc
High density lipoproteins (HDL) (α–lipoprotein band)	Low risk >60 mg/dL Moderate risk 35–60 mg/dL High risk <35 mg/dL	*Increased* in familial hyper–alpha–lipoproteinemia, alcohol intake, estrogens, ascorbic acid, treated diabetes, etc *Decreased* in familial hypo–alpha–lipoproteinemia, Tangier disease, hypertriglyceridemia, CHD, uremia, liver disease, malnutrition, AIDS, untreated diabetes, starvation, etc
Low density lipoproteins (LDL) (β–lipoprotein band)	Desirable level <130 mg/dL Borderline risk 130–159 mg/dL High risk level >160 mg/dL	*Increased* in familial hypercholesterolemia, hypothyroidism, hepatic disease, pregnancy, diabetes mellitus, chronic renal disease, nephrotic syndrome, etc *Decreased* in malnutrition, malabsorption, chronic anemias, hyperthyroidism, etc
Apolipoproteins		The protein portion of lipoproteins; four major classes identified (A,B,C,E)
Apo A	Major apoprotein of HDL	*Decreased* in CHD even when HDL is normal
Apo B	Major apoprotein of LDL	*Increased* in CHD even when LDL is normal
Apo C	Major apoprotein of VLDL	
Apo E	Found in all lipoprotein fractions	High affinity for macrophages; may play an important role in atherogenesis

NOTES

Lab Tips (continued)

TESTS USED TO ASSESS THE RISK OF CORONARY HEART DISEASE (continued)

LDL/HDL Ratio		Cholesterol/HDL Ratio	
Low risk	0.5–3.0	Low risk	3.3–4.4
Moderate risk	3.0–6.0	Average risk	4.4–7.1
High risk	>6.0	Moderate risk	7.1–11.0
		High risk	>11.0

A 40-Year-Old Woman With a Painful and Swollen Calf

▶ **Clinical History and Presentation**

A 40-year-old woman presented with pain and swelling of two days' duration in the right calf. Previous to this episode she had been in good health. She was married and the mother of a 16-year-old daughter. She was a frequent long-distance traveler and smoked a pack of cigarettes per day. She had had no significant past medical or surgical history. She was on no medications aside from oral contraceptives. Physical examination revealed an alert and oriented woman in no acute distress. Her blood pressure was 160/76 mmHg, heart rate was 64 per minute and regular, temperature was 99° F, and respiratory rate was 18 per minute. Pertinent physical findings included edema of the right calf with tenderness in the upper posterior portion and a positive Homan's sign (pain on dorsiflexion of the foot). Pulses were present in both lower extremities. The patient was admitted to the hospital.

Admission Data

TABLE 14–1. HEMATOLOGY		
WBC	8.1 thousand/μL	(4.5–11.0)
Neut	65%	(44–88)
Band	0%	(0–10)
Lymph	20%	(12–43)
Mono	12%	(2–11)
Eos	2%	(0–5)
Baso	1%	(0–2)
RBC	2.81 million/μL	(3.9–5.0)
Hgb	9.5 g/dL	(12.0–15.0)
HCT	29.2%	(36.0–44.0)
MCV	103.9 fL	(79.0–96.0)
MCH	33.8 pg	(26.0–32.0)
MCHC	32.5 g/dL	(32.5–36.0)
Plts	274 thousand/μL	(130–400)

TABLE 14–2. CHEMISTRY		
Glucose	85 mg/dL	(65–110)
Creatinine	0.9 mg/dL	(0.7–1.4)
BUN	7 mg/dL	(7–24)
Uric acid	3.3 mg/dL	(3.0–7.5)
Cholesterol	250 mg/dL	(150–240)
Calcium	9.4 mg/dL	(8.5–10.5)
Protein	7.1 g/dL	(6–8)
Albumin	4.2 g/dL	(3.7–5.0)
LDH	274 U/L	(100–250)
Alk Phos	70 U/L	(30–120)
AST	22 U/L	(0–55)
GGTP	31 U/L	(0–50)
Bilirubin	0.4 mg/dL	(0.0–1.5)
Bilirubin, direct	0.07 mg/dL	(0.02–0.18)

TABLE 14–3. ERYTHROCYTE SEDIMENTATION RATE

ESR	60 mm/hr	(0–15)

TABLE 14–4. COAGULATION

PT	12.5 sec	(11–14)
aPTT	21 sec	(19–28)

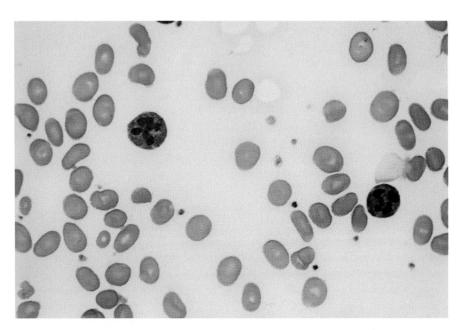

FIGURE 14–1. Peripheral blood smear. Wright/Giemsa stain. Original magnification ×197.

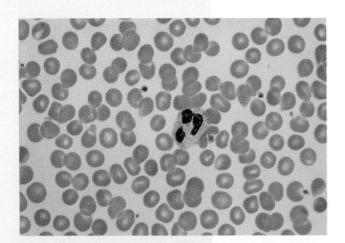

FIGURE 14–2. Normal blood smear. Wright/Giemsa stain. Original magnification ×252.

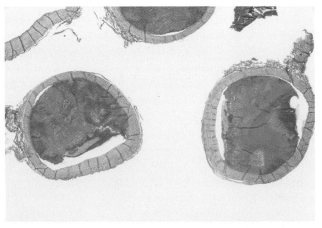

FIGURE 14–3. Portions of a vein from another patient with this disease (1–2 hours duration). Hematoxylin–eosin stain. Original magnification ×2.5.

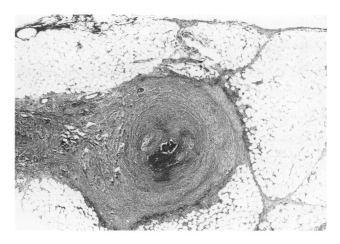

FIGURE 14–4. Portion of a vein from another patient with this disease (several days' duration). Hematoxylin–eosin stain. Original magnification ×5.

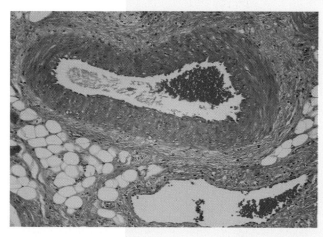

FIGURE 14–5. Normal artery and vein. Hematoxylin–eosin stain. Original magnification ×31.

► Questions

On the basis of the preceding information, you can best conclude the following:

1. All of the factors listed below could have contributed to this patient's acute condition EXCEPT:
   a. genetic factors
   b. long car trips (physical inactivity)
   c. delayed type hypersensitivity
   d. oral contraceptives
   e. smoking

2. The abnormal CBC can be explained by:
   a. the patient's acute condition
   b. vitamin deficiency
   c. acute loss of blood
   d. chronic loss of blood
   e. an acute inflammatory condition

3. Which of the following laboratory findings would best support your diagnosis of the abnormal CBC in this patient?
   a. increased serum LDH
   b. increased serum cholesterol
   c. increased erythrocyte sedimentation rate
   d. normal BUN
   e. normal serum calcium

4. All of the following statements about the lesion depicted in Figures 14–3 and 14–4 are correct EXCEPT:
   a. it may undergo complete resolution
   b. it may detach and form an embolus
   c. it may become organized and incorporated into the vessel wall
   d. it may persist essentially unchanged for years
   e. it may become organized and re-canalized

▶ Clinical Course

The diagnosis of the patient's acute problem was confirmed, and she was started on anticoagulant therapy with heparin. Five days later she was started on warfarin. Her aPTT (activated partial thromboplastin time) and PT (prothrombin time) were closely monitored (*see Table 14–5*). Several days after the initiation of therapy, the swelling of the leg subsided and she was able to walk without any discomfort. The patient was discharged several days after admission and given instructions to continue the warfarin treatment for several weeks. She was also advised to have a work-up of her abnormal CBC.

TABLE 14–5. COAGULATION

		Time After Admission								
		Heparin Therapy						Warfarin		
Test	Reference Range	6 Hrs	12 Hrs	24 Hrs	2 Day	3 Day	4 Day	5 Day	6 Day	7 Day
PT	11–14 sec	13	N/D	N/D	N/D	13	12	15	15	19
aPTT	19–28	54	34	42	62	51	59	47	52	42

N/D = not done

▶ **Questions**

5. All of the following statements about anticoagulant treatment are correct EXCEPT:
   a. heparin inhibits coagulation by binding to and activating antithrombin III
   b. warfarin decreases the levels of factors II, VII, IX, and X
   c. vitamin K is used to counteract bleeding due to warfarin
   d. the warfarin effect is immediate

6. Identify the INCORRECT statement:
   a. superficial venous thrombi may cause congestion, swelling, pain, and tenderness along the course of the involved vein
   b. deep venous thrombi in the leg cause congestion, swelling, pain, and tenderness
   c. superficial and deep venous thrombi of the leg have the same prognostic significance
   d. deep venous thrombi may be asymptomatic
   e. thrombosis may appear in healthy individuals without provocation or predisposition

7. Which of the following situations DOES NOT lead to hypercoagulability of blood?
   a. tissue damage
   b. chronic use of aspirin
   c. protein C deficiency
   d. protein S deficiency
   e. antithrombin III deficiency

8. The most serious complication of venous thrombosis in the deep veins of the leg is:
   a. pain and swelling
   b. impaired venous drainage
   c. skin ulceration
   d. pulmonary embolism

9. All of the following statements about this patient's condition are correct EXCEPT:
   a. it is pertinent to ask the whether she uses oral contraceptives
   b. there is a reason to ask the patient again about her alcohol consumption
   c. it could be explained to the patient that cigarette smoking has no effect on the development of her acute problem
   d. it should be recommended to the patient that she avoid prolonged trips with limited mobility
   e. it should be explained to the patient that work-up for the CBC abnormality might include determination of the serum B12 and folate levels

NOTES

▶ Figure Descriptions

Figure 14–1. Peripheral blood smear. Wright/Giemsa stain. Original magnification ×197.

The photomicrograph shows decreased numbers of red cells, anisocytosis, poikilocytosis with macrocytes (some of which are oval), and hypersegmented neutrophils. These findings are consistent with a macrocytic, hyperchromic anemia most likely due to a vitamin deficiency.

Figure 14–2. Normal blood smear. Wright/Giemsa stain. Original magnification ×252.

The red cells are much more even in size and shape, have normal central pallor, and are normal in numbers.

Figure 14–3. Portions of a vein from another patient with this disease (1–2 hours duration). Hematoxylin–eosin stain. Original magnification ×2.5.

These cross-sections of a stripped vein show a recent thrombus. It is too early for organization or inflammation.

Figure 14–4. Portion of a vein from another patient with this disease (several days' duration). Hematoxylin–eosin stain. Original magnification ×5.

With time, venous thrombosis invariably leads to inflammatory changes in the wall of the vein, as can be seen in this photomicrograph. The vein wall is markedly thickened due to inflammation. The clot is partially organized and undergoing partial resolution.

Figure 14–5. Normal artery and vein. Hematoxylin–eosin stain. Original magnification ×31.

The vessels shown in this image are normal in appearance. Their walls are not thickened, the lumens are patent, and no inflammation is present.

▶ Answers

1. **(c)** The patient had a deep venous thrombosis. The contributing factors for her deep venous thrombosis included oral contraceptives, smoking, and prolonged immobilization (long trips). Delayed hypersensitivity plays no role in the development of deep venous thrombosis.

2. **(b)** The patient had an increased MCV (mean corpuscular volume), a decreased erythrocyte count, increased mean corpuscular hemoglobin (MCH), and a normal mean corpuscular hemoglobin concentration (MCHC). These findings are compatible with a macrocytic anemia and are not related to the patient's acute condition (deep venous thrombosis), acute or chronic loss of blood, or acute inflammation. Vitamin B12 and folate deficiencies are common causes of macrocytic anemia.

3. **(a)** Increased serum cholesterol, increased erythrocyte sedimentation rate, or normal BUN and serum calcium do not play an important role in the diagnosis of macrocytic anemia. The increase in LDH, however, could reflect an increase in RBC hemolysis which is a feature of macrocytic (megaloblastic) anemia. In megaloblastic anemia, the LDH_1 isoenzyme is particularly increased.

4. (**d**) Figures 14–3 and 14–4 show thrombosed veins. The fate of venous thrombosis may include complete resolution or embolization. The thrombus may become organized and incorporated into the vessel wall or re-canalized. It will not, however, remain unchanged for a prolonged period of time.

5. (**d**) Anticoagulant drugs are used widely in the treatment of venous thrombosis. Heparin acts almost immediately, by activating antithrombin III, which forms complexes with activated serine protease coagulation factors (thrombin and factors IXa, Xa, and XIa) and inactivates them. Therapy should be monitored by aPTT. Warfarin is a vitamin K antagonist, which decreases the activity of factors II, VII, IX, and X. Factor VII levels fall considerably within 24 hours, but the prothrombin time rises after 3 days and only then is the patient fully anticoagulated. Vitamin K is the specific antidote if bleeding occurs after warfarin therapy.

6. (**c**) Venous thrombosis is an unpredictable phenomenon and may occur in otherwise healthy individuals. Both superficial and deep venous thrombi may cause congestion, swelling, pain, and tenderness. Deep venous thrombi may be asymptomatic. The prognostic significance of deep venous thrombi, however, is their potential for causing pulmonary embolism and infarction, which is not a feature of superficial thrombosis.

7. (**b**) Aspirin has an antithrombotic effect by suppressing platelet function. Tissue damage leads to the release of a pro-coagulant factor, which activates the extrinsic coagulation pathway. Protein C, protein S, and antithrombin III are powerful anticoagulants and any deficiency of one of them leads to a thrombotic tendency.

8. (**d**) Pulmonary embolism is the most serious complication of deep venous thrombosis of the leg. The other complications (pain, swelling, impaired venous drainage, and skin ulceration) are not life threatening.

9. (**c**) The use of oral contraceptives may predispose to thrombogenesis. The risk of developing thrombi is substantially increased when the use of oral contraceptives is combined with cigarette smoking. Prolonged immobility is another important risk factor in thrombogenesis. This patient also had macrocytic red blood cell indices. The question about alcohol consumption is an important one, since alcohol abuse is the most frequent cause of an increased MCV (mean corpuscular volume) in the absence of significant anemia. A deficiency of vitamin B12 or folate is a well-known cause of megaloblastic anemia. The macrocytic anemia work-up usually includes assays for vitamin B12 and folate levels.

▶ Final Diagnosis and Synopsis of the Case

- Deep Venous Thrombosis
- Macrocytic Anemia

This was a case of deep venous thrombosis in a healthy, middle-aged woman. She admitted to cigarette smoking, the use of oral contraceptives, and extensive travel by car. All of these factors may have contributed to the development of deep venous thrombosis. Routine laboratory tests revealed macrocytic red blood cells. She had a mild increase in LDH level and a high erythrocyte sedimentation rate. She was admitted to the hospital for anticoagulant treatment for her deep venous thrombosis. The patient's therapy was begun with intravenous heparin (monitored by aPTT) and maintained with oral warfarin (monitored by PT). She responded well, did not develop any complications, and was discharged after seven days. Her anticoagulation therapy, however, continued for several weeks. It was also recommended that she have a work-up for her macrocytic anemia. This case documents the development of a deep vein thrombosis as an unpredictable phenomenon which can affect otherwise healthy individuals.

LAB TIPS

Prothrombin Time (PT)

This test is performed by the addition of tissue extract to citrated plasma in the presence of an excess of calcium. The amount of time it takes for a fibrin clot to form is measured. This is a measurement of the extrinsic pathway (factors VII, X, V, II, and fibrinogen) and it is frequently used to screen for hemostatic disorders involving fibrin formation and to monitor warfarin therapy.

Activated Partial Thromboplastin Time (aPTT)

In this test, citrated plasma is incubated with a reagent containing phospholipid and a surface activator of factor XII. Calcium chloride is added and the time it takes for clot formation is measured. It is a measurement of the intrinsic pathway (prekallikrein, high molecular weight kininogen (HMWK), factors XII, XI, IX, VIII, X, V, II, and fibrinogen) and is usually used to screen for disorders of fibrin formation and to monitor heparin therapy. It may be prolonged by inhibitors, and when the PT is normal or nearly normal among hospitalized patients, a prolonged aPTT is most likely due to the lupus anticoagulant or heparin therapy.

Bleeding Time Test

The time it takes for bleeding to stop after a controlled small puncture is made in the patient's skin is measured. It is used as a screening test for platelet disorders and there is a good correlation between bleeding time and the platelet count. It should not be performed if the platelet count is <40 thousand μL, as it will likely be abnormal. The bleeding time can be significantly prolonged for up to a week following the ingestion of 600 mg of acetylsalicylic acid.

COAGULATION TESTS IN SELECTED CONDITIONS				
Condition	**Platelet Count**	**PT**	**aPTT**	**Bleeding Time**
Thrombocytopenia	Decreased	Normal	Normal	Prolonged
Hemophilia	Normal	Normal	Usually prolonged	Normal
von Willebrand's disease	Normal	Normal	Normal or prolonged	Normal or prolonged
Liver disease	Usually normal	Prolonged	Normal	Usually normal
Heparin therapy	Normal	May be prolonged	Prolonged	Normal or prolonged
Excess dicumarol therapy	Normal	Prolonged	Prolonged	Usually normal
Henoch–Schöenlein purpura	Normal	Normal	Normal	Normal
Platelet function disorders	Normal or increased	Normal	Normal	Prolonged

15

$Chapter$

A 20-Year-Old
Disoriented
Woman With
"Garbled"
Speech

▶ Clinical History and Presentation

A 20-year-old female college student was brought to the physician's office by her father because of disorientation and "garbled" speech of several hours' duration. The patient admitted to a suicidal attempt. She had swallowed a full bottle (24 tablets) of 500 mg Tylenol (acetaminophen) tablets earlier that morning. The patient's father reported that she was in good health, but had suffered from depression since a car accident 4 months previously in which she had broken her nose. At that time, the CT scan of the head was negative for any intracranial bleeding. She was on no medication and did not smoke or drink alcohol. Physical examination revealed a thin (50 kg) female in no acute distress. She was disoriented in time and place. The rest of the physical examination was unremarkable. She was admitted to the hospital.

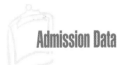 Admission Data

TABLE 15–1. HEMATOLOGY		
WBC	8.9 thousand/µL	(4.5–11.0)
Neut	87%	(44–88)
Band	0%	(0–10)
Lymph	8%	(12–43)
Mono	3%	(2–11)
Eos	1%	(0–5)
Baso	1%	(0–2)
RBC	4.4 million/µL	(3.9–5.0)
Hgb	12.7 g/dL	(12.0–15.0)
HCT	38.2%	(36.0–44.0)
MCV	86.7 fL	(79.0–96.0)
MCH	28.9 pg	(26.0–32.6)
MCHC	33.3 g/dL	(32.5–36.0)
Plts	314 thousand/µL	(130–400)

NOTES

TABLE 15–2. CHEMISTRY

Glucose	95 mg/dL	(65–110)
Creatinine	1.2 mg/dL	(0.7–1.4)
BUN	10 mg/dL	(7–24)
Uric acid	3.2 mg/dL	(3.0–8.5)
Cholesterol	191 mg/dL	(150–240)
Calcium	8.9 mg/dL	(8.5–10.5)
Protein	7.7 g/dL	(6–8)
Albumin	4.7 g/dL	(3.7–5.0)
LDH	168 U/L	(100–250)
Alk Phos	69 U/L	(0–120)
AST	30 U/L	(0–55)
GGTP	19 U/L	(0–50)
Bilirubin	0.3 mg/dL	(0.0–1.5)
Bilirubin, direct	0.09 mg/dL	(0.02–0.18)

TABLE 15–3. ELECTROLYTES

Na	134 mEq/L	(134–143)
K	3.6 mEq/L	(3.5–4.9)
Cl	99 mEq/L	(95–108)
CO_2	22 mEq/L	(21–32)

TABLE 15–4. COAGULATION

PT	13 sec	(11–14)
aPTT	22 sec	(22–31)

TABLE 15–5. ACETAMINOPHEN LEVEL

Tylenol	120 µg/mL	(10–30)

▶ **Questions**

On the basis of the preceding information, you can best conclude the following:

1. Which of the following statements concerning this patient at this time is correct?
   a. profound changes in CBC should have occurred
   b. there should be a significantly prolonged PT and aPTT
   c. an elevated plasma level of acetaminophen is usually the only abnormal laboratory finding
   d. one would expect the patient to develop acute pulmonary edema
   e. one would expect an elevated serum amylase and lipase

2. Which of the following tests would be LEAST useful in further evaluating this patient?
   a. chest X-ray
   b. acetaminophen plasma level
   c. PT and aPTT
   d. serum transaminase level
   e. blood glucose

3. Which of the following factors, if present, would adversely affect the outcome of acute acetaminophen poisoning?
   a. a history of asthma
   b. a history of frequent sore throat
   c. a history of frequent alcohol abuse
   d. a history of contact dermatitis
   e. recent blood transfusion

4. An acute acetaminophen overdose is best known to cause:
   a. acute liver failure
   b. a profound myelosuppression
   c. acute pancreatitis
   d. acute pulmonary edema
   e. cystitis

5. Laboratory signs of organ damage in acute acetaminophen poisoning usually reach their peak at which interval after ingestion?
   a. 0–4 hours
   b. 4–12 hours
   c. 12–24 hours
   d. 24–48 hours
   e. 2–4 days

▶ Clinical Course

The patient developed nausea and epigastric pain. She was treated with N-acetylcysteine (MUCOMYST). Blood chemistry, coagulation, and acetaminophen plasma levels were monitored. Her vital signs were stable and the EKG was normal. The patient was also seen by a psychiatrist to address her depression. Her condition improved and she was discharged five days later. Follow-up care for her depression was initiated.

TABLE 15–6. LABORATORY DATA

Test (Reference Range)		Hours After Tylenol Ingestion				
		24	48	72	96	120
Chemistry						
Glucose	(65–110 mg/dL)	91	125	127	119	94.0
Creatinine	(0.7–1.4 mg/dL)	1.0	1.0	0.8	0.8	0.8
BUN	(7–24 mg/dL)	10	6	3	3	4.0
Uric acid	(3.0–8.5 mg/dL)	3.6	3.5	3.0	1.8	2.2
Cholesterol	(150–240 mg/dL)	180	153	134	113	135
Calcium	(8.5–10.5 mg/dL)	9.3	8.6	8.5	8.2	9.2
Protein	(6–8 g/dL)	7.8	6.3	5.6	5.4	6.2
Albumin	(3.7–5.0 g/dL)	4.6	3.8	3.5	3.2	3.5
LDH	(100–250 U/L)	223	277	2740	255	191
Alk Phos	(0–120 U/L)	72	61	56	53	65
AST	(0–55 U/L)	149	234	2685	600	278
GGTP	(0–50 U/L)	30	31	26	54	98
Bilirubin	(0.0–1.5 mg/dL)	1.0	0.7	0.6	0.8	0.7
Bilirubin, direct	(0.02–0.18 mg/dL)	0.31	0.19	0.17	0.28	0.24
Electrolytes						
Na	(134–143 mEq/L)	138	138	141	142	141
K	(3.5–4.9 mEq/L)	4.1	4	3.2	3.2	4.2
Cl	(95–108 mEq/L)	105	101	105	106	107
CO$_2$	(21–32 mEq/L)	19	28	24	25	30
Acetaminophen level						
Tylenol	(10–30 μg/mL)	53	10	N/D	N/D	N/D
Coagulation						
PT	(11–14 sec)	15.5	16.5	17	15	13
aPTT	(22–31 sec)	26	26	28	26	25

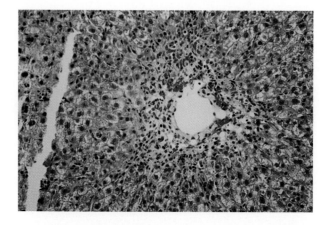

FIGURE 15–1. Liver biopsy from another patient with this condition (96 hours after ingestion). Hematoxylin–eosin stain. Original magnification ×50.

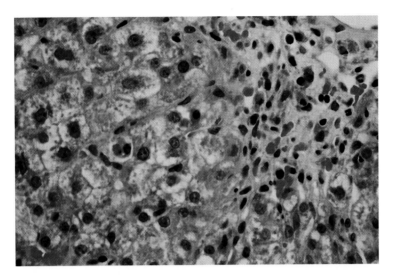

FIGURE 15–2. Liver biopsy from another patient with this condition (96 hours after ingestion). Hematoxylin–eosin stain. Original magnification ×125.

▶ Questions

6. All of the following statements about N-acetylcysteine (MUCOMYST) are correct EXCEPT:
   a. it is most effective when given within 10 hours after ingestion of acetaminophen
   b. its major therapeutic effect is the prevention of absorption of acetaminophen from the stomach
   c. it provides cysteine for glutathione synthesis
   d. it helps to reduce the severity of liver necrosis in acetaminophen poisoning

7. All of the following statements about the hepatotoxicity of acetaminophen are correct EXCEPT:
   a. it is dose-dependent
   b. it causes an idiosyncratic type of reaction
   c. the injury is caused by a toxic metabolite of acetaminophen
   d. the activity of the cytochrome P-450 mixed-function oxidase system plays an important role in its pathogenesis
   e. availability of glutathione plays an important role in its pathogenesis

8. Which of the following situations most clearly predisposes to acetaminophen hepatic toxicity?

LIVER P-450 ACTIVITY	LIVER GLUTATHIONE STORE
a. normal	increased
b. increased	increased
c. decreased	increased
d. increased	decreased
e. decreased	decreased

9. The liver biopsy (Figures 15–1 and 15–2) is representative of the liver status approximately 96 hours after ingestion of a toxic dose of acetaminophen. It shows:
   a. micronodular cirrhosis
   b. bridging necrosis
   c. pure cholestasis
   d. centrilobular necrosis
   e. a liver abscess

▶ Figure Descriptions

Figure 15–1. Liver biopsy from another patient with this condition (96 hours post-ingestion). Hematoxylin–eosin stain. Original magnification ×50.

This is an example of centrilobular necrosis due to acetaminophen ingestion. A number of hepatocytes around the central vein have disappeared, and in their place are inflammatory cells and pigment-laden Kupffer cells. Some sinusoidal congestion is also present.

Figure 15–2. Liver biopsy from another patient with this condition (96 hours post-ingestion). Hematoxylin–eosin stain. Original magnification ×125.

At higher magnification, some hepatocytes show evidence of ballooning degeneration. The increased number of Kupffer cells contain abundant lipofuchsin pigment. The inflammatory cells include lymphocytes, plasma cells, and neutrophils.

▶ Answers

1. **(c)** The question refers to findings approximately 10 hours after ingestion of over 10 g of acetaminophen. At this early time, the only abnormal test is usually an increased plasma level of acetaminophen. This level is the major guide to therapy. Pulmonary edema is not a feature of acute acetaminophen poisoning.

2. **(a)** Changes in the lung parenchyma or vasculature are not features of early acute acetaminophen poisoning, therefore a chest x-ray is the least useful diagnostic tool in providing information about the patient's status. All other tests are important in the follow-up. The acetaminophen level correlates with the severity of hepatic injury, transaminase levels, coagulation tests, and blood glucose levels also reflect the severity of liver damage.

3. **(c)** Frequent alcohol abuse potentiates the hepatic toxicity of acetaminophen by stimulating the P-450 mixed-function oxidase system and reducing the hepatic glutathione level. The other factors (asthma, sore throat, contact dermatitis, and recent blood transfusion) do not play any significant role in the recovery from acute acetaminophen poisoning.

4. **(a)** Acute acetaminophen poisoning leads to acute liver failure due to necrosis of the liver parenchyma. The other conditions listed (profound myelosuppression, acute pancreatitis, acute pulmonary edema, and cystitis) are not features of the acute phase of acetaminophen poisoning.

5. **(e)** During the first 12–24 hours, the increased serum drug level is the only abnormal laboratory finding. In the following 24 hours, liver function test abnormalities appear and reach their peak at 2–4 days after acetaminophen ingestion.

6. **(b)** The main therapeutic effect of N-acetylcysteine is in providing cysteine for the synthesis of glutathione, which becomes rapidly depleted in acetaminophen poisoning. Glutathione detoxifies the toxic metabolite of acetaminophen by binding to it, thus preventing it from reacting with essential cellular components. N-acetylcysteine is most effective when given during the first 10 hours after acetaminophen ingestion. N-acetylcysteine is not used to prevent absorption of acetaminophen from the stomach.

7. **(b)** The hepatotoxicity of acetaminophen is not due to an idiosyncratic reaction, which is a dose-independent and unpredictable phenomenon. The degree of liver damage depends on the dose ingested, and the activity of the cytochrome P-450 mixed-function oxidase

system, which influences the quantity of the toxic metabolite formed. Liver damage also depends on the stores of glutathione, which has the capacity to detoxify this metabolite.

8. (**d**) The hepatotoxicity of acetaminophen is potentiated by conditions in which there is a combination of an increased activity of cytochrome P-450 mixed-function oxidase system, which leads to an increased formation of the toxic acetaminophen metabolite of and depleted stores of glutathione, since the metabolite cannot be efficiently detoxified in the absence of glutathione. Chronic alcoholism is the best example of such a condition.

9. (**d**) The liver biopsy performed on another patient with this condition approximately 96 hours after acetaminophen ingestion shows a centrilobular necrosis. There is no fibrosis, and there is no suggestion of abscess formation. Morphological features of cholestasis, such as bile plugs and "bile lakes", are not present.

▶ Final Diagnosis and Synopsis of the Case

• Acetaminophen Poisoning
• Centrilobular Necrosis of Liver

This a case of acute acetaminophen poisoning in a young, depressed college student. The patient reported that she had swallowed at least 10 g of acetaminophen, and was admitted to the hospital approximately 10 hours after ingestion. Her major symptoms were disorientation and "garbled speech." Upon admission, the only laboratory abnormality was an increased plasma level of acetaminophen (120 g/μL). She was treated with N-acetylcysteine to reduce the severity of liver damage. N-acetylcysteine provides cysteine for the synthesis of glutathione, which has the capacity to detoxify the toxic acetaminophen metabolite. The extent of the liver damage was monitored, as was the plasma level of acetaminophen. The maximum elevation of serum LDH and AST levels occurred 72 hours after ingestion of the drug, at which time the PT also reached its peak. Five days after ingestion, the LDH and PT values returned to normal, and the AST level had significantly declined. With the exception of the presenting symptoms and some gastrointestinal discomfort during the first day, the patient had no other clinical symptoms, and her vital signs remained stable. She was expected to recover fully without any residual liver damage. She did require, however, follow-up care for her depression.

NOTES

LAB TIPS

Acetaminophen Toxicity

ACETAMINOPHEN LEVELS OVER TIME VERSUS HEPATOTOXICITY

Time from Ingestion	Blood Levels	Liver Damage
4 hours	<150 μg/mL	Not probable
	>200 μg/mL	Possible
8 hours	<80 μg/mL	Not probable
	>100 μg/mL	Possible
12 hours	<40 μg/mL	Not probable
	>50 μg/mL	Possible
24 hours	<5 μg/mL	Not probable
	>6 μg/mL	Possible

Clinical History and Presentation

A 47-year-old woman was admitted to the hospital with chief complaints of increasing shortness of breath and extreme fatigue. Her past medical history included cardiac arrhythmias and heavy consumption of alcohol for over twenty years. Physical examination revealed an alert and oriented woman. Blood pressure was 100/65 mmHg, heart rate was 96 per minute, temperature was 97.5° F, and respiratory rate was 23 per minute. Examination of the neck showed distended jugular veins. Abdominal examination showed a protuberant abdomen with ascites. The liver and spleen were not palpable. Pitting edema of the lower extremities was noted. The chest x-ray is depicted in Figure 16–1. The EKG showed sinus tachycardia and non-specific S-T segment changes.

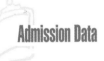

Admission Data

TABLE 16–1. HEMATOLOGY		
WBC	10.0 thousand/µL	(3.3–11.0)
Neut	63%	(44–88)
Band	0%	(0–10)
Lymph	21%	(12–43)
Mono	10%	(2–11)
Eos	4%	(0–5)
Baso	2%	(0–2)
RBC	3.94 million/µL	(3.9–5.0)
Hgb	11.8 g/dL	(11.6–15.6)
HCT	35.9%	(37.0–47.0)
MCV	91.2 fL	(79.0–99.0)
MCH	29.9 pg	(26.0–32.6)
MCHC	32.8 g/dL	(31.0–36.0)
Plts	326 thousand/µL	(130–400)

TABLE 16–2. CHEMISTRY

Glucose	92 mg/dL	(65–110)
Creatinine	1.2 mg/dL	(0.7–1.4)
BUN	18 mg/dL	(7–24)
Uric acid	6.7 mg/dL	(3.0–7.5)
Cholesterol	210 mg/dL	(150–240)
Calcium	9.1 mg/dL	(8.5–10.5)
Protein	6.2 g/dL	(6–8)
Albumin	3.0 g/dL	(3.7–5.0)
Alk Phos	183 U/L	(20–120)
AST	250 U/L	(10–30)
ALT	100 U/L	(5–30)
GGTP	360 U/L	(0–50)
Bilirubin	0.7 mg/dL	(0.0–1.5)
Bilirubin, direct	0.18 mg/dL	(0.02–0.18)

TABLE 16–3. ELECTROLYTES

Na	128 mEq/L	(134–143)
K	4.0 mEq/L	(3.5–4.9)
Cl	90 mEq/L	(95–108)
CO_2	25 mEq/L	(21–32)

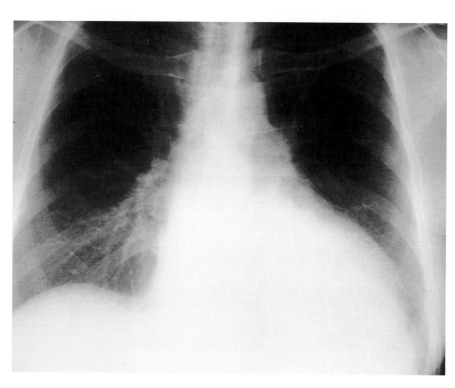

FIGURE 16–1. Admission chest x-ray.

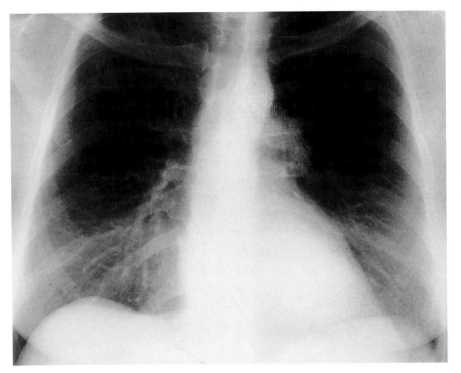

FIGURE 16–2. Patient's chest x-ray from three years previously.

▶ Questions

On the basis of the preceding information, you can best conclude the following:

1. The patient's history, clinical presentation, and laboratory findings are LEAST compatible with:
   a. complete extra-hepatic biliary obstruction
   b. fatty liver
   c. alcoholic hepatitis
   d. passive congestion of the liver

2. The patient's chest x-ray depicted in Figure 16–1 shows:
   a. pneumonia
   b. cardiomegaly
   c. bronchogenic carcinoma
   d. pulmonary abscess

3. All of the following statements concerning this patient's ascites are correct EXCEPT:
   a. congestive heart failure may have played a contributory role in its development
   b. total body sodium in this patient was most likely increased
   c. her ascitic fluid most likely had the characteristics of an exudate
   d. the aldosterone level in this patient was most likely increased

▶ Clinical Course

The patient developed severe hypotension and bradycardia of 35 per minute. After the patient was stabilized, a bedside echocardiogram was done, and showed left atrial and right ventricular hypokinesis. The next morning, the patient again developed severe hypotension and bradycardia progressing to asystole. Resuscitation efforts failed and the patient expired. An autopsy limited to the chest and abdomen was performed.

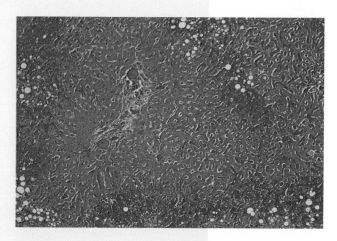

FIGURE 16–3. Patient's liver. Hematoxylin–eosin stain. Original magnification ×12.

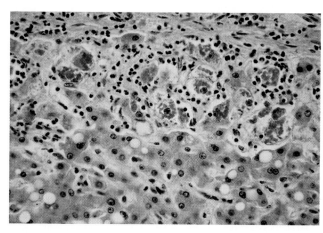

FIGURE 16–4. Patient's liver. Hematoxylin–eosin stain. Original magnification ×78.

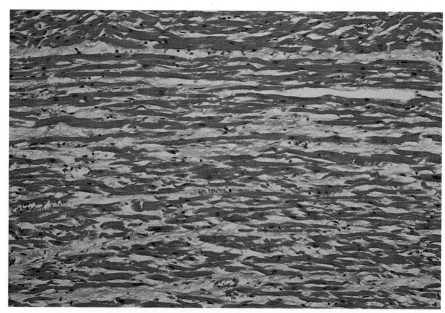

FIGURE 16–5. Patient's myocardium. Hematoxylin–eosin stain. Original magnification ×31.

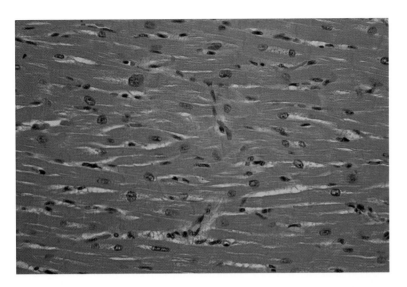

FIGURE 16–6. Normal myocardium. Hematoxylin–eosin stain. Original magnification ×78.

▶ Questions

4. Some of the hepatocytes depicted in Figure 16–3 show fatty change. This is primarily due to accumulation of:
   a. free fatty acids
   b. LDL
   c. triglyceride
   d. HDL
   e. cholesterol

5. The eosinophilic structures depicted in Figure 16–4 are composed of:
   a. aggregates of intermediate filaments
   b. aggregates of microtubules
   c. amyloid fibrils
   d. lipofuscin
   e. aggregates of endoplasmic reticulum

6. Which of the following histological findings is pathognomonic for this heart condition?
   a. myocardial edema
   b. fatty changes in the heart
   c. myofiber swelling
   d. mononuclear cell infiltration of myofibrils
   e. none of the above

7. Which of the following statements concerning this patient is correct?
   a. congestive heart failure could have contributed to the ascites formation
   b. the patient had alcoholic liver disease
   c. alcohol could have contributed to this patient's cardiac problem
   d. all of the above
   e. none of the above

NOTES

Figure Descriptions

Figure 16–1. Admission chest x-ray.

There is moderate cardiac enlargement. Pulmonary vascular congestion and mild pulmonary edema are present.

Figure 16–2. Patient's chest x-ray 3 years ago.

This chest x-ray of the patient 3 years ago shows the heart to be normal in size and the lung fields clear.

Figure 16–3. Patient's liver. Hematoxylin–eosin stain. Original magnification ×12.

The liver weighed 1440 grams (mean normal weight is 1300 grams) and the cut surface had a nutmeg pattern. The photomicrograph shows centrilobular congestion and necrosis consistent with acute passive congestion. Fatty change is also present.

Figure 16–4. Patient's liver. Hematoxylin–eosin stain. Original magnification ×78.

Foci of inflammation and hepatocyte degeneration were present in some sections of the liver. A number of the hepatocytes contained amorphous, eosinophilic inclusions consistent with Mallory bodies. Following the death of a hepatocyte containing Mallory bodies, the bodies usually remain, appearing extracellular, and are often surrounded by neutrophils, as can be seen in this photomicrograph. Fatty change is also present. These findings are consistent with alcoholic liver disease.

Figure 16–5. Patient's myocardium. Hematoxylin–eosin stain. Original magnification ×31.

The patient's heart weighed 570 grams (average normal weight is 250 grams) and appeared flabby. No gross evidence of scarring was present. This photomicrograph of the myocardium shows a fine fibrosis with thinning of the myocytes, some of which show enlarged nuclei. Other areas showed fatty change.

Figure 16–6. Normal myocardium. Hematoxylin–eosin stain. Original magnification ×78.

The myocardial fibers appear uniform with unremarkable nuclei. No inflammation or fatty infiltration is present.

Answers

1. **(a)** Complete extra-hepatic biliary obstruction leads to a marked increase of serum alkaline phosphatase, serum aspartate aminotransferase (AST), and gamma-glutamyl transpeptidase (GGTP), as well as an increase in total and direct bilirubin. The other three listed options (fatty liver, alcoholic hepatitis, and passive congestion of the liver) lead to a less pronounced increase in the above enzymes. The patient's long history of alcohol abuse is consistent with alcoholic hepatitis and her cardiac arrhythmia and congestive heart failure are consistent with passive congestion of the liver.

2. **(b)** The patient's x-ray, depicted in Figure 16–1, shows an enlarged heart. There are no pulmonary infiltrates, cavitary lesion of the lung, or pulmonary mass to suggest pneumonia, lung abscess, or bronchogenic carcinoma, respectively.

3. (**c**) Congestive heart failure was most likely the main factor underlying this patient's generalized edema and ascites (other findings pointing to congestive heart failure include distended jugular veins, cardiomegaly, and shortness of breath). The accumulation of ascitic fluid is associated with a state of total body excess of water and sodium due to an activation of the renin-angiotensin-aldosterone system. In congestive heart failure, the ascitic fluid has the characteristics of a transudate, rather than an exudate.

4. (**c**) Alcohol abuse alters hepatic fatty acid uptake and metabolism of fatty acids by the liver and leads to cytoplasmic accumulation of triglycerides in hepatocytes, as depicted in Figure 16–3.

5. (**a**) The eosinophilic structures depicted in Figure 16–4 represent Mallory bodies (*see Figure description*). Mallory bodies (also known as "alcoholic hyalin") are cytoplasmic aggregates of intermediate filaments (cytokeratin) and represent a type of cell injury to the cellular cytoskeleton. Mallory bodies can be seen in a variety of liver diseases such as Wilson's disease, primary biliary cirrhosis, focal nodular hyperplasia, and hepatocellular carcinoma, as well as alcoholic hepatitis.

6. (**e**) In the dilated (congestive) cardiomyopathy that is associated with alcohol toxicity, the histological findings are variable. Myocardial edema, fatty changes in the heart, myofiber swelling, fibrosis, and mononuclear cell infiltration of myofibrils may be seen in the dilated cardiomyopathy, though none of them is pathognomonic of this condition.

7. (**d**) This patient's two primary problems were dilated cardiomyopathy and alcoholic liver disease. She presented with ascites and pitting edema of the extremities. These physical findings could have been induced by congestive heart failure, alcoholic liver disease, or both conditions in combination. Alcohol may also have been a contributing factor for her cardiomyopathy, although proof of a cause and effect relationship is lacking.

▶ Final Diagnosis and Synopsis of the Case

- Dilated Cardiomyopathy
- Congestive Heart Failure
- Alcoholic Liver Disease With Acute and Chronic Passive Congestion

A middle-aged woman was admitted to the hospital because of increasing shortness of breath. She was found to be in severe congestive heart failure with marked generalized edema. A diagnosis of dilated cardiomyopathy was made on the basis of echocardiographic studies and was confirmed by the autopsy findings. The dilated cardiomyopathy was attributed to the effects of her chronic alcoholism, which was also a cause of her liver disease. The patient developed severe hypotension and bradycardia progressing to asystole. Efforts at resuscitation failed and the patient expired.

LAB TIPS

SELECTED LABORATORY PARAMETERS IN ALCOHOL ABUSE[a]

Parameter	Reference Range	Effect of Alcohol	Comment
γ-Glutamyl transpeptidase (GGTP, GGT)	0–50 U/L	Increased with chronic ingestion	A microsomal enzyme induced by alcohol; useful to identify occult alcoholism; also elevated in obstructive jaundice, infiltrative disease of liver
Aspartate amino-transferase (AST, SGOT)	0–55 U/L	Increased When AST <300 U/L, AST/ALT ratio > 1 strongly suggests alcoholic liver disease	May be markedly increased in alcoholic hepatitis; Alanine aminotransferase (ALT, SGPT) usually normal
Serum albumin	3.7–5.0 g/dL	Decreased in chronic or severe disease	Decreased levels usually due to poor nutrition, but may indicate cirrhosis; often seen with polyclonal increase in immuno-globulins
White blood cell count	3.3–11.0 thousand/μL	Leukocytosis 1/3 of patients have WBC > 15,000/μL with a left shift	
Mean corpuscular volume	81–99 fL	Macrocytosis >50% of chronic alcoholics	Alcoholism is one of the most common causes of macrocytic anemia; folic acid, vitamin B$_{12}$, and iron deficiency anemias may also be present

[a]The changes in these parameters are not specific for alcohol abuse and can be seen in a number of other conditions. While chronic alcohol abuse may also lead to increases in serum phosphorus, hemoglobin, mean corpuscular hemoglobin, and alkaline phosphatase and to decreases in total protein and blood urea nitrogen, these changes are usually within the reference range.

A 32-Year-Old Man With Persistent Fever and Cough

▷ **Clinical History and Presentation**

A 32-year-old man was admitted for the investigation of persistent fever and an unproductive cough of two weeks' duration. He had immigrated to the United States from Taiwan 7 years previously, and had lived in California and Michigan. Physical examination revealed a normally developed, alert, and apprehensive man. His temperature was 103° F, heart rate was 100 per minute and regular, and blood pressure was 110/52 mmHg. The physical examination was unremarkable except for rales at both lung bases.

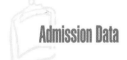 **Admission Data**

TABLE 17–1. HEMATOLOGY		
WBC	13.5 thousand/μL	(3.3–11.0)
Neut	83%	(44–88)
Band	0%	(0–10)
Lymph	8%	(12–43)
Mono	5%	(2–11)
Eos	3%	(0–5)
Baso	2%	(0–2)
RBC	4.37 million/μL	(3.9–5.0)
Hgb	12.4 g/dL	(11.6–15.6)
HCT	38.2%	(37.0–47.0)
MCV	87.5 fL	(79.0–99.0)
MCH	28.4 pg	(26.0–32.6)
MCHC	32.4 g/dL	(31.0–36.0)
Plts	246 thousand/μL	(130–400)

TABLE 17–2. CHEMISTRY		
Glucose	105 mg/dL	(65–110)
Creatinine	1.1 mg/dL	(0.7–1.4)
BUN	11 mg/dL	(7–24)
Uric acid	4 mg/dL	(3.0–7.5)
Cholesterol	114 mg/dL	(150–240)
Calcium	8.5 mg/dL	(8.5–10.5)
Protein	6.3 g/dL	(6–8)
Albumin	3.3 g/dL	(3.7–5.0)
LDH	179 U/L	(100–250)
Alk Phos	70 U/L	(0–120)
AST	32 U/L	(0–55)
GGTP	21 U/L	(0–50)
Bilirubin	0.4 mg/dL	(0.0–1.5)
Bilirubin, direct	0.13 mg/dL	(0.02–0.18)

TABLE 17–3. MICROBIOLOGY
Blood cultures: pending

TABLE 17–4. URINALYSIS
Within normal limits

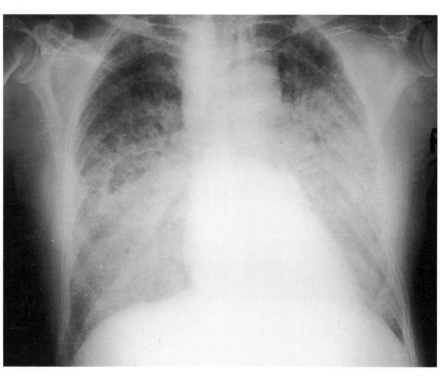

FIGURE 17–1. Patient's chest x-ray.

> **Questions**

On the basis of the preceding information, you can best conclude the following:

1. Figure 17-1 is an x-ray of the patient's chest. The LEAST likely cause of his pulmonary disease is:
   a. histoplasmosis
   b. tuberculosis
   c. sarcoidosis
   d. cytomegalovirus infection
   e. coccidiomycosis

2. In this case, the patient's residence in California may be considered to be uniquely relevant to which of the following possible diagnoses?
   a. histoplasmosis
   b. blastomycosis
   c. coccidiomycosis
   d. tuberculosis
   e. aspergillosis

3. Which of the following tests would you consider helpful in the diagnosis of the pulmonary problem of this patient?
   a. a PPD (purified protein derivative) tuberculin test
   b. determination of the angiotensin converting enzyme (ACE) blood level
   c. fungal serology
   d. all of the above

▶ Clinical Course

Blood cultures were reported as "no growth." Sputum was obtained for smears and cultures (Figure 17–2). The results of additional tests are listed below. A purified protein derivative (PPD) tuberculin test was performed and resulted in an area of induration approximately 20 mm in diameter. The patient was begun on multiple antibiotic therapy and discharged to be followed on an outpatient basis. His blood chemistry pattern prior to his discharge is shown.

TABLE 17–5. SEROLOGY AND IMMUNOLOGY

Mycoplasma	Neg	(Neg)
Legionella	Neg	(Neg)
Blastomyces	Neg	(Neg)
Coccididoides	Neg	(Neg)
Aspergillus	Neg	(Neg)
Candida albicans, Ab	Neg	(Neg)

TABLE 17–6. SPECIAL STUDIES

Angiotensin–1–conv. enz	24.7 U/L	(12–50)

TABLE 17–7. CHEMISTRY (DAY 11)

Glucose	101 mg/dL	(65–110)
Creatinine	1.0 mg/dL	(0.7–1.4)
BUN	11 mg/dL	(7–24)
Uric acid	12.7 mg/dL	(3.0–7.5)
Cholesterol	141 mg/dL	(150–240)
Calcium	8.6 mg/dL	(8.5–10.5)
Protein	6.9 g/dL	(6–8)
Albumin	3.2 g/dL	(3.7–5.0)
LDH	145 U/L	(100–250)
Alk Phos	79 U/L	(0–120)
AST	26 U/L	(0–55)
GGTP	27 U/L	(0–50)
Bilirubin	0.4 mg/dL	(0.0–1.5)
Bilirubin, direct	0.12 mg/dL	(0.02–0.18)

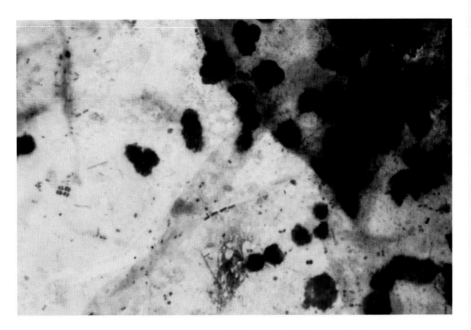

FIGURE 17–2. Patient's sputum smear. Acid-fast stain. Original magnification ×315.

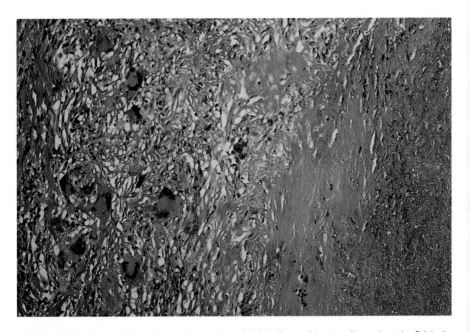

FIGURE 17–3. Portion of lung from another patient with this disease. Hematoxylin–eosin stain. Original magnification ×31.

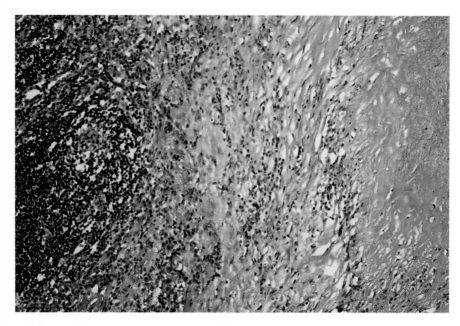

FIGURE 17–4. Portion of lung from another patient with this disease. Hematoxylin–eosin stain. Original magnification ×31.

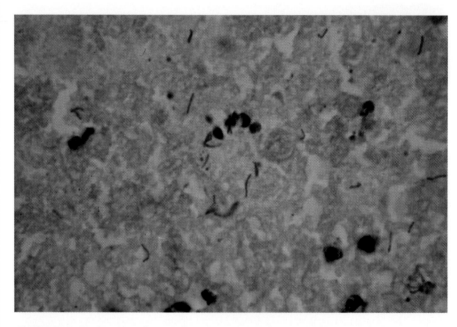

FIGURE 17–5. Portion of lung from another patient with this disease. Acid-fast stain. Original magnification ×320.

▶ Questions

4. The pertinent organism seen in the sputum smear (Figure 17–2) is:
   a. *Candida* species
   b. a mycobacterium
   c. *Klebsiella pneumoniae*
   d. none of the above

5. The level of circulating angiotensin converting enzyme (ACE) was found to be within normal limits in this patient. Which of the following diseases most often shows an increased level of this enzyme?
   a. sarcoidosis
   b. tuberculosis
   c. histoplasmosis
   d. coccidiomycosis
   e. cytomegalovirus infection

6. Which of the following statements concerning a positive reaction to an intracutaneous injection of PPD tuberculin is correct?
   a. it is generally a reliable indication of prior infection with *Mycobacterium tuberculosis*
   b. it may be negative in persons with *Mycobacterium tuberculosis* infections
   c. false positive reactions to non-pathogenic mycobacteria may occur
   d. all of the above statements are correct

7. All of the following statements concerning *Mycobacterium tuberculosis* are correct EXCEPT:
   a. it is an aerobic microorganism
   b. it grows slowly in culture
   c. it is pathogenic by virtue of the release of a known endotoxin
   d. it prevents the fusion of phagosomes with lysosomes in macrophages
   e. it fails to stimulate a respiratory burst when phagocytosed by macrophages

8. All of the following statements about the lesion depicted in Figures 17–3, 17–4, and 17–5 are true EXCEPT:
   a. it is characteristically evoked by a slowly-dividing infectious agent
   b. it requires the presence of T cell mediated immune response
   c. it can be highly infectious
   d. it can undergo fibrosis and calcification
   e. it is an abscess

9. The killing of intracellular *Mycobacterium tuberculosis* is associated with the activity of:
   a. CD4+ helper T cells
   b. interferon-γ
   c. reactive oxides of nitrogen
   d. epithelioid cell granulomas
   e. all of the above

10. Cell-mediated hypersensitivity to *Mycobacterium tuberculosis* is associated with:
    a. the activity of CD8+ suppressor T cells
    b. the death of infected macrophages
    c. caseation of granulomas
    d. a positive PPD (tuberculin) reaction
    e. all of the above

11. On day 11, the chemistry panel of this patient showed a marked increase in the serum uric acid level as compared to his admission value. Which of the following statements about this hyperuricemia is correct?
    a. the patient may be asymptomatic
    b. the patient may develop a gouty arthritis
    c. it is most likely a consequence of his drug therapy
    d. all of the above statements are correct

NOTES

▶ **Figure Descriptions**

Figure 17–1. Patient's chest x-ray.

There is an interstitial infiltrate throughout both lung fields. Hilar lymphadenopathy is also present. The impression of the radiologist included pneumonia, tuberculosis, or other granulomatous disease.

Figure 17–2. Patient's sputum smear. Acid-fast stain. Original magnification ×315.

Organisms present in this photomicrograph include dark-staining cocci and rods, and slender, pink, acid-fast positive, slightly curved rods consistent with *Mycobacteria*. A number of inflammatory cells are also present.

Figure 17–3. Portion of lung from another patient with this disease. Hematoxylin–eosin stain. Original magnification ×31.

This is the edge of a tuberculous granuloma and shows epithelioid cells, fibroblasts, and several Langhans' giant cells. Note the hyaline fibrosis in the wall and the granular, caseous necrosis on the right side of the image.

Figure 17–4. Portion of lung from another patient with this disease. Hematoxylin–eosin stain. Original magnification ×31.

At the edge of this granuloma, a moderately intense inflammatory infiltrate (chiefly lymphocytes) is present, in addition to the epithelioid histiocytes and fibroblasts. Hyaline fibrosis and necrosis are again present on the right side of the image.

Figure 17–5. Portion of lung from another patient with this disease. Acid-fast stain. Original magnification ×320.

This photomicrograph is from the center of a granuloma and shows the presence of slender, acid-fast positive, slightly curved and beaded bacilli, suggestive of *Mycobacteria*.

▶ **Answers**

1. (**d**) The x-ray shows pulmonary hilar lymphadenopathy, as well as parenchymal lesions. Hilar lymphadenopathy is a common feature of primary pulmonary tuberculosis, of histoplasmosis, coccidiomycosis, and sarcoidosis, but not of cytomegalic pneumonitis. *(See description of Figure 17–1).*

2. (**c**) A diagnosis of coccidiomycosis was specifically considered because of the patient's residence in California, where coccidiomyces is a common soil saprophyte, and coccidiomycosis is endemic (eg, San Joaquin Valley fever). The other options have no particular association with California.

3. (**d**) The differential diagnosis includes tuberculosis, sarcoidosis, and pulmonary mycoses. A PPD tuberculin test would be used to identify tuberculosis, angiotensin converting enzyme (ACE) blood levels are most commonly found to be increased in sarcoidosis, and fungal serology is used to identify a pulmonary mycosis. *(See also the answer to Question 5).*

4. (**b**) The sputum smear shows bacilli stained red with an acid-fast stain. Such bacterial staining is specific for mycobacteria. In this case, it is specific for *Mycobacterium tuberculosis*. *Candida* is a fungus, which may show a yeast-like or pseudohyphal morphology, and does not stain with acid-fast stains. *Klebsiella pneumoniae,* which is a Gramnegative bacterium, will also not stain.

5. (**a**) Serum levels of angiotensin converting enzyme (ACE) are elevated in 50%–80% of cases of active sarcoidosis. This discovery has been found useful in distinguishing between active and inactive sarcoidosis, and between sarcoidosis and other granulomatous diseases. The test, however, is not highly specific. In 5%–20% of cases, ACE values are raised in the absence of sarcoidosis. These include tuberculosis and active histoplasmosis, Gaucher's disease, Hodgkin's disease, and cirrhosis.

6. (**d**) All of the statements listed are correct. A positive reaction to the intracutaneous injection of PPD tuberculin is, in general, a reliable indication of prior infection with *Mycobacterium tuberculosis.* However, immunosuppressed persons, especially those with AIDS, may be anergic, and react negatively. This may also occur in persons with newly-active lung disease, or with miliary tuberculosis. In warm and humid climates, exposure to non-pathogenic mycobacteria may occur, and lead to non-specific positive reactions. As a practical matter, reactions ≥5 mm in diameter are usually regarded as positive in persons also having AIDS, reactions of ≥10 mm are usually regarded as positive in persons from population groups at high risk of developing tuberculosis, and reactions of ≥15 mm in diameter are usually regarded as positive in low-risk population groups.

7. (**c**) The virulence of *Mycobacterium tuberculosis* is complex; it is not related to the effects of a known endotoxin or exotoxin. Virulent strains can prevent the fusion of phagosomes and lysosomes when the organisms are engulfed by macrophages, and prevent the respiratory burst necessary to kill them. The organism is strictly aerobic, which accounts for its predilection for the pulmonary apices, and grows slowly, which raises problems for timely diagnosis by culture.

8. (**e**) The lesion is a granuloma with caseation necrosis, which is a typical lesion of tuberculosis. It represents a form of chronic inflammatory reaction to *Mycobacterium tuberculosis* (a slowly dividing infectious agent) in the presence of a T cell mediated immune response. The mycobacteria are present within the lesion (Figure 17–5). The presence of mycobacteria in early lesions makes those lesions highly infectious. The fibrosis and calcification of a granuloma usually occur after the mycobacterial growth has been controlled. The caseation helps in this regard, since mycobacteria cannot grow within the acidic, necrotic, extracellular environment, which lacks oxygen. The lesion is not an abscess, which is a localized collection of pus.

9. (**e**) All of the options listed are correct. CD4 positive T lymphocytes secrete interferon-γ, which activates macrophages to kill ingested mycobacteria by generating the reactive nitrogen compounds NO, NO_2, and HNO_3. This process is accompanied by a change in appearance of the macrophages to that of "epithelioid" cells, to form granulomas. These reactions form an example of the protective aspect of the classic cell-mediated type IV hypersensitivity.

10. (**e**) All of the options listed are correct. This question addresses the destructive aspect of cell-mediated type IV hypersensitivity to *Mycobacterium tuberculosis.* CD8+ suppressor T cells kill infected macrophages. The dead cells form the basis of caseation necrosis. With the appearance of a positive PPD (tuberculin) skin reaction, cell-mediated (type IV) hypersensitivity can be assumed to be established.

11. (**d**) All statements are correct. The hyperuricemia in this patient was most likely due to the effect of one of the drugs used in the treatment of tuberculosis (pyrazinamide), which is known to inhibit the renal excretion of urates. The patient may remain asymptomatic, or he may develop gouty arthritis. If the patient develops gouty arthritis, the drug should be discontinued.

▶ Final Diagnosis and Synopsis of the Case

• Tuberculous Pneumonia

The patient, a 32-year-old man who had immigrated to the United States about seven years previously, was admitted for the investigation of fever and an unproductive cough of two weeks' duration. A chest x-ray showed pneumonia with interstitial infiltration in both lung fields, and hilar lymphadenopathy. Serological studies were negative for fungi, *Legionella*, mycoplasma, and cytomegalovirus. Normal levels of circulating angiotensin converting enzyme were thought to make sarcoidosis less likely as an etiology for hilar lymphadenopathy. An acid-fast stain of sputum was positive for acid-fast organisms, which subsequently proved to be *Mycobacterium tuberculosis* on culture. A diagnosis of tuberculosis, probably of primary type, was made, and triple antibiotic therapy (isoniazid, rifampin, and pyrazinamide) was instituted. The patient improved remarkably and was discharged on the eleventh hospital day to continue therapy on an out-patient basis. The pyrazinamide component of his drug regimen apparently caused an asymptomatic hyperuricemia.

LAB TIPS

The Laboratory Diagnosis of Mycobacterial Infections

Organisms from the genus *Mycobacterium* are widespread in the environment and include the major human pathogens *Mycobacterium tuberculosis*, *Mycobacterium leprae*, and the *Mycobacterium avium intracellulare* complex. They are aerobic, Gram-positive rods that demonstrate the ability, when stained with carbol-fuchsin, to resist decolorization with acid alcohol. This property of acid-fastness provides a simple technique to detect their presence in specimens, and given the unusually long culture times for these organisms, provides an opportunity for a rapid diagnosis.

Tissue Samples

In surgical pathology specimens, the granulomatous inflammation characteristic of tuberculosis is readily apparent with routine hematoxylin–eosin staining. When discovered, it will result in the addition of an acid-fact stain for the detection of mycobacteria. Since fungal infections may also result in this type of tissue response, stains for these organisms, also, are usually done. In severely immunocompromised patients, the tissue response to infection from these organisms may be atypical and the addition of acid-fast and fungal stains may be necessary because of the clinical setting, alone.

Cytologic Specimens

With the increasing use of bronchial washings, alveolar lavages, and fine needle aspiration techniques, material can be obtained from virtually any organ. Smears can be quickly made, stained, and searched for organisms.

Cultures

Identification of individual species from cultures depends on rate of growth, pigment production, the ideal temperature for growth, and biochemical testing. Recently, new technologies, such as DNA probes and radiometric instruments, have been introduced to increase the speed of recovery and identification of mycobacteria.

NOTES

▶ Clinical History and Presentation

A 70-year-old man was admitted to the hospital with a chief complaint of hematemesis of several hours' duration. He woke during the night with nausea and vomiting of bloody material. Subsequently, he vomited several times and was brought to the emergency room by his wife. He reported that he had taken one aspirin daily for several years, and in the last few days had taken ibuprofen for leg pain. The patient also recalled passing a dark stool for several consecutive days. He denied alcohol consumption and he had quit smoking 10 years previously. There was no other medical or surgical history and the patient claimed to be otherwise in good health. Physical examination revealed a well nourished man in acute distress due to persistent nausea. Blood pressure was 130/90 mmHg in supine position and 100/75 mmHg on standing, heart rate was 104 per minute, temperature was 97.6° F, and respiratory rate was 16 per minute. The abdomen was soft and nontender with active bowel sounds. No masses were felt. Rectal examination showed black stool, which was guaiac positive. An esophago-gastro-duodenoscopy was performed in the emergency room. It revealed a large amount of old blood, and some fresh blood was noted in the body and cardia of the stomach. The bleeding lesion, however, was not identified. The esophagus and duodenum were normal.

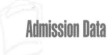

Admission Data

TABLE 18-1. HEMATOLOGY		
WBC	10.6 thousand/μL	(3.6–11.2)
Neut	77%	(44–88)
Band	0%	(0–10)
Lymph	16%	(12–43)
Mono	5%	(2–11)
Eos	1%	(0–5)
Baso	1%	(0–2)
RBC	2.8 million/μL	(4.0–5.6)
Hgb	7.8 g/dL	(12.6–17.0)
HCT	34%	(37.0–50.4)
MCV	85.7 fL	(80.5–102.0)
MCH	27.9 pg	(27.0–35.6)
MCHC	32.5 g/dL	(30.7–36.7)
Plts	195 thousand/μL	(130–400)

NOTES

TABLE 18–2. CHEMISTRY

Glucose	98 mg/dL	(65–110)
Creatinine	1.1 mg/dL	(0.7–1.4)
BUN	45 mg/dL	(7–24)
Uric acid	3.7 mg/dL	(3.0–8.5)
Cholesterol	171 mg/dL	(150–240)
Calcium	8.0 mg/dL	(8.0–10.0)
Protein	5.6 g/dL	(6–8)
Albumin	3.4 g/dL	(3.2–4.6)
LDH	125 U/L	(100–220)
Alk Phos	67 U/L	(0–120)
AST	12 U/L	(10–30)
GGTP	15 U/L	(10–40)
Bilirubin	0.2 mg/dL	(0.1–1.0)
Bilirubin, direct	0.05 mg/dL	(0.02–0.18)
Amylase	85 U/L	(23–85)
Lipase	20 U/L	(4–24)

TABLE 18–3. ELECTROLYTES

Na	135 mEq/L	(134–143)
K	3.8 mEq/L	(3.5–4.9)
Cl	101 mEq/L	(95–108)
CO_2	21 mEq/L	(21–32)

TABLE 18–4. COAGULATION

PT	11.5 sec	(11–14)
aPTT	22 sec	(22–31)

TABLE 18–5. URINALYSIS

Normal

▶ **Questions**

On the basis of the preceding information, you can best conclude the following:

1. In your evaluation of this patient prior to the endoscopy, which of the following causes of bleeding would you consider to be LEAST likely?
   a. duodenal carcinoma
   b. duodenal ulcer
   c. gastric carcinoma
   d. gastric ulcer
   e. gastritis

2. The increase in blood urea nitrogen (BUN) in this patient is LEAST likely caused by:
   a. gastrointestinal tract hemorrhage
   b. primary kidney disease
   c. vomiting and dehydration
   d. hypovolemia due to acute blood loss

3. In general, dark stool is LEAST likely due to:
   a. esophageal bleeding
   b. gastric bleeding
   c. duodenal bleeding
   d. ruptured hemorrhoids
   e. consumption of iron-rich food

4. All of the following statements about this patient's anemia are correct EXCEPT:
   a. the RBC count, Hgb, and HCT will further decrease upon hydration of the patient
   b. it is at least of six months' duration and only became exacerbated by the acute hemorrhage
   c. it is a normocytic anemia
   d. the RBCs will most likely not show any abnormalities on microscopic examination

5. Which of the following indicators would point to acute blood loss in this patient?
   a. orthostatic hypotension
   b. increased blood urea nitrogen (BUN) level
   c. low RBC count, hematocrit (HCT), and hemoglobin (Hgb)
   d. all of the above
   e. none of the above

NOTES

▶ Clinical Course

The patient was begun on intravenous fluid and his hemoglobin and hematocrit were closely monitored. After blood typing and cross matching, he received three units of packed red blood cells. The bleeding continued and the patient underwent a laparotomy and gastrotomy. The bleeding gastric lesion was excised and blood clots were removed from the stomach. The patient tolerated the procedure well and received three more units of packed red blood cells. Figures 18–1 through 18–6 show the histological appearance of the gastric lesion and surrounding mucosa. The patient's hematocrit and hemoglobin values are summarized in Table 18–6. The post-operative course was uneventful and the patient was discharged two weeks later. He was given medication and was scheduled for a follow-up endoscopy.

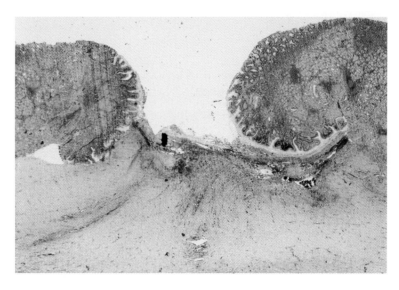

FIGURE 18–1. Gastric lesion. Hematoxylin–eosin stain. Original magnification ×3.

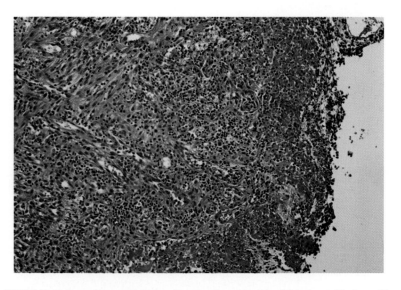

FIGURE 18–2. Base of the gastric lesion. Hematoxylin–eosin stain. Original magnification ×31.

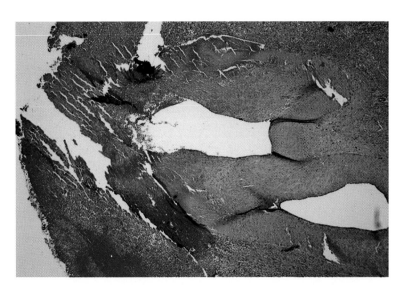

FIGURE 18–3. Another section of the gastric lesion. Hematoxylin–eosin stain. Original magnification ×8.

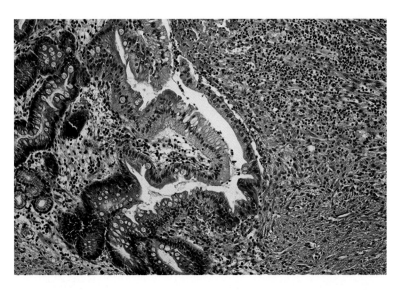

FIGURE 18–4. Edge of the gastric lesion. Hematoxylin–eosin stain. Original magnification ×31.

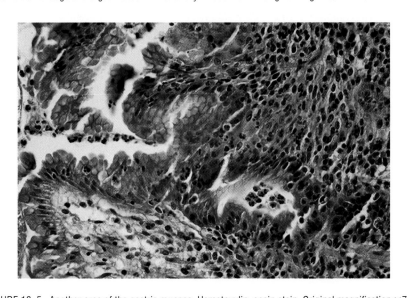

FIGURE 18–5. Another area of the gastric mucosa. Hematoxylin–eosin stain. Original magnification ×78.

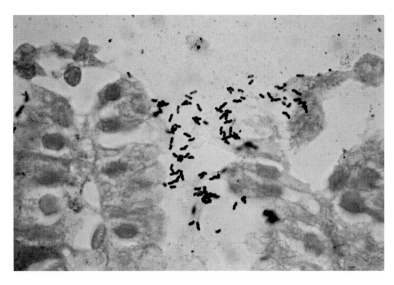

FIGURE 18–6. Gastric mucosa. Warthin-Starry stain. Original magnification ×315.

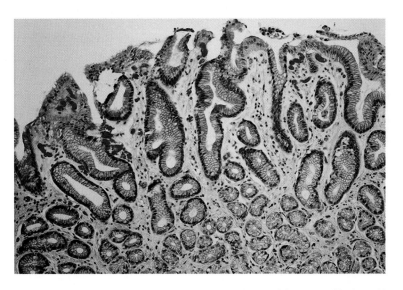

FIGURE 18–7. Normal gastric mucosa. Hematoxylin–eosin stain. Original magnification ×31.

TABLE 18–6. HEMATOLOGY

Test	Reference Values	Post–Endoscopy and 3 Units of PRBCs	Post–Operative and 3 Units of PRBCs		
		Day 1	Day 2	Day 3	Day 4
Hgb	12.6–17	8.6 g/dL	11 g/dL	10 g/dL	11.2 g/dL
HCT	37.2–50.4	26.3%	31.9%	29.2%	34%

► Questions

6. The excised gastric lesion depicted in Figures 18–1 through 18–3 is:
   a. a malignant gastric ulcer
   b. a lymphoma penetrating the gastric wall
   c. a benign gastric ulcer
   d. a gastric polyp
   e. a granulomatous gastritis

7. All of the following features are present in the gastric lesion illustrated in Figures 18–1 through 18–6 EXCEPT:
   a. microbial organisms
   b. an inflammatory cell infiltrate
   c. a small artery with erosion of the wall
   d. cells with a "signet ring" appearance

8. All of the following statements concerning this gastric lesion are correct EXCEPT:
   a. at the time of the diagnosis it has usually metastasized and the treatment is mostly symptomatic and palliative
   b. it typically affects middle-aged and older patients
   c. it often appears without an obvious precipitating factor
   d. gastritis is often associated with the lesion
   e. in the majority of patients, there is usually a solitary lesion

9. The lesion depicted in Figures 18–1 through 18–6 is often associated with:
   a. the presence of *Helicobacter pylori*
   b. an increased prostaglandin concentration in the gastric mucosa
   c. an uncontrolled growth of cells
   d. granuloma formation
   e. a similar lesion in the liver

10. Transfusion of one unit of packed red blood cells (PRBC) should increase the hemoglobin concentration in a non-bleeding, 70 kg male by approximately:
    a. 50 mg/dL
    b. 100 mg/dL
    c. 1 g/dL
    d. 3 g/dL
    e. none of the above

NOTES

▶ Figure Descriptions

Figure 18–1. Gastric lesion. Hematoxylin–eosin stain. Original magnification ×3.

The lesion was grossly an oval-shaped, sharply defined defect on the lesser curvature of the stomach. Microscopically, the base is fairly level and the margins are not appreciably elevated above the adjacent mucosa. The ulcer extends into the muscular wall and is close to an underlying blood vessel.

Figure 18–2. Base of the gastric lesion. Hematoxylin–eosin stain. Original magnification ×31.

The surface of the ulcer (right side of image) shows a thin layer of fibrinoid debris and acute inflammatory cells. Beneath this is active granulation tissue composed of proliferating small blood vessels, fibroblasts, and acute and chronic inflammatory cells in a loose stroma.

Figure 18–3. Another section of the gastric lesion. Hematoxylin–eosin stain. Original magnification ×8.

This shows an eroded artery that was the source of bleeding in this patient. A large mass of fibrin and inflammatory cells is present at the site of erosion.

Figure 18–4. Edge of the gastric lesion. Hematoxylin–eosin stain. Original magnification ×31.

The base of the ulcer is present on the right side of the image and shows a surface layer of fibrin with underlying active granulation tissue. Note the adjacent gastric mucosa containing scattered mucous goblet cells and the lamina propria showing an inflammatory cell infiltrate consisting of lymphocytes and plasma cells. These findings are consistent with chronic gastritis.

Figure 18–5. Another area of gastric mucosa. Hematoxylin–eosin stain. Original magnification ×78.

In addition to lymphocytes and plasma cells in the lamina propria, neutrophils can be seen within the epithelium above the basement membrane. Their presence indicates active gastritis.

Figure 18–6. Gastric mucosa. Warthin-Starry stain. Original magnification ×315.

A number of plump, black, curved, S-shaped bacilli are present on the luminal surface of the gastric epithelial cells but are not present within the tissue itself. Their morphologic appearance is consistent with *Helicobacter pylori*.

Figure 18–7. Normal gastric mucosa. Hematoxylin–eosin stain. Original magnification ×31.

The gastric mucosa is intact. No inflammatory cells are present within the epithelium or the lamina propria.

▶ Answers

1. (**a**) Cancers of the small intestine are very uncommon. Erosive gastritis, duodenal ulcer, gastric ulcer, and esophagogastric mucosal tears account for 90% of cases of upper gastrointestinal hemorrhage.

2. (**b**) Urea is formed in the liver and represents an end-product of protein catabolism. It is excreted by the kidneys. As a result, the rate of protein catabolism and the rate at which the kidney excretes urea are the decisive factors determining the level of blood urea nitrogen (BUN). The least likely cause of increased blood urea nitrogen (BUN) in this patient is a primary kidney disease; the patient has no history or indication of a primary renal disease and his serum creatinine is normal. On the other hand, gastrointestinal tract hemorrhage leads to increased protein catabolism and to an increased BUN. Acute hypovolemia (blood loss and vomiting) leads to renal hypoperfusion and to impaired excretion of urea, which causes an increased level of BUN.

3. (**d**) Bleeding from ruptured hemorrhoids characteristically leaves small amounts of blood on the surface of the stool or on toilet tissue. The dark or black color of the stool indicates upper gastrointestinal bleeding (the change in the color is caused by hematin, which results from the contact of blood with hydrochloric acid). Such a stool is also described as "tarry," which refers to its stickiness. Consumption of iron-rich food also leads to dark stools, though it does not cause a "tarry" appearance.

4. (**b**) The patient had a normocytic anemia due to acute blood loss. It is characterized by low RBC count, low hemoglobin (Hgb), and low hematocrit (HCT). Other red blood cell indices are within the normal range. If the anemia were of six months' duration, the RBC indices would be abnormal (hypochromic and microcytic). The RBC count, Hgb, and HCT will further decrease upon fluid replacement because of the dilution factor. The peripheral blood smear should show normocytic, normochromic red blood cells.

5. (**d**) Acute blood loss from the gastrointestinal tract leads to a decreased RBC count, decreased HCT and Hgb, increased BUN level, and orthostatic hypotension (a fall in blood pressure greater than 30/20 mmHg on standing upright from a supine position, due to volume loss).

6. (**c**) The lesion depicted in Figures 18–1 through 18–3 is a benign ulcer (*see Figure description*). There is no granuloma present and the lesion clearly is not a polyp (a mass that projects into the lumen, above the level of the mucosa). No neoplastic glandular epithelium or "signet ring" cells (typical of the diffuse variant of gastric adenocarcinoma) are present. The lymphocytes present in the base of the ulcer are a part of the inflammatory response to the ulcer and do not represent malignancy.

7. (**d**) Features seen in Figures 18–1 through 18–6 include *Helicobacter pylori* on the mucosal surface of the stomach and inflammatory cells infiltrating the mucosa and the submucosa and eroding the wall of a small blood vessel in the submucosa, which was most likely the cause of bleeding. Malignant "signet ring" cells are not present.

8. (**a**) Since the lesion represents a benign gastric ulcer, it does not have metastatic potential. Gastric ulcers typically affect middle-aged and older individuals and may appear without any previous warning and in the absence of known precipitating factors. A gastric ulcer is usually a solitary lesion and gastritis is commonly present in addition to the ulcer.

9. (**a**) Benign gastric ulcer is known to be associated with *Helicobacter pylori* infection (90%–100%). Granuloma formation is not a feature of peptic ulcers. The ulcer heals in an organized fashion (an uncontrolled growth of cells is not a feature of the ulcer or of its healing process), and its recurrence in some patients is linked to a decreased (not increased) level of prostaglandin concentration in the gastric mucosa. Since gastric ulcer is a benign lesion, it does not metastasize.

10. **(c)** Let us assume the following data:
- the total volume of blood of a 70 kg male is about 5 L
- one unit of blood contains 0.5 L (5 dL)
- hemoglobin concentration in a unit of PRBC is approximately 12 g/dL
- total amount of hemoglobin in a unit of PRBC is 60 g (12 g $\times$ 5 dL)
- transfusion of one unit of packed red blood cells represents transfusion of 60 g of hemoglobin into a volume of 5 L

Therefore, transfusion of one unit of packed red blood cells should increase the hemoglobin concentration in a non-bleeding, 70 kg male by approximately 60 g/5 L = 12 g/1 L = 1.2 g/dL.

▶ Final Diagnosis and Synopsis of the Case

- Peptic Ulcer
- *Helicobacter Pylori* Infection

A 70-year-old man presented with severe hematemesis and a history of "tarry stools." He was a chronic user of low doses of aspirin and an occasional user of ibuprofen. Endoscopy in the emergency room failed to identify the bleeding lesion because of an excessive amount of blood clot in the stomach. Transfusion of three units of packed red blood cells failed to raise his hemoglobin and hematocrit. He then began to bleed again and he was taken to surgery. A benign ulcer eroding a submucosal artery was found and excised. Histologic examination confirmed the benign character of the lesion and the presence of *Helicobacter pylori*. The excision of the lesion was curative and the bleeding stopped. Additional transfusions improved the patient's Hgb and HCT levels and the post-operative course was uneventful. The patient was begun on therapy with H-2 receptor antagonists and antibiotics for his *Helicobacter pylori* infection.

LAB TIPS

Blood Transfusion

The decision to transfuse should be based primarily on the patient's clinical condition, not the level of hemoglobin or hematocrit. There are occasions when a patient may need to be transfused even in the face of a normal hemoglobin and hematocrit. It may take an hour following an acute blood loss for a patient's hemoglobin and hematocrit to reflect that loss. On the other hand, in patients with chronic anemia, mechanisms develop to help compensate for the decreased hemoglobin levels, and the emphasis should be placed on correcting the cause of the anemia, not on transfusing the patient to "normalize" the laboratory values.

BLOOD TRANSFUSION

Condition	Blood Product of Choice	Effects of Transfusion
Acute blood loss—>25% of blood volume	Stored whole blood	Blood volume expansion is greater than increase in hemoglobin. 1 unit whole blood leads to (about): a. 10% expansion in blood volume[a] b. .5 g/dL rise in hemoglobin[b] c. 1.5 % rise in hematocrit
Acute blood loss—<25% of blood volume	Usually not indicated	Volume expansion corrected by electrolyte solutions
Chronic blood loss, decompensated patient	Packed red blood cells	To increase oxygen-carrying capacity with minimal expansion of blood volume 1 unit of packed red blood cells leads to (about): a. 6% expansion in blood volume[a] b. 1 g/dL rise in hemoglobin[b] c. 3% rise in hematocrit
Chronic blood loss, compensated patient	Usually not indicated	Efforts should be directed at determining and correcting the source of the blood loss

[a]These are immediate effects; at 24 hours post–transfusion, the patient's blood volume returns to the pretransfusion level if hypovolemia was not present before transfusion.
[b]These are also immediate effects; at 24 hours post-transfusion both units will result in a 1 g/dL rise in the hemoglobin.

▶ **Clinical History and Presentation**

A 63-year-old woman was admitted to the hospital with a chief complaint of generalized abdominal pain which was most severe in the left lower quadrant, chills, and watery diarrhea of ten days' duration. She had been recently diagnosed with Lyme disease and had been treated with a cephalosporin for the previous two weeks. She had no other significant medical or surgical history. Physical examination revealed an alert woman in mild distress. Blood pressure was 114/80 mmHg, heart rate was 90 per minute and regular, temperature was 101° F, and respiratory rate was 20 per minute. Examination of the chest was unremarkable. Abdominal examination showed mild tenderness in the upper abdomen and remarkable tenderness in the left lower quadrant. The rest of the abdominal examination, including rectal examination, was unremarkable. Samples for blood and stool cultures were obtained. A flat plate of the abdomen was taken (Figure 19–1). A sigmoidoscopy and a colonic biopsy were performed (Figure 19–3).

Admission Data

TABLE 19–1. HEMATOLOGY		
WBC	36 thousand/μL	(3.3–11.0)
Neut	60%	(44–88)
Band	30%	(0–10)
Lymph	9%	(12–43)
Mono	1%	(2–11)
Eos	0%	(0–5)
Baso	0%	(0–2)
RBC	4.3 million/μL	(3.9–5.0)
Hgb	13.1 g/dL	(11.6–15.6)
HCT	41.1%	(37.0–47.0)
MCV	95 fL	(79.0–99.0)
MCH	30.3 pg	(26.0–32.6)
MCHC	32 g/dL	(31.0–36.0)
Plts	322 thousand/μL	(130–400)

TABLE 19–2. CHEMISTRY		
Glucose	173 mg/dL	(65–110)
Creatinine	0.8 mg/dL	(0.7–1.4)
BUN	20 mg/dL	(7–24)
Uric acid	4 mg/dL	(3.0–7.5)
Cholesterol	195 mg/dL	(150–240)
Calcium	8.4 mg/dL	(8.5–10.5)
Protein	5.9 g/dL	(6–8)
Albumin	3.7 g/dL	(3.7–5.0)
LDH	179 U/L	(100–250)
Alk Phos	97 U/L	(0–120)
AST	34 U/L	(0–55)
GGTP	15 U/L	(0–50)
Bilirubin	0.6 mg/dL	(0.0–1.5)
Bilirubin, direct	0.12 mg/dL	(0.02–0.18)

TABLE 19–3. ELECTROLYTES

Na	137 mEq/L	(134–143)
K	3.3 mEq/L	(3.5–4.9)
Cl	99 mEq/L	95–108)
CO_2	25 mEq/L	(21–32)

TABLE 19–4. EXAMINATION OF STOOL

The stool was watery.

Blood	Neg	(Neg)
WBC	14/HPF	(<5)
Mucus	++	(Neg)

TABLE 19–5. SPECIAL STUDIES

Pending

TABLE 19–6. MICROBIOLOGY

Stool culture: pending
Blood culture: pending

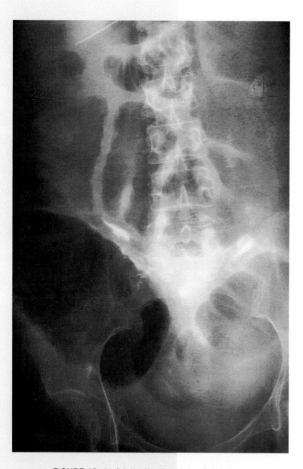

FIGURE 19–1. Admission flat plate of abdomen.

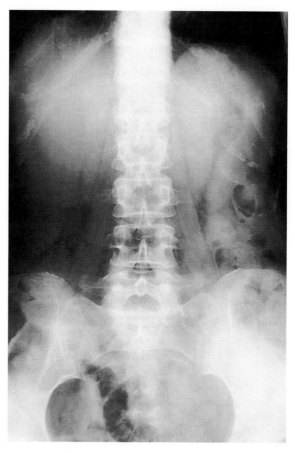

FIGURE 19–2. Normal flat plate of abdomen.

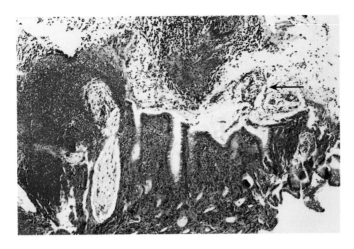

FIGURE 19–3. Colonic biopsy. Hematoxylin–eosin stain. Original magnification ×20.

▶ Questions

On the basis of the preceding information, you can best conclude the following:

1. The abdominal x-ray (Figure 19–1) is LEAST consistent with:
   a. toxic megacolon
   b. Crohn's disease
   c. Chagas' disease
   d. colonic perforation
   e. intestinal pseudo-obstruction

2. The clinical presentation of this patient is LEAST consistent with:
   a. acute diverticulitis
   b. pseudomembranous colitis
   c. *Campylobacter enterocolitis*
   d. complete intestinal obstruction

3. All of the following microscopic findings are present in Figure 19–3 EXCEPT:
   a. intense, predominantly mononuclear cell infiltration
   b. focal necrosis of the colonic mucosa
   c. leukocyte-rich exudate
   d. crypt abscess

4. The lesion indicated by the arrow in Figure 19–3 is composed of:
   a. necrotic debris
   b. fibrin
   c. mucus
   d. inflammatory cells
   e. all of the above

5. All of the following antibiotics are known to be implicated as the cause of this patient's condition EXCEPT:
   a. clindamycin
   b. ampicillin
   c. vancomycin
   d. cephalosporin

NOTES

▶ Clinical Course

The stool was positive for *Clostridium difficile* toxin. Blood cultures were negative for any bacterial growth. The patient was begun on a specific antibiotic therapy. On the second day after admission, her blood pressure had fallen to 50 mmHg systolic and became 90/60 with appropriate therapeutic measures. Her temperature was 102.2° F, and her vital signs were unstable. The abdomen became distended and diminished bowel sounds were present. The following night, her systolic blood pressure fell rapidly to 30 mmHg despite the use of pressors and intravenous fluids. The patient expired on the third day after admission. A postmortem examination was performed.

TABLE 19–7. PERTINENT LABORATORY DATA FROM SECOND AND THIRD HOSPITAL DAYS

	Normal Value	Day 2	Day 3
Hematology			
Plts	130–400 thousand/μL	120 thousand/μL	32 thousand/μL
Electrolytes			
Na	134–143 mEq/L	121 mEq/L	115 mEq/L
K	3.5–4.9 mEq/L	5.6 mEq/L	6.0 mEq/L
Cl	95–108 mEq/L	98 mEq/L	93 mEq/L
CO_2	21–32 mEq/L	8 mEq/L	8 mEq/L
Chemistry			
Creatinine	0.7–1.4 mg/dL	1.6 mg/dL	2.0 mg/dL
BUN	7–24 mg/dL	45 mg/dL	56 mg/dL
Calcium	8.5–10.5 mg/dL	9 mg/dL	7.5 mg/dL
Protein	6–8 g/dL	4 g/dL	2.1 g/dL
Albumin	3.7–5.0 g/dL	1.9 g/dL	0.9 g/dL
LDH	100–250 U/L	350 U/L	1136 U/L
LDH_1	17–28%	n/d	9%
LDH_2	30–36%	n/d	16%
LDH_3	19–25%	n/d	18%
LDH_4	10–16%	n/d	18%
LDH_5	6–13%	n/d	39%
Alk Phos	0–120 U/L	115 U/L	128 U/L
Arterial Blood Gases			
pH	7.35–7.45	7.27	6.93
$PaCO_2$	32–45 mm Hg	31 mm Hg	21 mm Hg
HCO_3^-	19–24 mEq/L	15 mEq/L	4 mEq/L
Coagulation			
Bleeding time	3–9.5 min	n/d	17 min
PT	11–16 sec	n/d	18 sec
aPTT	19–28 sec	n/d	40 sec
Fibrin degradation products	<10 μg/mL	n/d	>40 μg/mL
Fibrinogen	150–450 mg/dL	n/d	50 mg/dL

n/d = Not done

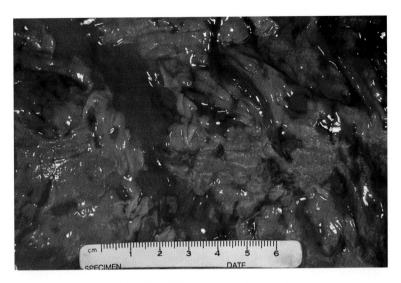

FIGURE 19–4. Colon at autopsy. Gross photo.

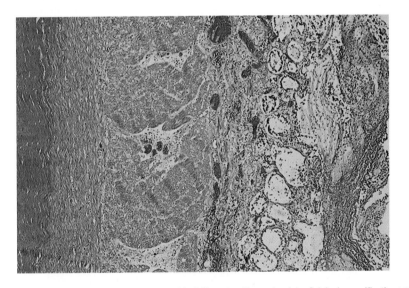

FIGURE 19–5. Portion of colon seen in Figure 19–4. Hematoxylin–eosin stain. Original magnification ×12.

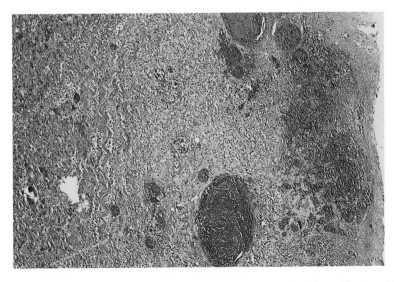

FIGURE 19–6. Another area of colon at autopsy. Hematoxylin–eosin stain. Original magnification ×12.

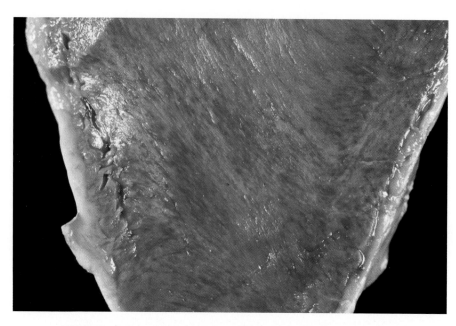

FIGURE 19–7. Cut surface of ventricular septum of heart at autopsy. Gross photo.

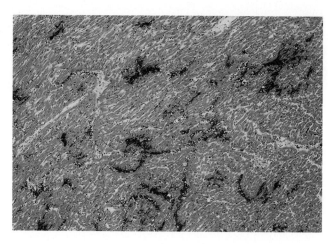

FIGURE 19–8. Myocardium at autopsy. Hematoxylin–eosin stain. Original magnification ×12.

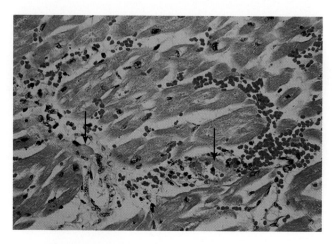

FIGURE 19–9. Myocardium at autopsy. Hematoxylin–eosin stain. Original magnification ×78.

► **Questions**

6. The intestinal disorder with which this patient presented may be associated with:
   a. a previously normal colonic mucosa
   b. a hemorrhagic colonic mucosa
   c. pseudomembrane formation
   d. all of the above
   e. none of the above

7. The lactate dehydrogenase (LDH) value and its isoenzyme pattern in this patient on the third hospital day are consistent with injury of which of the following organs or tissues?
   a. red blood cells
   b. myocardium
   c. brain
   d. kidney
   e. skeletal muscle

8. This patient's blood gas values on the third hospital day indicate:
   a. metabolic acidosis without respiratory compensation
   b. metabolic acidosis with partial respiratory compensation
   c. metabolic acidosis with complete respiratory compensation
   d. respiratory acidosis
   e. mixed metabolic and respiratory acidosis

9. All of the following statements regarding this patient's condition and laboratory findings are true EXCEPT:
   a. the admission CBC shows leukocytosis with a "left" shift
   b. diarrhea is the most common presenting symptom in this intestinal disorder
   c. the rapid fall of blood pressure during the second and third hospital days was most likely due to septic shock
   d. this intestinal condition may lead to the development of toxic megacolon and colonic perforation
   e. this intestinal condition is usually caused by *Clostridium sordelli*

10. The underlying mechanisms of the patient's abnormal coagulation profile and the findings in Figures 19–7, 19–8, and 19–9 include all of the following EXCEPT:
    a. the release of tissue factor into the circulation
    b. the activation of the intrinsic coagulation pathway
    c. the activation of the extrinsic coagulation pathway
    d. severe epithelial cell injury

▶ Figure Descriptions

Figure 19–1. Flat plate of abdomen.

There is moderate dilatation of the colon. The dilation is greater on the patient's right side (left side of figure). No fluid levels or pneumoperitoneum were present. Marked fecal retention is present.

Figure 19–2. Normal flat plate of abdomen.

The colon is not dilated and there is no evidence of a pneumoperitoneum or fluid levels within the bowel.

Figure 19–3. Colonic biopsy. Hematoxylin–eosin stain. Original magnification ×20.

This photomicrograph shows a portion of colonic mucosa containing a crypt distended by a mass of inflammatory cells and mucus. The purulent necrotic debris and fibrin suspended above the epithelium in this image (ie, the pseudomembrane, indicated by the arrow) was formed by the material ejected from numerous swollen crypts as they ruptured. These features are characteristic of pseudomembranous colitis.

Figure 19–4. Colon. Gross photo.

At autopsy, the colon was markedly dilated (toxic megacolon). The cecum measured 12 cm in diameter and contained several liters of semi-solid fecal material. Here, the bowel wall itself was flabby and friable but no perforations were present. This photograph is from an area of the colon that was less dilated and shows a red mucosa with irregular masses of friable greyish-green pseudomembrane scattered over the surface.

Figure 19–5. Portion of colon seen in Figure 19–4. Hematoxylin–eosin stain. Original magnification ×12.

The findings are similar to those seen in the biopsy material. There is a pseudomembrane composed of fibrin, necrotic debris, and neutrophils, with underlying distended colonic crypts. In this portion of the colon, the layers of the bowel wall can still be identified.

Figure 19–6. Another area of colon. Hematoxylin–eosin surface. Original magnification ×12.

In an area of marked dilatation, the epithelium appears denuded, the bowel wall appears necrotic, and the normal layers are no longer visible. The muscle fibers on the left side of the image are still viable and are becoming fragmented and infiltrated by acute inflammatory cells. If this patient had survived longer, the entire thickness of the bowel wall in this area would have become necrotic and probably resulted in a perforation.

Figure 19–7. Cut surface of ventricular septum of heart. Gross photo.

Multiple petechial hemorrhages are present throughout the myocardium. Similar findings were noted in the lungs and kidneys.

Figure 19–8. Myocardium. Hematoxylin–eosin stain. Original magnification ×12.

This is the microscopic appearance of the petechial hemorrhages that were noted grossly in Figure 19–7.

Figure 19–9. Myocardium. Hematoxylin–eosin stain. Original magnification ×78.

In one of these areas of hemorrhage, at higher magnification, we can see fibrin thrombi in some of the capillaries (arrows). The histologic findings here and in Figure 19–8 are consistent with a diagnosis of disseminated intravascular coagulation (DIC).

▶ **Answers**

1. (**d**) The abdominal x-ray (Figure 19–1) shows colonic dilatation *(see Figure description).* Toxic dilatation of the colon occurs with ulcerative colitis and, to a lesser extent, Crohn's disease. Toxic megacolon is also a known complication of severe pseudomembranous colitis. In addition, toxic megacolon can be seen with various congenital and acquired conditions such as Hirschsprung's disease (aganglionic megacolon), in a chronic idiopathic megacolon that occurs in late infancy at the beginning of toilet training, and in Chagas' disease due to destruction of the colonic ganglion cells by *Trypanosoma cruzi.* Megacolon is also observed with intestinal pseudo-obstruction (an acute or chronic motility disorder). In colonic perforation, a plain abdominal x-ray shows pneumoperitoneum (free air in the peritoneal cavity).

2. (**d**) Complete intestinal obstruction does not present with diarrhea. The differential diagnosis of this case includes diverticulitis, pseudomembranous colitis, *Campylobacter* enterocolitis, and many other diseases that lead to diarrhea and lower abdominal pain.

3. (**a**) The lesion depicted in Figure 19–3 is consistent with pseudomembranous colitis. The first microscopical finding in pseudomembranous colitis is focal necrosis of the colonic mucosa. This necrosis is accompanied by severe neutrophilic infiltration, but not by a mononuclear cell infiltrate of the lamina propria. Crypt abscesses, mucus, and leukocyte-rich exudates erupting to form larger abscesses ("minivolcanos") are usually seen.

4. (**e**) The arrow in Figure 19–3 points to a pseudomembrane, a typical feature of pseudomembranous colitis. The pseudomembrane is composed of necrotic debris, fibrin, mucus, and inflammatory cells.

5. (**c**) Pseudomembranous colitis is principally caused by the toxins of *Clostridium difficile.* Onset of the symptoms usually occurs during antibiotic therapy or within one month after the therapy. All antibiotics except vancomycin and streptomycin have been implicated in this disease. Vancomycin is the treatment of choice for pseudomembranous colitis.

6. (**d**) Morphologically, pseudomembranous colitis may exhibit normal, hemorrhagic, or friable colonic mucosa. It may also show mild congestion and edema of the colonic mucosa or pseudomembrane formation.

7. (**e**) The patient developed septic shock as a consequence of toxic megacolon. The LDH was markedly elevated, with the LDH_5 fraction comprising 39% of the total LDH (normal values are 6%–13% of the total). This pattern is seen with anoxic injury of striated muscle. Injury to red blood cells, such as hemolysis, leads to a predominant increase of LDH_1. Injury of myocardium, such as myocardial infarction, characteristically shows increase of LDH_1 and LDH_2, with a more marked increase of the LDH_1 proportion. This leads to a "flipped" LDH_1/LDH_2 ratio. Injury to brain and kidney leads to an increase in the proportions of LDH_3 and LDH_4. *(See Lab Tip in Chapter 28).*

8. (**b**) The patient's arterial blood gases indicate an acidotic status (pH < 7.35). The reduction in HCO_3^- (<23) in the presence of a low pH points to metabolic acidosis. This patient has a severe metabolic acidosis (a pH of 6.93) and a low $PaCO_2$, which indicates a partial respiratory compensation. In uncompensated metabolic acidosis, the $PaCO_2$ is usually within the normal range (35–45). With complete respiratory compensation (hyperventilation), the pH would increase to approach normal values and the $PaCO_2$ would decrease. Mixed respiratory and metabolic acidosis is characterized by a low pH and HCO_3^- with a high $PaCO_2$ level (>45).

9. (**e**) The patient was admitted with pseudomembranous colitis. The markedly elevated WBC count and the presence of a high proportion of immature myeloid cells ("bands") suggested a leukemoid reaction ("left" shift). Diarrhea is the most common presenting symptom in pseudomembranous colitis. One of the complications of pseudomembranous colitis is toxic megacolon, which may lead to colonic perforation, hypoalbuminemia, electrolyte disturbances, and septic shock. Patients in a decompensated stage of septic shock have severe hypotension, an increased heart rate, respiratory insufficiency, generalized anoxia, rapid deterioration of renal function, and metabolic acidosis. *Clostridium sordelli* does not cause pseudomembranous colitis.

10. (**d**) The coagulation profile of this patient reflects the presence of disseminated intravascular coagulation (DIC) *(see Figures 19–7, 19–8, and 19–9)*. The PT, aPTT, bleeding time, and fibrin degradation products are increased, the platelet count and fibrinogen level are significantly reduced. The underlying mechanisms of disseminated intravascular coagulation (DIC) include prolonged activation of the extrinsic or intrinsic coagulation pathways and/or severe endothelial cell injury. The release of tissue factor leads to activation of the extrinsic pathway. Activation of factor XII by contact with a negatively charged substance (collagen) triggers the intrinsic coagulation pathway. Both extrinsic and intrinsic pathways lead to the production of thrombin, which converts fibrinogen to fibrin. This process is balanced by the formation of plasmin and the clearance of clotting factors. Endothelial, not epithelial, cell injury leads to the activation of the intrinsic coagulation pathway and platelet aggregation.

▶ Final Diagnosis and Synopsis of the Case

- Severe Pseudomembranous Colitis
- Toxic Megacolon
- Disseminated Intravascular Coagulation
- Septic Shock

This was a case of severe pseudomembranous colitis which developed as a complication of cephalosporin therapy. The patient presented with abdominal pain, fever, and diarrhea, which are the most common presenting features of pseudomembranous colitis. The stool was watery, and on microscopic examination was found to contain WBCs and mucus. The diagnosis was confirmed by the presence of *Clostridium difficile* toxins in the stool and the findings on the colonic biopsy. The CBCs showed a significant leukocytosis with "left" shift (increased proportion of immature myeloid cells). The patient developed toxic megacolon, which is one of the most feared complications of pseudomembranous colitis. Toxic megacolon led to the development of septic shock and disseminated intravascular coagulation (DIC), and the patient expired.

LAB TIPS

TESTS FOR *CLOSTRIDIUM DIFFICILE*

Stool culture for *Clostridium difficile*	Very sensitive but not specific as it may be present in 25% of hospitalized adults without evidence of disease; found in stools of 3% of healthy, non-hospitalized adults; frequently isolated from stool of healthy infants.
Assay for *Clostridium difficile* toxins by tissue culture cytoxicity	Stool extracts are inoculated into tissue culture tubes some of which have added antitoxin. A positive test is the observance of a cytopathic effect in those tubes without the antitoxin and no cytopathic effect in those tubes with the antitoxin. This method correlates well with sigmoidoscopic evidence of pseudomembranous colitis.
Immunoassay for *Clostridium difficile* toxins	These immunoassays show good sensitivity and, because they are rapid, make good screening procedures. *Clostridium difficile* produces two exotoxins: Toxin A—an enterotoxin Toxin B—a cytotoxin

▶ Clinical History and Presentation

A 41-year-old farmer from southern New Jersey presented with fever, chills, headache, generalized muscle ache, and a rash on his legs of approximately five days' duration. He had smoked 2 packs of cigarettes daily for many years and did not drink alcohol. The patient had been in good health, and took no medication. Physical examination revealed an alert and oriented man in no acute distress. His blood pressure was 120/84 mmHg, heart rate was 88 per minute and regular, temperature was 101.2° F, and respiratory rate was 20 per minute. The pertinent physical findings included several circular skin lesions on his legs. The largest lesion measured 7 cm in diameter (Figure 20–1). This lesion was warm and flat with red outer borders. It was not painful or itchy. The patient recalled that about 10 days earlier he had removed a tick from the popliteal area. There were no other skin lesions, lymphadenopathy, or joint abnormalities present. The rest of the physical examination was unremarkable. A polymerase chain reaction from the affected tissue is shown in Figure 20–2.

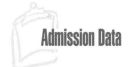

Admission Data

TABLE 20–1. HEMATOLOGY		
WBC	4.7 thousand/μL	(4.5–11.0)
Neut	75%	(44–88)
Band	0%	(0–10)
Lymph	19%	(12–43)
Mono	4%	(2–11)
Eos	1%	(0–5)
Baso	1%	(0–2)
RBC	4.5 million/μL	(4.4–5.8)
Hgb	14.9 g/dL	(14.0–17.0)
HCT	42.0%	(40.0–49.0)
MCV	93.3 fL	(80.0–94.0)
MCH	33.0 pg	(27.0–32.0)
MCHC	35.4 g/dL	(32.0–36.5)
Plts	168 thousand/μL	(130–400)

TABLE 20–2. CHEMISTRY		
Glucose	87 mg/dL	(65–110)
Creatinine	1.1 mg/dL	(0.7–1.4)
BUN	10 mg/dL	(7–24)
Uric acid	3.1 mg/dL	(3.0–8.5)
Cholesterol	132 mg/dL	(150–240)
Calcium	9.0 mg/dL	(8.5–10.5)
Protein	6.7 g/dL	(6–8)
Albumin	4.1 g/dL	(3.7–5.0)
LDH	196 U/L	(100–250)
Alk Phos	61 U/L	(30–120)
AST	32 U/L	(0–55)
GGTP	29 U/L	(0–50)
Bilirubin	0.4 mg/dL	(0.0–1.5)
Bilirubin, direct	0.12 mg/dL	(0.02–0.18)

TABLE 20–3. SEROLOGY AND IMMUNOLOGY

RF	19 IU/mL	(0–40)
RPR	nonreactive	(NR)
ANA	Neg	(Neg)
Lyme Ab	2.8 au/mL	(<20)

RF = Rheumatoid factor; RPR = Rapid plasma reagin; ANA = Anti-nuclear antibodies; Lyme Ab = Antibodies to *Borrelia burgdorferi* (ELISA)

TABLE 20–4. ELECTROLYTES

Na	135 mEq/L	(134–143)
K	3.9 mEq/L	(3.5–4.9)
Cl	98 mEq/L	(95–108)
CO_2	27 mEq/L	(21–32)

TABLE 20–5. COAGULATION

PT	12 sec	(11–14)
aPTT	27 sec	(22–31)

TABLE 20–6. URINALYSIS

Normal

TABLE 20–7. MICROBIOLOGY

Blood cultures: pending

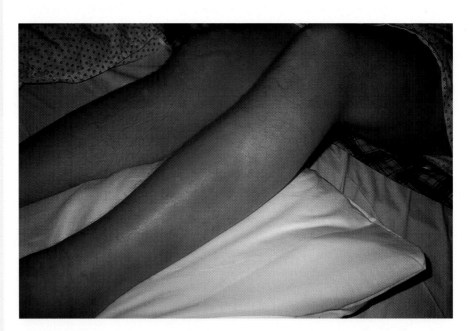

FIGURE 20–1. Skin lesions on legs.

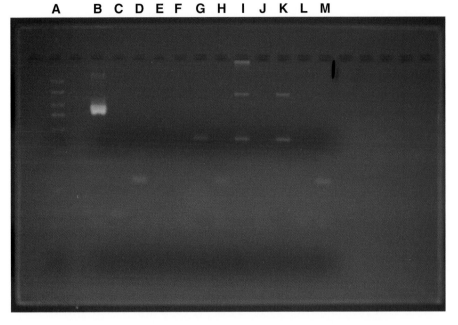

FIGURE 20–2. Polymerase chain reaction (PCR) for *Borrelia burgdorferi* DNA.

▶ **Questions**

On the basis of the preceding information, you can best conclude the following:

1. The gross appearance of the skin lesions (Figure 20–1) is most characteristic of:
   a. a furuncle
   b. erythema chronicum migrans (ECM)
   c. basal cell carcinoma
   d. dermatitis herpetiformis

2. At this stage, all of the following statements are correct EXCEPT:
   a. most of the patient's symptomatology can be characterized as "flu-like"
   b. the skin lesion is highly suggestive of the diagnosis
   c. a normal CBC and serology-immunology tests exclude any causal relationship between the tick bite and the patient's symptoms
   d. the positive polymerase chain reaction (PCR) provides direct evidence of the etiology of this patient's symptoms

3. Which of the following treatment modalities would you recommend?
   a. local antibiotics for the skin lesion
   b. the "wait and watch" approach
   c. systemic antibiotics
   d. excision of the skin lesion
   e. irradiation of the skin lesion

► Clinical Course

Blood cultures were negative. The patient was begun on oral medication and instructed to take it for three weeks. He was assured that he would most likely be cured without any sequelae. His fever subsided in two days. The CBC, chemistry, and other laboratory tests, with the exception of PCR, were repeated at the end of the treatment and were normal.

▶ **Questions**

4. If untreated, this patient would be at risk of developing any of the following problems EXCEPT:
   a. lymphadenopathy
   b. chronic obstructive lung disease
   c. Bell's palsy
   d. arthritis
   e. cardiac conduction abnormalities

5. If untreated, the patient would be expected to show positivity for which assays if tested 6 months after the onset of his symptoms?
   a. HIV antibodies
   b. antibodies to *Borrelia burgdorferi*
   c. VDRL
   d. IgA granular deposits in the tips of the dermal papillae, by direct immunofluorescence
   e. anti-nuclear antibodies (ANA)

6. The major goal of therapy in this patient was:
   a. to prevent metastasis
   b. to treat the "flu-like" symptoms
   c. to suppress the immune system
   d. to eradicate the causative organism
   e. to prevent further transmission by sexual contact

7. If the patient wanted to be informed about his prognosis after he completed his course of therapy, which of the following statements should have been avoided?
   a. the patient will be immune to the causative agent
   b. it is unlikely that there will be a recurrence of his presenting symptoms
   c. the patient's condition will not be contagious
   d. his original problem is not likely to spread to other tissues
   e. the patient will not be immunodeficient as a result of this disease

▶ Figure Descriptions

Figure 20–1. Skin lesions on legs.

Several erythematous, annular lesions can be seen on the legs of the patient. There is slight central pallor and a minimally raised area near the center of the lesion on the lateral aspect of the left knee.

Figure 20–2. Polymerase chain reaction (PCR) for Borrelia burgdorferi *DNA.*

The polymerase chain reaction (PCR) is used to detect the presence of a specific nucleotide sequence delineated by a primer pair. The polymerase repeatedly transcribes the nucleotide stretch between the two primers. For valid testing, both positive (known to contain the sequence to be amplified) and negative (known not to contain such a nucleotide sequence) controls must be included. The quality of the specimen processing (the quality of DNA extraction) is controlled by screening for the presence of "amplifiable DNA." This is done by use of one of the "housekeeping genes" present in all cells, such as β-globin. The photograph of the gel shows DNA size markers in LANE A, negative controls for *Borrelia burgdorferi* DNA in LANES B and C, and positive controls for *Borrelia burgdorferi* DNA in LANES D and M. Patient samples (not our patient's) negative for *Borrelia burgdorferi* DNA are shown in LANES F and J. The presence of amplifiable DNA (β-globin gene) for these patients' samples is shown in LANES G and K. Our patient's sample is shown in LANE H. It clearly shows the presence of *Borrelia burgdorferi* DNA. LANE I shows amplification of the β-globin gene in our patient's sample.

▶ Answers

1. **(b)** The skin lesion has a typical appearance of erythema chronicum migrans (ECM) of Lyme disease (it is painless, not itchy, and mostly flat with a red outer border). A furuncle represents a deep *Staphylococcus aureus* infection of the hair follicle which presents as a red, painful nodule with central necrosis. Basal cell carcinoma presents as a red plaque that may be eroded and crusted. Dermatitis herpetiformis is an extremely pruritic lesion that presents as urticarial plaques and vesicles and is often associated with celiac disease.

2. **(c)** The patient presented with "flu-like" symptoms and a skin lesion characteristic of early Lyme disease. The history of a tick bite at the site of the lesion further points to the diagnosis. The detectable specific antibodies (IgM) appear and their titer peaks between 3–6 weeks after the onset of the disease, so it is not surprising that the test is negative in our patient, whose symptoms are less than a week in duration. Other, non-specific, laboratory abnormalities often seen include an elevated erythrocyte sedimentation rate and SGOT (AST) level, or an elevated white cell count. These changes affect only some patients. In others there may be no changes in the laboratory profile. The detection of *Borrelia burgdorferi* DNA in the skin specimen by the polymerase chain reaction (PCR) provides direct evidence of infection by this organism.

3. **(c)** An early stage of Lyme disease is treated with oral antibiotics (several different regimens are used currently). About 10% of treated patients develop, within the first 24 hours of the treatment, worsening of their symptoms (higher fever, increased aches and pains, and a worsening rash). This is a reaction similar to Jarisch-Herxheimer reaction, seen in the treatment of syphilis. The pathogenesis of such reactions is unclear. All other treatment modalities are inappropriate and have no place in the treatment of Lyme disease.

4. **(b)** Patients with unrecognized and/or untreated early Lyme disease are likely to develop any or all of the manifestations of "early" through "late" stages of the disease. In addition to early skin lesions, a lymphadenopathy (regional or generalized) is a common finding. Neurologic involvement (meningitis, encephalitis, peripheral radiculoneuropathy, etc) is common and usually resolves completely. Cardiac involvement, most commonly fluctuating degrees of atrioventricular block, occur in later stages of Lyme disease. About 60% of patients develop arthritis, which primarily affects large joints. The attacks of arthritis seem to recur for years. Chronic obstructive pulmonary disease, however, is not a feature of Lyme disease.

5. **(b)** About 6 weeks after the onset of the disease, the untreated patient should test positively for IgM specific antibody against *Borrelia burgdorferi*. It takes months to develop specific antibodies of IgG type. The finding of specific antibodies to *Borrelia burgdorferi* is particularly useful in patients in whom the early diagnosis was missed. Patients with Lyme disease should not test positively for ANA, VDRL, and HIV (unless there is a co-existent problem for which these tests are positive). Granular deposits of IgA at the tips of dermal papillae are not a feature of Lyme disease, but are typical of dermatitis herpetiformis.

6. **(d)** The goal of the therapy of Lyme disease is to eradicate *Borrelia burgdorferi* and prevent the development of "later" and "late" manifestations of Lyme disease. The best chance of doing so is in the early stages of the disease. Therefore, prompt treatment with antibiotics is important. A cured patient is, however, susceptible to reinfection. Lyme disease is not a malignancy, therefore metastatic potential is not considered; symptomatic treatment of "flu-like" symptoms is only a supportive measure and not a cure. A suppression of immunity would impede the eradication of *Borrelia burgdorferi* and is not indicated. Lyme disease is not considered to be a sexually transmitted disease.

7. **(a)** The patient will not be immune to another infection by *Borrelia burgdorferi*. The combination of his original symptoms will not recur unless the patient is infected again. The patient is expected to be cured (ie, *Borrelia burgdorferi* will be eradicated from his system), therefore there should not be any continuity of the disease. Lyme disease is very responsive to treatment in the early stage of the disease, which was the case in this patient. Lyme disease is not known to lead to immunodeficiency.

▶ Final Diagnosis and Synopsis of the Case

• Lyme Disease

A 41-year-old farm worker presented with nonspecific "flu-like" symptoms of less than one week's duration and a skin lesion typical of erythema chronicum migrans. He recalled removing a tick from the site of the skin lesion about 10 days previously. His laboratory findings, including specific serology tests, were normal. A skin biopsy (not routinely done for diagnostic purposes) showed a mononuclear cell infiltrate, a non-specific change consistent with the diagnosis of erythema chronicum migrans. A polymerase chain reaction (not routinely indicated in such a case) provided direct evidence of *Borrelia burgdorferi* DNA in the tissue. The patient was treated with oral antibiotics and was expected to be cured. He will most likely remain seronegative for specific antibodies against *Borrelia burgdorferi*. He was not expected to develop any further manifestations of Lyme disease. This was a case of early diagnosed Lyme disease, a disease which can easily be overlooked in the absence of a typical skin lesion. The serology is not helpful at this stage, since it takes several weeks for the specific IgM antibody titer to become detectable. A polymerase chain reaction test provides direct evidence of *Borrelia burgdorferi* DNA in the tissue, but is not routinely done, particularly in the presence of the erythema chronicum migrans lesion. The early stage of Lyme disease is very amenable to antibiotic treatment.

LAB TIPS

Lyme Disease Testing

The diagnosis depends on serologic studies and clinical findings, as the organism is difficult to culture. The table below shows various methods of detection.

LYME DISEASE TESTING	
Method	**Usefulness**
Enzyme-linked immunosorbent assay (ELISA)	IgM antibodies—develop over 3–6 weeks; detected in about 50% of patients with acute infection IgG antibodies—develop over 8–12 weeks; high titers seen in patients with cardiac, nervous system, or joint involvement. False positives—rheumatoid factor, infectious mononucleosis False negatives—test may have been done too soon; retest
Western blot test	More sensitive and specific than ELISA; sometimes used in early disease when ELISA is inconclusive
Polymerase chain reaction (PCR) for *Borrelia burgdorferi* DNA	Extremely specific and sensitive
Cerebrospinal fluid (CSF) analysis	When neurologic involvement is present, CSF may show increased protein, lymphocytes, IgG; the presence of CSF antibody is highly sensitive for neurologic disease.
Joint fluid analysis	When arthritis is present, there are increases in synovial fluid protein and white blood cells (mainly neutrophils)

A 60-Year-Old Woman With Generalized Weakness and Stiff Knees

▶ Clinical History and Presentation

A 60-year-old woman was admitted to the hospital with a chief complaint of generalized weakness of two weeks' duration, morning stiffness of both knees, which was aggravated by movement, and mild fever. The patient stated that she had lost 10 pounds since the previous month. She had no other significant medical or surgical history, except for two similar episodes the previous year involving the joints of the wrists and hands, for which she was taking anti-inflammatory medications. Physical examination revealed an alert female in mild distress. Blood pressure was 120/80 mmHg, heart rate was 85 per minute and regular, temperature was 100° F, and respiratory rate was 20 per minute. The abdomen was soft with mild splenomegaly. Both knees were swollen, warm, and painful with movement. Mild atrophy of the muscles of the forearms and small subcutaneous firm nodules in the back of forearms were noted. Swelling of the metacarpal-phalangeal joints was noted and a plain x-ray of the hand was taken (Figure 21–1).

 Admission Data

TABLE 21–1. HEMATOLOGY		
WBC	11.5 thousand/μL	(3.3–11.0)
Neut	55%	(44–88)
Band	0%	(0–10)
Lymph	35%	(12–43)
Mono	8%	(2–11)
Eos	1%	(0–5)
Baso	1%	(0–2)
RBC	3.75 million/μL	(3.9–5.0)
Hgb	10.6 g/dL	(11.6–15.6)
HCT	33.9%	(37.0–47.0)
MCV	91.5 fL	(79.0–99.0)
MCH	28.5 pg	(26.0–32.6)
MCHC	31.2 g/dL	(31.0–36.0)
Plts	553 thousand/μL	(130–400)
Erythrocyte Sedimentation Rate		
ESR	53 mm/hr	(0–15)

TABLE 21–2. CHEMISTRY

Glucose	110 mg/dL	(65–110)
Creatinine	0.9 mg/dL	(0.7–1.4)
BUN	18 mg/dL	(7–24)
Uric acid	2.8 mg/dL	(3.0–7.5)
Cholesterol	254 mg/dL	(150–240)
Calcium	8.7 mg/dL	(8.5–10.5)
Protein	6.7 g/dL	(6–8)
Albumin	3.4 g/dL	(3.7–5.0)
LDH	137 U/L	(100–250)
Alk Phos	76 U/L	(0–120)
AST	14 U/L	(0–55)
GGTP	19 U/L	(0–50)
Bilirubin	0.2 mg/dL	(0.0–1.5)
Bilirubin, direct	0.05 mg/dL	(0.02–0.18)

TABLE 21–3. IMMUNOLOGY

RF	103 IU/mL	(0–40)
ANA	Neg	(Neg)

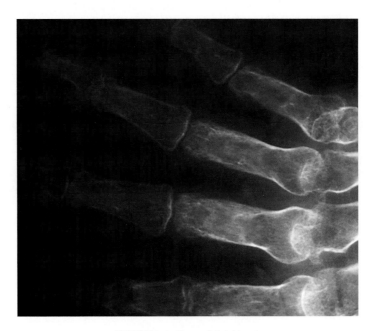

FIGURE 21–1. X-ray of distal hand.

▶ Questions

On the basis of the preceding information, you can best conclude the following:

1. The pain in this patient's knees was most likely due to all of the following EXCEPT:
   a. stretching of the joint capsule
   b. accumulation of synovial fluid
   c. osteophyte formation
   d. synovial hypertrophy
   e. thickening of the joint capsule

2. Conditions such as those seen in this patient most typically develop in which of the following joints?
   a. knee
   b. elbow
   c. proximal interphalangeal and metacarpophalangeal joints of the hand
   d. wrist
   e. ankle

3. The active stage of the disease affecting this patient is known to be typically associated with all of the following findings EXCEPT:
   a. thrombocytosis
   b. elevated erythrocyte sedimentation rate (ESR)
   c. normocytic anemia
   d. hypoalbuminemia
   e. swollen, warm joints

4. The plain x-ray of the hand (Figure 21–1) shows:
   a. joint space narrowing
   b. bone destruction
   c. periarticular osteoporosis
   d. all of the above
   e. none of the above

▶ Clinical Course

The patient was begun on anti-inflammatory medication. During her hospital stay, a biopsy of a subcutaneous nodule (Figure 21–7) and synovial fluid aspiration were performed (Figures 21–2, 21–3, and 21–4). A rheumatoid factor (RF) assay was repeated. Her condition improved and she was discharged to be followed up as an outpatient.

TABLE 21–4. SYNOVIAL FLUID ANALYSIS

Property	Normal	Patient
Volume	3.5 mL	6 mL
Appearance	Clear	Turbid
Color	Colorless	Yellow
Viscosity	High	Decreased
Fibrin clot	Absent	Positive
Mucin clot	Good	Poor
WBC	<200/μL	3000/μL
Neut	<25%	90%

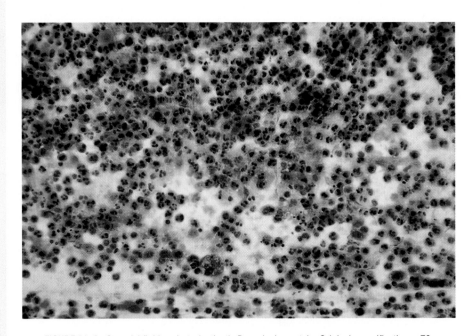

FIGURE 21–2. Synovial fluid aspirate (patient). Papanicolaou stain. Original magnification ×78.

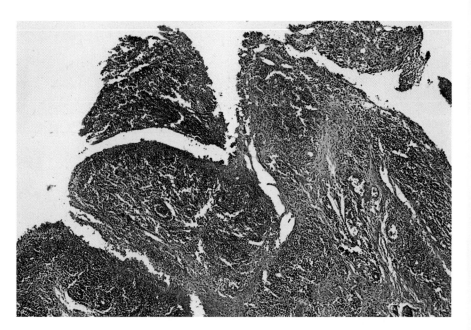

FIGURE 21–3. Portion of synovium from patient. Hematoxylin–eosin stain. Original magnification ×12.

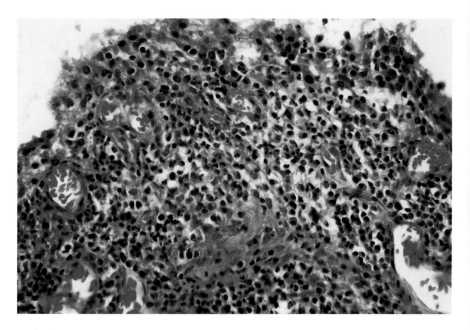

FIGURE 21–4. Portion of synovium from patient. Hematoxylin–eosin stain. Original magnification ×78.

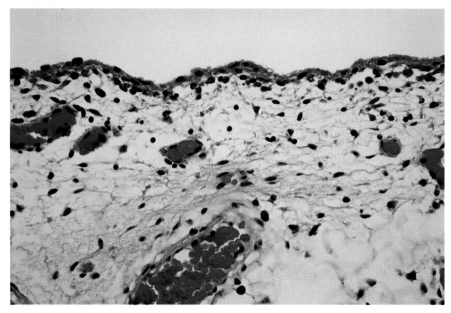

FIGURE 21–5. Essentially normal synovial lining. Hematoxylin–eosin stain. Original magnification ×78.

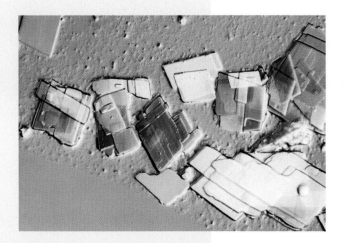

FIGURE 21–6. Material present in subcutaneous nodule from patient. Unstained. DIC microscopy. Original magnification ×150.

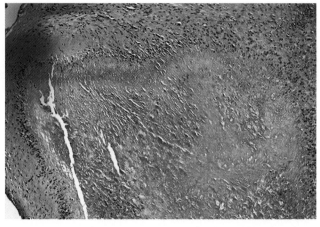

FIGURE 21–7. Subcutaneous nodule from patient. Hematoxylin–eosin stain. Original magnification ×20.

▶ **Questions**

5. The accumulation of the predominant cell type in the synovial fluid seen in Figure 21–2 is primarily due to:
   a. an elevated level of interleukin-2 (IL-2)
   b. complement fragment C5a
   c. complement fragment C3b
   d. an elevated level of interleukin-4 (IL-4)
   e. activation of cell-mediated immunity

6. All of the following statements about rheumatoid factor (RF) are correct EXCEPT:
   a. it is an IgM auto-antibody against the Fc fraction of the IgG molecule
   b. it forms immune complexes in the serum, synovial fluid, and synovial membrane
   c. it is detected only in patients with active rheumatoid arthritis
   d. it is a product of activated B lymphocytes

7. In this patient, synovial fluid findings alone are helpful to rule out:
   a. degenerative joint disease
   b. rheumatic fever
   c. tuberculous arthritis
   d. septic arthritis
   e. gonococcal arthritis

8. If a flow cytometric analysis of this patient's peripheral blood were performed, it would show:
   a. an increased proportion of hematopoietic stem cells
   b. a reversed CD4/CD8 ratio
   c. monoclonal restriction of B cells
   d. an increased proportion of activated T lymphocytes
   e. monoclonal restriction of T cells

9. Lesions such as the one depicted in Figure 21–7 are least likely to be found in the:
   a. lung
   b. spleen
   c. diaphysis of long bone
   d. myocardium
   e. aorta

10. The center of the lesion depicted in Figure 21–7 is characteristic of:
    a. caseous necrosis
    b. fibrinoid necrosis
    c. an abscess
    d. fat necrosis

NOTES

▶ Figure Descriptions

Figure 21–1. X-ray of distal hand.

This x-ray shows some of the characteristic radiographic changes of rheumatoid arthritis. The ulnar deviation of the fingers is a result of the contractures and subluxations secondary to involvement of the joint ligaments by the disease process. Periarticular osteoporosis can be seen as a clearing of the ends of the bones. Especially prominent at the phalangeal-metacarpal joints are areas of bone and cartilage destruction with resulting narrowing of the joint space.

Figure 21–2. Joint aspiration (patient). Papanicolaou stain. Original magnification ×78.

This is a photomicrograph of the fluid obtained by aspiration of the left knee joint. The predominant cells are neutrophils, but scattered macrophages are also identifiable. Early involvement of a joint in rheumatoid arthritis characteristically produces a neutrophil-rich exudate.

Figure 21–3. Portion of synovium from patient. Hematoxylin–eosin stain. Original magnification ×12.

The synovial villi are thickened with a heavy inflammatory cell infiltrate and increased vascularity (granulation tissue). Superficial areas of necrosis are present and masses of inflammatory cells can be seen free above the synovial surface.

Figure 21–4. Portion of synovium from patient. Hematoxylin–eosin stain. Original magnification ×78.

The nature of the inflammatory changes may be seen better at higher magnification. Neutrophils, lymphocytes, plasma cells, macrophages, and fibroblasts are responsible for the increased cellularity. Capillaries are increased in number, the synovial lining cells are hypertrophic and hyperplastic, and a small area of superficial necrosis can be seen near the top center of the image. With time, numerous lymphoid follicules will appear.

Figure 21–5. Essentially normal synovial lining. Hematoxylin–eosin stain. Original magnification ×78.

The lining epithelium is thin and lies on top of a loose connective tissue layer. Some scattered lymphocytes and plasma cells are present. The slightly prominent capillaries discount this as a completely normal synovium.

Figure 21–6. Material present in subcutaneous nodule from patient. Unstained. DIC microscopy. Original magnification ×150.

The resected nodule contained an area of partially liquefied material. Upon examination as a wet preparation, it showed numerous flat, notched plates consistent with cholesterol crystals. This is not an uncommon finding in rheumatoid nodules.

Figure 21–7. Subcutaneous nodule from patient. Hematoxylin–eosin stain. Original magnification ×20.

A portion of the subcutaneous nodule is shown in this photomicrograph. It has an eosinophilic center of fibrinoid necrosis surrounded by palisading histiocytes. Peripheral to this is an inflammatory cell infiltrate of lymphocytes and plasma cells, as well as some fibrosis.

▶ Answers

1. **(c)** This patient has rheumatoid arthritis (RA). In this disease, the joint pain is due to synovial inflammation, which leads to accumulation of synovial fluid, synovial hypertrophy, and thickening and stretching of the joint capsule. The sensory (pain) nerve fibers supplying the joint capsule are markedly sensitive to stretching. Osteophyte formation is usually seen with osteoarthritis due to degenerative changes in the articular cartilage.

2. **(c)** In the early stages, rheumatoid arthritis often leads to synovial joint disease that typically involves the proximal interphalangeal and metacarpophalangeal joints of the hand. Other joints may also be involved.

3. **(d)** In active rheumatoid arthritis, normocytic normochromic anemia, thrombocytosis, and an elevated erythrocyte sedimentation rate (ESR) are frequently present. Swollen, red, and warm joints are signs of acute inflammation. Hypoalbuminemia is not a typical feature of RA in its active stage.

4. **(d)** The plain x-ray of the wrist (Figure 21–1) shows changes typically found in joints affected by rheumatoid arthritis (periarticular osteoporosis, bone and cartilage destruction, and joint space narrowing).

5. **(b)** The predominant inflammatory cells in the synovial fluid are neutrophils. They were attracted to this location by chemotactic agents, such as fragments of the complement system (primarily fragment C5a). Arachidonic acid metabolites, such as leukotriene B_4 (LB_4), some cytokines, and bacterial products, also have a chemotactic effect on neutrophils. Interleukin-2 (IL-2) is a cytokine that mainly activates lymphocytes. Interleukin-4 (IL-4) is crucial for the activation of IgE-producing B lymphocytes, which mediate type I hypersensitivity. Complement fragment C3b is an opsonin. Cell-mediated immunity is activated in RA, but plays no role in attracting neutrophils to the inflammation site.

6. **(c)** Rheumatoid factor (RF) is usually an IgM auto-antibody to IgG, though occasionally it may be an IgG, IgA, or IgE auto-antibody. It is produced by activated B cells and forms an immune complex by binding to the Fc fraction of IgG molecules. Rheumatoid factor (RF) may be present in healthy individuals and may be absent in some patients with rheumatoid arthritis.

7. **(a)** The synovial fluid in this patient had an increased volume (6 mL) and was turbid and yellow in color. It also had a decreased viscosity and a WBC count of 3000/μL with 90% neutrophils. It formed a definite fibrin clot, and its mucin clot formation was poor. These findings may be seen in a variety of conditions: rheumatic fever, tuberculous arthritis, septic arthritis, gonococcal arthritis, and rheumatoid arthritis. These findings, however, would rule out the diagnosis of degenerative joint disease (DJD), which is not associated with severe inflammatory changes. The synovial fluid findings in DJD show increased volume, clear color, high viscosity, and good mucin, but no fibrin clot formation.

8. **(d)** Flow cytometric analysis of the peripheral blood is not routinely used in the diagnosis or management of rheumatoid arthritis. However, it has been established that the majority of T cells are activated and express the class II major histocompatibility gene complex product HLA-DR. In active RA, the T cell subsets show an increased CD4/CD8 ratio (helper/inducer to suppressor/cytotoxic). RA is not a lymphoproliferative disorder and there is no clonal T or B cell restriction.

9. **(c)** Figure 21–7 shows the typical appearance of a rheumatoid nodule. Rheumatoid nodules are present in 20%–30% of people with RA. They are usually found on pressure areas (periarticular) such as the elbow. In addition, they are occasionally seen in lung, spleen, myocardium, cardiac valves, pericardium, and aorta.

10. **(b)** Rheumatoid nodules are non-tender nodules, usually less than 2 cm in diameter. They show central fibrinoid necrosis surrounded by a "palisade" of histiocytes (macrophages) and chronic inflammatory cells (lymphocytes and plasma cells). Caseous necrosis is typical of tuberculous granulomas and deep mycoses. The lesion depicted in Figure 21–7 has none of the features of an abscess or fat necrosis.

▶ Final Diagnosis and Synopsis of the Case

• Active Rheumatoid Arthritis

This was a case of a 60-year-old woman with active rheumatoid arthritis (RA). The manifestation of RA began in her wrist and hand one year before her current presentation. Symmetrical joint pain, swelling, and morning stiffness are the typical complaints of rheumatoid arthritis patients. The x-ray findings, synovial fluid analysis, and presence of rheumatoid nodules, combined with the typical clinical presentation and elevated serum rheumatoid factor (RF), confirmed the diagnosis of rheumatoid arthritis. Thrombocytosis, mild normocytic anemia, and elevated ESR are typically seen in the active stage. This case demonstrates most of the typical clinical and laboratory findings in rheumatoid arthritis.

LAB TIPS

Synovial Fluid Analysis

Arthrocentesis is the aspiration of synovial fluid by the insertion of a sterile needle into a joint space (eg, knee, shoulder, elbow, etc) under strictly sterile conditions. Though it may differ with the joint, the amount of synovial fluid normally present is not large, and ranges between 0.1–3.5 mL. Unless an effusion is present, the aspiration will yield little material. The fluid is collected with a sterile needle and plastic syringe and placed into sterile heparinized (sodium heparin) tubes for microbiological examination, microscopy, and chemical studies. Other anticoagulants, such as potassium oxalate, ethylene diamine tetracetic acid (EDTA), and lithium heparin, may cause artifacts during the microscopic analysis and should be avoided in this procedure.

The examination of synovial fluid for the presence or absence of organisms and crystals is the most important part of the analysis. When limited in fluid amount or by available resources, these determinations should be given priority. When fluid is abundant, a full analysis can be performed and would include:

1. gross examination for viscosity, color, and appearance

2. microscopical examination to determine the total number of cells present, the type of cells, and the presence and type of crystals

3. chemical analyses such as a mucin clot test, synovial fluid glucose and protein determinations, and immunologic studies (rheumatoid factor, antinuclear antibodies, complement, etc)

4. microbiologic studies, including a Gram stain and appropriate cultures.

It must be remembered that except for the presence of specific crystals or organisms, most of the synovial fluid findings are nonspecific and can be found in a number of disease entities. In addition, several processes may be occurring in the same joint simultaneously (eg, gout and rheumatoid arthritis, septic arthritis, and rheumatoid arthritis, etc).

(Continued)

NOTES

Lab Tips (continued)

SELECTED SYNOVIAL FLUID FINDINGS IN VARIOUS CONDITIONS

Condition	Color/Clarity	Viscosity
Normal	Yellow/clear	High
Osteoarthritis	Yellow/clear	High
Traumatic arthritis	Yellow to bloody/ clear to cloudy	High
SLE	Yellow/clear to slightly cloudy	Decreased
Rheumatoid arthritis	Yellow/cloudy	Low
Gout (acute attack)	Yellow/cloudy	Low
Pseudogout	Yellow/clear to slightly cloudy	Low
Bacterial arthritis, acute	Yellow to bloody/cloudy to purulent	Low
Tuberculous arthritis	Yellow/cloudy	Low

Condition	Total WBCs (% Neut)
Normal	0–200/μL (0–25)
Osteoarthritis	200–2000/μL (0–25)
Traumatic arthritis	200–5000/μL (0–50[a])
SLE	2000–5000/μL (25–50)
Rheumatoid arthritis	5000–50,000/μL (50–90)
Gout (acute attack)	5000–50,000 μL (50–90)
Pseudogout	5000–50,000/μL (35–85)
Bacterial arthritis, acute	>50,000/μL (90–100)
Tuberculous arthritis	2000–100,000/μL (30–90)

Condition	Formed Elements	Mucin Clot
Normal	None	Good
Osteoarthritis	Collagen fibrils[b] Cartilage fragments[b]	Good
Traumatic arthritis	Many RBCs[a]	Good
SLE	LE cells	Good to fair
Rheumatoid arthritis	Cholesterol crystals (occasionally)	Fair to poor
Gout (acute attack)	Urate crystals[c]	Fair to poor
Pseudogout	Calcium pyrophosphate crystals[c]	Fair to poor
Bacterial arthritis, acute	Bacteria usually present on gram stain[d]	Poor
Tuberculous arthritis	Gram stain—20% positive Cultures—80–90% positive	Poor

[a]Leukocytes and RBC usually low in traumatic arthritis unless hemorrhage is present.
[b]Best seen with phase microscopy.
[c]Easily identified and differentiated with polarized light microscopy utilizing a first-order red plate.
[d]Gram stains of synovial fluid in septic arthritides are positive in 70 to 95% of Gram-positive infections and in about 30 to 50% of Gram negative infections.

▶ **Clinical History and Presentation**

A 28-year-old woman, known to be positive for human immunodeficiency virus (HIV) for 6 years, was admitted to the hospital because of jaundice and a fever of 102° F. She had contracted HIV from a boyfriend, who had died of AIDS eight years previously, and her HIV positivity was discovered incidentally during a mortgage insurance physical examination. She was married, though her husband refused to be tested for HIV. Her clinical course had been protracted and managed on an outpatient basis. She had been treated with an anti-retroviral agent, which she tolerated poorly. She had developed a progressive wasting syndrome and anemia, and had suffered one episode of prolonged fever, which was treated with antibiotics. Her most recent problem had been progressive liver failure with elevated liver enzymes and jaundice, which within the previous five days had been accompanied by fever. Physical examination revealed a cachectic female, fully oriented. Her blood pressure was 100/40 mmHg, heart rate was 88 per minute and regular; temperature was 101.8° F. Her skin and sclerae were icteric, and there was no lymphadenopathy. Her chest was clear. She had a protuberant abdomen with ascites. The liver and spleen were markedly enlarged. The lower extremities were edematous.

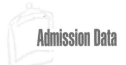

Admission Data

TABLE 22–1. HEMATOLOGY		
WBC	3.09 thousand/μL	(3.3–11.0)
Neut	56%	(44–88)
Band	37%	(0–10)
Lymph	3%	(12–43)
Mono	2%	(2–11)
Eos	1%	(0–5)
Baso	1%	(0–2)
RBC	3.04 million/μL	(3.9–5.0)
Hgb	8 g/dL	(11.6–15.6)
HCT	26.4%	(37.0–47.0)
MCV	86.7 fL	(79.0–99.0)
MCH	26.4 pg	(26.0–32.6)
MCHC	30.4 g/dL	(31.0–36.0)
Plts	55 thousand/μL	(130–400)

TABLE 22–2. CHEMISTRY		
Glucose	100 mg/dL	(65–110)
Creatinine	0.7 mg/dL	(0.7–1.4)
BUN	12 mg/dL	(7–24)
Uric acid	3.5 mg/dL	(3.0–7.5)
Cholesterol	145 mg/dL	(150–240)
Calcium	7.6 mg/dL	(8.5–10.5)
Protein	4 g/dL	(6–8)
Albumin	2 g/dL	(3.7–5.0)
LDH	223 U/L	(100–250)
Alk Phos	1620 U/L	(0–120)
AST	75 U/L	(0–55)
GGTP	862 U/L	(0–50)
Bilirubin	8.8 mg/dL	(0.0–1.5)
Bilirubin, direct	5.67 mg/dL	(0.02–0.18)
Amylase	12 U/L	(23–85)

NOTES

TABLE 22–3. URINALYSIS

pH	6	(5.0–7.5)
Protein	Neg	(Neg)
Glucose	Neg	(Neg)
Ketone	Neg	(Neg)
Bile	Neg	(Neg)
Occult blood	1+	(Neg)
Color	Yellow	(Yellow)
Clarity	Clear	(Clear)
Sp.grav	1.004	(1.010–1.055)
WBC	1/HPF	(0–5)
RBC	0/HPF	(0–2)
Epith. cell	0/HPF	(0)
Bacteria	0	(0)
Urobilinogen	Neg	(Neg)
Bilirubin	2+	(Neg)

TABLE 22–4. COAGULATION

PT	15 sec	(11–14)
aPTT	34 sec	(19–28)

TABLE 22–5. ELECTROLYTES

Na	134 mEq/L	(134–143)
K	3.5 mEq/L	(3.5–4.9)
Cl	95 mEq/L	(95–108)
CO_2	24 mEq/L	(21–32)

TABLE 22–6. SEROLOGY

HBc Ab IgM	Neg
HBs Ag	Neg
HBs Ab	Pos
HC Ab	Neg
HA Ab	Neg

TABLE 22–7. MICROBIOLOGY

Blood cultures: pending
Urine cultures: pending

TABLE 22–8. T LYMPHOCYTE SUBSETS

	Patient	Normal
Percent T Lymphocytes		
CD3+	63%	68 ± 7%
CD3+/CD4+	1%	45 ± 7%
CD3+/CD8+	59%	27 ± 6%
T Lymphocytes Absolute Count		
CD3+	58 cell/μL	1554 ± 355
CD3+/CD4+	1 cell/μL	1026 ± 233
CD3+/CD8+	55 cell/μL	621 ± 192

► Questions

On the basis of the preceding information, you can best conclude the following:

1. This patient:
   a. is considered to be in the early, acute, phase of HIV infection
   b. is considered to be in the chronic, middle phase of HIV infection
   c. this patient has developed AIDS
   d. none of the above statements about this patient is correct

2. Which of the following cytopenias is most likely to occur at the early, asymptomatic stage of HIV infection?
   a. thrombocytopenia
   b. neutropenia
   c. T cell lymphopenia
   d. B cell lymphopenia
   e. anemia

3. This patient's cytopenia could be caused by:
   a. the effects of HIV infection
   b. anti-retroviral chemotherapy
   c. a so far undiagnosed secondary neoplasm
   d. opportunistic infections
   e. all of the above

4. The damage to the liver of this patient could have been induced by:
   a. chemotherapy
   b. infection with *Mycobacterium avium intracellulare* (MAI)
   c. cytomegalovirus (CMV) infection
   d. all of the above

5. Identify the INCORRECT statement about this patient:
   a. her hypocalcemia is associated with her low serum albumin level
   b. low serum albumin and hypoproteinemia could result from a decreased synthesis in the liver
   c. her hyperbilirubinemia is caused predominantly by hemolysis
   d. her prolonged PT and aPTT reflect hepatocellular damage or the presence of biliary obstruction
   e. portal hypertension should be considered in this patient

6. The hepatitis serology profile suggests all of the following EXCEPT:
   a. the patient may have been vaccinated against hepatitis B earlier in her life
   b. the patient's current liver condition is not due to acute hepatitis B infection
   c. the patient is not a chronic carrier for hepatitis B virus
   d. the patient is most likely highly infectious for hepatitis B virus
   e. the patient does not have acute hepatitis A

▶ Clinical Course

The patient was treated empirically for cytomegalovirus (CMV) and *Mycobacterium avium intracellulare* (MAI) hepatitis. She was also treated with diuretics and salt-poor albumin for her ascites. Her condition did not improve. The patient's liver function continued to deteriorate and she developed an electrolyte imbalance, which needed correction (Table 22–9). Her cytopenia worsened (Table 22–10), and she required transfusion of several units of packed red blood cells. Blood and urine cultures were negative. One week after admission, the patient developed oral and esophageal lesions, for which specific treatment was begun. The extremely grim prognosis at this stage of the disease was discussed with the patient and her family. The patient wished to go home. She expired at home two days later. An antemortem stool culture was positive for the organism seen in Figure 22–2. An autopsy was performed, and selected findings can be seen in Figures 22–1, 22–2, 22–3, 22–4, 22–5, and 22–6.

TABLE 22–9. LABORATORY DATA

	Reference	Day 2	Day 4	Day 5
Chemistry				
Glucose	56–110 mg/dL	93	89	86
BUN	7–24 mg/dL	13	15	14
Creatinine	0.7–1.4 mg/dL	0.6	0.8	0.9
Uric acid	3.0–7.5 mg/dL	3	3	2.7
Cholesterol	150–240 mg/dL	117	151	130
Calcium	8.5–10.5 mg/dL	7.3	5.8	5.8
Protein	6–8 g/dL	3.5	3.5	3.2
Albumin	3.7–5.0 g/dL	1.8	1.9	1.7
LDH	100–225 U/L	222	370	319
Alk Phos.	30–120 U/L	1255	1740	1154
AST	0–55 U/L	63	65	41
GGTP	0–50 U/L	797	1023	807
Bilirubin	0.0–1.5 mg/dL	12.6	15.6	15.8
Bilirubin, direct	0.02–0.18 mg/dL	9.57	11.2	11.6
Electrolytes				
Na	134–143 mEq/L	134	139	137
K	3.5–4.9 mEq/L	3.1	2.2	3.3
Cl	95–108 mEq/L	95	100	100
CO_2	21–32 mEq/L	24	23	21

TABLE 22–10. HEMATOLOGY

	Reference	Day 5
WBC	4.5–11.0 thousand/μL	2.59
Neut	44–88%	75
Band	0–10%	15
Lymph	12–43%	1.2
Mono	2–11%	7.8
Eos	0–5%	1
Baso	0–2%	1
RBC	3.9–5.0 million/μL	2.76
Hgb	12.0–15.0 g/dL	7.2
HCT	36–44%	24.4
Plts	150–400 thousand/μL	105

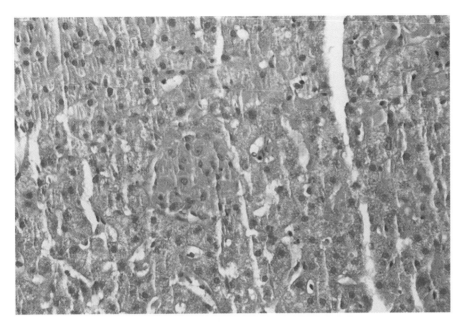

FIGURE 22–1. Patient's liver. Hematoxylin–eosin stain. Original magnification ×120.

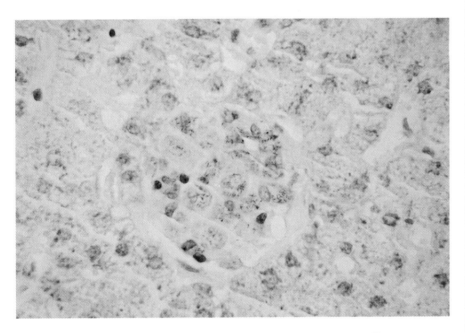

FIGURE 22–2. Patient's liver. Acid-fast stain. Original magnification ×160.

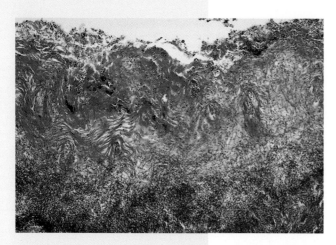

FIGURE 22–3. Portion of patient's esophagus. Hematoxylin–eosin stain. Original magnification ×31.

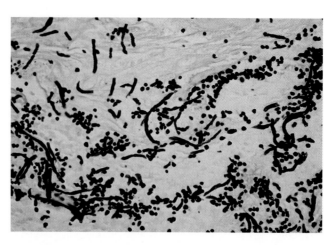

FIGURE 22–4. Portion of patient's esophagus. Gomori's methenamine silver stain. Original magnification ×100.

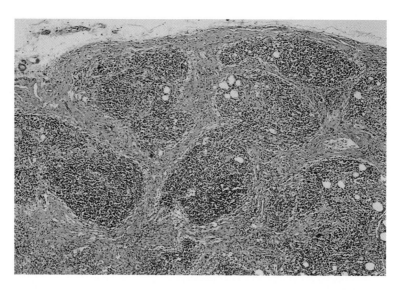

FIGURE 22–5. Patient's lymph node. Hematoxylin–eosin stain. Original magnification ×31.

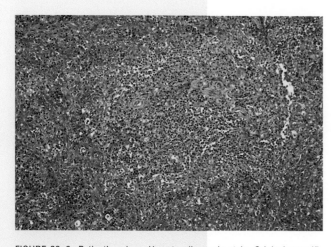

FIGURE 22–6. Patient's spleen. Hematoxylin–eosin stain. Original magnification ×31.

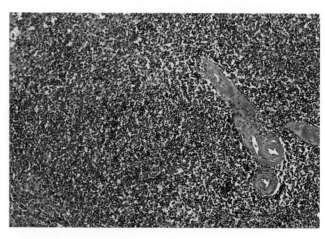

FIGURE 22–7. Normal spleen. Hematoxylin–eosin stain. Original magnification ×31.

▷ Questions

7. The most likely cause of hypokalemia in this patient was:
   a. diuretic treatment
   b. an increased serum level of conjugated bilirubin
   c. intravascular hemolysis
   d. fever
   e. blood transfusion

8. The organisms depicted in Figure 22–2 are:
   a. streptococci
   b. *Neisseria gonorrheae*
   c. staphylococci
   d. candida
   e. mycobacteria

9. The section of the liver (Figure 22–1) shows which of the following?
   a. multiple abscesses
   b. a granuloma
   c. cholestasis
   d. fatty change

10. The lesion depicted in Figures 22–3 and 22–4:
    a. may appear in HIV-infected, asymptomatic patients
    b. may cause dysphagia
    c. indicates a defect in cell mediated immunity
    d. is often coexistent in mouth and esophagus
    e. all of the above statements are correct

11. The section of the lymph node (Figure 22–5) shows all of the following EXCEPT:
    a. generalized atrophy
    b. partially hyalinized germinal centers
    c. depletion of lymphocytes in mantle zone
    d. marked follicular hyperplasia

12. In the terminal stages of this patient's disease, all of the following can be expected EXCEPT:
    a. a higher level of viremia than that seen in the middle, chronic phase of the disease
    b. lower numbers of CD4+ cells in the peripheral blood than those seen in the middle, chronic phase of the disease
    c. a negative tuberculin test
    d. increased activity of natural killer cells
    e. serious opportunistic infections

NOTES

▶ Figure Descriptions

Figure 22–1. Patient's liver. Hematoxylin–eosin stain. Original magnification ×120.

A poorly defined granuloma composed of epithelioid histiocytes is present in the center of the photomicrograph. There are no other significant histologic changes.

Figure 22–2. Patient's liver. Acid-fast stain. Original magnification ×160.

The granuloma seen in Figure 22–1 shows numerous filamentous, acid-fast organisms consistent with *Mycobacterium avium intracellulare*.

Figure 22–3. Portion of esophagus from patient. Hematoxylin–eosin stain. Original magnification ×31.

At autopsy, large areas of the esophagus were covered by an adherent, grey-white membrane. This photomicrograph of one of these areas shows numerous fungal organisms as a bluish wavy band across the bottom of the image. Inflammatory cells, necrotic debris, and several collections of bacteria are present towards the lumen, at the top of image.

Figure 22–4. Portion of esophagus from patient. Gomori's methenamine silver stain. Original magnification ×100.

When the membrane is stained for fungi, numerous yeast and pseudohyphal forms are present consistent with a *Candida* species.

Figure 22–5. Lymph node from patient. Hematoxylin–eosin stain. Original magnification ×12.

As AIDS progresses, striking changes take place in the lymph nodes, as shown in this patient. This lymph node is atrophic, with marked depletion of lymphocytes in both the mantle zone and the germinal centers, which are small and show areas of hyalinization. Viewing this lymph node demonstrates why this patient produced a poor inflammatory response to her infections.

Figure 22–6. Spleen from patient. Hematoxylin–eosin stain. Original magnification ×31.

Lymphoid depletion of the spleen was severe, as this photomicrograph of the white pulp illustrates. Note the difficulty in identifying this as white pulp.

Figure 22–7. Normal spleen. Hematoxylin–eosin stain. Original magnification ×31.

The white pulp contains numerous lymphocytes and is clearly delineated from the surrounding red pulp.

▶ **Answers**

1. (**c**) This patient has AIDS. Current guidelines of the Center for Disease Control (CDC) state that any HIV-infected person with fewer than 14% of CD4+ cells in the peripheral blood and/or fewer than 200 of CD4+ cells/μL is considered to have AIDS. The "acute phase" of HIV infection follows 3–6 weeks after initial infection, usually presents with nonspecific symptoms (fever, rash, myalgia, etc) and usually resolves spontaneously. The "middle phase" is a period of clinical latency, during which patients are asymptomatic and present with mild constitutional symptoms and lymphadenopathy. The last, or "crisis" stage, which is AIDS, occurs due to a breakdown of immune defenses, and is characterized by fever, loss of weight, diarrhea, and the appearance of opportunistic infections and secondary neoplasms. The CD4+ percentage and absolute count are decreased.

2. (**a**) Thrombocytopenia is known to be one of the presenting laboratory findings in the early stage of HIV infection in otherwise asymptomatic individuals. All other cytopenias tend to occur with the deterioration of the immune function in the late stage of HIV infection, or in AIDS.

3. (**e**) Cytopenia in HIV infection and AIDS can be due to multiple etiologies and/or their combinations. HIV infection, opportunistic infections, chemotherapy, and secondary neoplasms are considered major factors in the etiology of cytopenia.

4. (**d**) Chemotherapy (AZT-Zidovudine) is known to cause hepatic transaminase elevation. *Mycobacterium avium intracellulare* (MAI) and cytomegalovirus (CMV) are known to cause hepatitis. All of these factors have been considered in the work-up of this patient.

5. (**c**) The hyperbilirubinemia in this patient was predominantly of conjugated type, due to impaired hepatic excretion of conjugated bilirubin. Hemolytic anemia leads to excess production of unconjugated bilirubin. This patient's hypocalcemia was most likely associated with her hypoalbuminemia. About 50% of the blood calcium is ionized, and the rest is protein-bound. A decrease in serum albumin level will result in a decrease of the total serum calcium (0.8 mg of calcium is bound to 1.0 g of albumin). A low serum albumin and protein in this patient were likely to have been caused by a decrease in their production by the liver, owing to hepatic parenchymal cell damage, and also by malnutrition. Prolonged PT and aPTT in patients with hepatic failure result from reduced synthesis and secretion of clotting factors, and from the malabsorption of vitamin K. Ascites and splenomegaly are common in patients with portal hypertension.

6. (**d**) The presence of HBs Ab, as the only positive marker, suggests that the patient may have been immunized, was in the convalescent phase, or had recovered from hepatitis B infection. It indicates the absence of infectivity. HBs Ab persists for many years, or for life, in the great majority of patients. The presence of HBs Ab excludes the acute phase of hepatitis B infection, since it does not rise until the acute phase is over, and after the disappearance of HBs Ag. The absence of HBs Ag excludes the carrier status for hepatitis B virus.

7. (**a**) Hypokalemia in this patient appeared after diuretic treatment was started. Furosemide (a loop diuretic) was one of the diuretics used. It is known to lead to potassium loss. The serum level of conjugated bilirubin does not affect the level of serum potassium; intravascular hemolysis and blood transfusion would more likely be associated with hyperkalemia. Fever, if accompanied by sweating, could contribute to the hypokalemia.

8. (**e**) Figure 22–2 shows macrophages filled with acid-fast bacilli. Macrophages phagocytosed these bacilli, but were unable to kill them. The depletion of T lymphocytes leads to the lack of a cell-mediated immune response, which is necessary to activate macrophages. *Mycobacterium* is a bacillus, therefore it is morphologically distinct from cocci (*Streptococcus, Staphylococcus,* and *Neisseria*). Candida could be seen in tissue sections or cytological preparations as a yeast (round or oval cells reproducing by budding), or as pseudo-hyphae.

9. (**b**) The section of the liver (Figure 22–1) shows a poorly defined granuloma. Cholestasis, fatty change, and abscesses are not present.

10. (**e**) The lesion is esophageal candidiasis. It often coexists in the mouth and esophagus and causes dysphagia. It may occur in asymptomatic HIV infected patients, and its presence signifies worsening of the patient's immune competence. It should be treated.

11. (**d**) The section of the lymph node (Figure 22–5) shows generalized atrophy with poorly developed germinal centers, some of which show areas of hyalinization. Lymphocyte depletion is prominent in the mantle zone.

12. (**d**) With the progression of the disease, there is an accelerated loss of CD4+ cells infected with HIV and an increased spill-over of HIV into the plasma. The tuberculin test in HIV-positive patients infected with mycobacteria would be most likely negative, owing to the defective function and the low number of T lymphocytes. The activity of natural killer cells is severely decreased; this could contribute to the appearance of certain malignant tumors. The profound immunosuppression at this stage of HIV infection leads to opportunistic infections.

▷ Final Diagnosis and Synopsis of the Case

- AIDS
- Liver Failure
- *Mycobacterium Avium Intracellulare* infection
- Esophageal Candidiasis

A 28-year-old woman who was HIV-positive presented with a wasting syndrome, fever, and progressively deteriorating liver function of unknown etiology. She had pancytopenia and virtually no CD4 positive T lymphocytes. Routine cultures were negative; she had ascites, hepatosplenomegaly, edema of the legs, and was icteric. The most likely causes of her liver failure were anti-retroviral chemotherapy, infection with *Mycobacterium avium intracellulare* (MAI), and cytomegalovirus (CMV) infection. The hepatitis virus serology was positive only for HBs Ab. She was admitted for the treatment of liver failure, which included treatment for CMV and MAI infection. The patient received diuretics and low-salt albumin for her ascites, and required packed red blood cell transfusion. She developed hypocalcemia (most likely associated with her hypoalbuminemia), and hypokalemia (most likely a consequence of her diuretic therapy). Her cytopenia deteriorated further, and she had virtually no lymphocytes. She developed thrush and *Candida esophagitis,* which required treatment. She remained febrile and her condition deteriorated rapidly. She was discharged at her wish and expired two days later at home. Stool culture grew *Mycobacterium avium intracellulare* (MAI). Autopsy revealed a cirrhotic liver, congested splenomegaly, and esophageal varices due to portal hypertension.

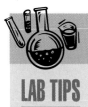

LAB TIPS

NONSEROLOGIC METHODS FOR THE DETECTION OF CYTOMEGALOVIRUS

Method	Advantages	Disadvantages
Identification in tissue sections by light microscopy	Relatively rapid; intranuclear and intracytoplasmic forms fairly easy to locate	Presumptive identification; requires tissue biopsy
Isolation of virus by cell culture and observation of cytopathic effect	Identification can be made within days (50% of total positive cases of CMV detected in 10 days); virus availale for further study; 100% specificity, high sensitivity	Presumptive identification; confirmation of a specific virus requires an immunologic method; faster methods now available; specimen collection requirements strict; cell culture laboratory must be available
Shell vial centrifugation followed by viral antigen staining with monoclonal antibodies	Rapid detection of virus (with CMV 50% of total positives detected in 1 day, 90% in 2 days)	Specimen collection requirements strict; cell culture laboratory must be available
Viral antigen staining on patient specimen using immunofluorescence assay, enzyme immuno-assay, or radioimmuno-assay	Results may be available within hours; assays can be arranged to detect antiviral antibody; specimen collection requirements less strict; cell culture laboratory not necessary	Test is less specific and may be less sensitive than viral isolation; patient specimens must contain sufficient numbers of infected cells
Electron microscopy	With CMV, it may be used to detect the virus in brain tissue; viral particles can be detected within hours	Procedure expensive; not generally available

A 60-Year-Old
Woman With
Fever and
Epistaxis

▷ Clinical History and Presentation

A 60-year-old woman was admitted to the hospital with a fever of 102° F of two days' duration and reported multiple episodes of nasal bleeding over the previous week. She also stated that she had noted multiple bluish areas over her knees and elbows. Over the previous few months, she had felt tired and unable to perform her normal household work. Her past medical history was unremarkable. Physical examination revealed a thin, pale female in no acute distress. Blood pressure was 120/85 mmHg, heart rate was 90 per minute and regular, and temperature was 102° F. The chest was clear. Abdominal examination revealed an enlarged spleen, but no other remarkable findings. Multiple areas of ecchymoses and petechiae were seen over the chest, abdomen, knees, and elbows. There was no lymphadenopathy.

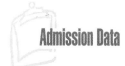

Admission Data

TABLE 23–1. HEMATOLOGY		
WBC	56.2 thousand/μL	(3.3–11.0)
Neut	2%	(44–88)
Band	1%	(0–10)
Lymph	4%	(12–43)
Mono	0%	(2–11)
Eos	0%	(0–5)
Baso	0%	(0–2)
Myelocyte	1%	(00)
Promyelocyte	2%	(00)
Blasts	84%	(00)
RBC	2.33 million/μL	(3.9–5.0)
Hgb	6.9 g/dL	(11.6–15.6)
HCT	20.5	(37.0–47.0)
MCV	87.7 fL	(79.0–99.0)
MCH	29.4 pg	(26.0–32.6)
MCHC	33.5 g/dL	(31.0–36.0)
Plts	41 thousand/μL	(130–400)

TABLE 23–2. CHEMISTRY

Glucose	107 mg/dL	(65–110)
Creatinine	0.8 mg/dL	(0.7–1.4)
BUN	10 mg/dL	(7–24)
Uric acid	8.1 mg/dL	(3.0–7.5)
Cholesterol	112 mg/dL	(150–240)
Calcium	8.6 mg/dL	(8.5–10.5)
Protein	6.0 g/dL	(6–8)
Albumin	3.1 g/dL	(3.7–5.0)
LDH	559 U/L	(100–250)
Alk Phos	116 U/L	(0–120)
AST	30 U/L	(0–55)
GGTP	50 U/L	(0–50)
Bilirubin	0.6 mg/dL	(0.0–1.5)
Bilirubin, direct	0.19 mg/dL	(0.02–0.18)

TABLE 23–3. URINALYSIS

Within normal range

TABLE 23–4. MICROBIOLOGY

Blood culture: pending

TABLE 23–5. COAGULATION

PT	13.5 sec	(11–14)
aPTT	25 sec	(19–28)

TABLE 23–6. ELECTROLYTES

Na	140 mEq/L	(134–143)
K	4.7 mEq/L	(3.5–4.9)
Cl	103 mEq/L	(95–108)
CO_2	25 mEq/L	(21–32)

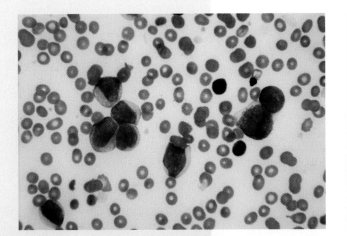

FIGURE 23–1. Admission peripheral blood smear. Wright/Giemsa stain. Original magnification ×197.

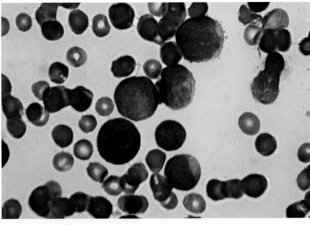

FIGURE 23–2. Admission peripheral blood smear. Wright/Giemsa stain. Original magnification ×315.

▶ **Questions**

On the basis of the preceding information, you can best conclude the following:

1. This patient's clinical presentation and laboratory findings suggest the presence of:
   a. an acute inflammatory disorder
   b. a genetically determined metabolic disorder
   c. a chronic inflammatory disorder
   d. a neoplastic disorder
   e. none of the above

2. This patient's peripheral blood smear (Figures 23–1 and 23–2) and CBC are most consistent with:
   a. acute lymphoblastic leukemia
   b. a megaloblastic anemia
   c. chronic lymphocytic leukemia
   d. leukemoid reaction
   e. none of the above

3. The elevated uric acid in this patient is most likely due to:
   a. acute renal failure
   b. high protein diet
   c. accelerated nucleic acid turnover
   d. deficiency of hypoxanthine guanine phosphoribosyl transferase (HGPRT)
   e. none of the above

4. The multiple ecchymoses and petechiae in this patient are most probably due to
   a. thrombocytopenia
   b. the presence of antibodies against a specific coagulation factor
   c. qualitative platelet abnormalities
   d. all of the above
   e. none of the above

5. The elevated serum level of lactate dehydrogenase (LDH) in this patient is most likely associated with:
   a. damage to the liver
   b. underlying hematological problem
   c. renal failure
   d. none of the above

NOTES

▶ Clinical Course

The patient was transfused with ten units of random donor platelets. Bone marrow biopsy was performed and submitted for histological, cytogenetic, and flow cytometric examination. Blood cultures were negative for any bacterial growth after 5 days. The patient was started on the appropriate therapy.

TABLE 23–7. FLOW CYTOMETRIC ANALYSIS OF THE BONE MARROW[a]

Cluster Designation	Percent Positive
CD45 (pan–leukocyte antigen)	95
CD14 (monocytes)	0.4
CD2 (T lymphocytes)	8
CD4 (T cell helper)	4
CD3 (T cell receptor)	6
CD8 (T cell suppressor)	2
CD19 (B lymphocytes)	2
CD10 (pre–B lymphocytes)	0.1
Surface immunoglobulin (mature B cells)	2
Kappa light chain (mature B cells)	1.4
Lambda light chain (mature B cells)	0.6
HLA-DR (B cell, macrophages, activated T cell)	91
CD13 (myelomonocytic antigen)	45
CD33 (myelomonocytic antigen)	92
CD34 (stem cell)	90

[a]One cell cluster is identified.

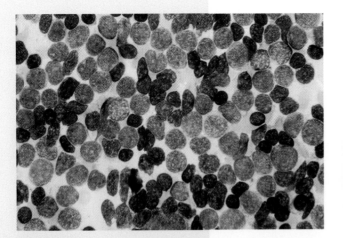

FIGURE 23–3. Bone marrow aspirate from this patient. Wright/Giemsa stain. Original magnification ×197.

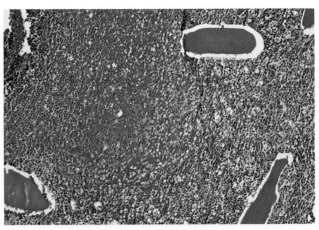

FIGURE 23–4. Bone marrow biopsy. Hematoxylin–eosin stain. Original magnification ×78

▶ **Questions**

6. This patient's bone marrow:
   a. is hypocellular
   b. shows multiple granulomas
   c. is hypercellular
   d. shows a normal myeloid to erythroid ratio

7. The cells seen in Figures 23–3 and 23–4 are most likely negative for:
   a. myeloperoxidase stain
   b. Sudan Black stain
   c. non specific esterase
   d. TdT (terminal deoxynucleotidyl transferase)
   e. CD13 antigen

8. The occurrence of the disease process manifested in this patient has been associated with:
   a. chronic myelogenous leukemia
   b. refractory anemia with excess blasts
   c. myelodysplastic syndromes
   d. agnogenic myeloid metaplasia
   e. all of the above

9. Flow cytometric analysis of this patient's bone marrow shows all of the following EXCEPT:
   a. a normal CD4/CD8 ratio
   b. a decreased proportion of B lymphocytes
   c. a decreased proportion of cells of myeloid origin
   d. a significant increase in the proportion of stem cells
   e. that all B lymphocytes are mature

10. The LEAST likely chromosomal abnormality expected in this case is:
    a. t(9;22)
    b. t(8;21)
    c. monosomy 5
    d. monosomy 7
    e. del 13q14

▶ **Figure Descriptions**

Figure 23–1. Admission peripheral blood smear. Wright/Giemsa stain. Original magnification ×197.

Several cells with the features of myeloblasts are present in this photomicrograph, and are representative of the majority of white blood cells seen in this patient's peripheral smear. Note the absence of cytoplasmic granules, and the prominent nucleoli and moderate amount of cytoplasm. The blasts seen in acute lymphoblastic leukemia are smaller, with much less cytoplasm, and indistinct nucleoli.

Figure 23–2. Admission peripheral blood smear. Wright/Giemsa stain. Original magnification ×315.

One of the cells near the center of the photomicrograph contains an Auer rod, which is a rod-shaped, reddish inclusion.

Figure 23–3. Bone marrow. Wright/Giemsa stain. Original magnification ×197.

This is an aspiration smear from the bone marrow. Almost all of the cells in the photomicrograph are similar in appearance to those seen in Figure 23–1 and have the morphologic features of myeloblasts. Definitive identification would require cytochemical staining.

Figure 23–4. Bone marrow. Hematoxylin–eosin stain. Original magnification ×78.

In the biopsy, the nature of the cells is harder to define. What can be noted is that the marrow is markedly hypercellular (absence of fat cells) and that the population of cells appears to be fairly uniform. It is apparent from the aspirate slide that the cells are myeloblasts. The normal heterogeneity of the bone marrow is not present.

▶ **Answers**

1. (**d**) This patient's presentation with fever, splenomegaly, thrombocytopenia, and an abnormal peripheral blood smear is consistent with acute myelogenous leukemia (AML), which is a neoplastic process. None of the other options (acute or chronic inflammatory disorders or genetically determined metabolic disorders) typically present with these clinical and laboratory features.

2. (**e**) The patient's CBC shows a significant increase in the WBC (leukocytosis). The majority of cells shown in Figures 23–1 and 23–2 are blasts, probably myeloblasts, owing to the presence of Auer rods (as demonstrated in Figure 23–2). One would not expect such a high number of blasts in a leukemoid reaction. The presence of a high number of myeloblasts in the peripheral blood suggests the diagnosis of AML. Further studies are needed to establish the class of AML (M1, M2, etc). There is no evidence to suggest the diagnosis of acute lymphoblastic leukemia (no lymphoblasts are present). The low number of mature lymphocytes and the presence of myeloblasts rule out chronic lymphocytic leukemia. There are no features of megaloblastic anemia in this smear.

3. (**c**) All the choices listed are associated with elevated uric acid. In a leukemic patient, an increase in uric acid is usually due to accelerated nucleic acid turnover, which will increase the production of free purine bases. In this patient, there are no signs or symptoms of acute renal failure and no evidence of consumption of a high protein diet. A

complete lack of hypoxanthine guanine phosphoribosyl transferase (HGPRT), as occurs in the x-linked Lesch-Nyhan syndrome, would lead to increased synthesis of purine nucleotides. Partial deficiency of hypoxanthine guanine phosphoribosyl transferase (HGPRT) is a very rare inborn error of metabolism. None of these other options are evident in this patient.

4. (a) The multiple ecchymoses and petechiae in this patient are probably due to thrombocytopenia (a platelet count of 41 thousand). There is no evidence of the presence of antibodies against a specific coagulation factor or qualitative platelet abnormalities, and these are not features of acute myelogenous leukemia.

5. (b) Over 95% of patients with acute myelogenous leukemia have an increased serum LDH. The liver and renal functions in this patient appear to be normal, therefore there is no reason to consider liver and renal diseases as the cause for elevated serum LDH level.

6. (c) This patient's bone marrow is hypercellular (almost 100% cellularity). In a section of normal bone marrow from a 60-year-old individual, 40% of its area would be occupied by hematopoietic cells and 60% by fat cells. The normal myeloid to erythroid ratio is about 2 to 1 or 3 to 1.

7. (d) The morphological diagnostic challenge in cases of acute leukemia is in distinguishing undifferentiated myeloblasts (M0, M1, M2) from lymphoblasts. Cytochemical stains such as myeloperoxidase and/or Sudan black are usually positive in M1, M2, and M3. In addition, blasts with monocytic differentiation (M4 and M5) are positive for non-specific esterase. On the other hand, TdT is negative in about 95% of AML blasts. The CD13 antigen is expressed primarily on the surface of cells of myelomonocytic origin.

8. (e) Factors associated with the development of acute myelogenous leukemia (AML) include radiation, myelotoxic agents (benzene compounds), chromosomal abnormalities, myelodysplastic syndromes, myeloproliferative syndromes, aplastic anemia, and paroxysmal nocturnal hemoglobinuria. Myelodysplastic syndromes include refractory anemia (RA), RA with ring sideroblasts, RA with excess blasts, and chronic myelomonocytic leukemia.

9. (c) Flow cytometric analysis shows one cell cluster. The vast majority of cells in this cluster express the early myeloid antigen CD33. These cells are also immature, since they express the hematopoietic stem cell (CD34) antigen. The proportions of T cells and B cells are decreased. T lymphocytes show a normal helper (CD4) to suppressor (CD8) ratio (2 to 1). All B lymphocytes are mature (ie, express surface immunoglobulin light chains).

10. (e) Deletion of 13q14 is seen in retinoblastomas, not in acute myelogenous leukemia (AML). The other chromosomal abnormalities are seen in a great proportion of AML cases: t(9;22) is mostly seen in the M1 class and carries a poor prognosis; t(8;21) is seen with M2 and indicates a good prognosis. Additional chromosomal abnormalities (not listed) observed in acute myelogenous leukemia (AML) are: t(5;17) in class M3; abnormalities in chromosome 16 and 11 observed with M4 and M5 respectively; and abnormalities in chromosome 5 and 7, variably seen in AML and especially in cases induced by environmental or occupational carcinogens.

NOTES

▶ Final Diagnosis and Synopsis of the Case

- Acute Myelogenous Leukemia (AML) Class M1
- Splenomegaly
- Increased Bleeding Tendency Due to Thrombocytopenia

A 60-year-old female presented with fever, fatigue, an increased bleeding tendency, and splenomegaly. Her CBC showed a significant thrombocytopenia and leukocytosis with a high percentage of blasts. The blasts on the peripheral blood smear were undifferentiated and some showed Auer rods (myeloblasts), consistent with the diagnosis of acute myelogenous leukemia without maturation (AML, M1). The patient's bleeding tendency due to her severe thrombocytopenia (platelet count of 41 thousand) and her anemia were primarily due to bone marrow replacement by undifferentiated myeloblasts. Her fever was associated with neutropenia. Flow cytometric analysis of this patient's bone marrow showed the presence of highly immature cells of myelomonocytic origin (CD33+, HLA-DR+, and partially CD13+), which also expressed the human progenitor cell antigen CD34.

LAB TIPS

The Classification of Acute Myeloblastic Leukemias (AML)

Acute leukemia in adults is usually myeloid in nature. Because it arises from a multipotential stem cell, a number of different morphologic expressions are possible. In 1976, the French-American-British (FAB) Co-operative Group proposed a classification system for the acute leukemias based on morphologic and cytochemical criteria (ie, special stains such as Sudan black B, myeloperoxidase, nonspecific esterase, alpha-naphthylbutyrate esterase, and NASD-acetate esterase) that allowed them to categorize a number of cases of acute leukemia. This scheme was recently modified to reflect both the degree of maturation and the predominant line of differentiation of the leukemic cells. It can be divided into two major categories: acute lymphocytic leukemia (ALL) and acute non-lymphocytic, or myeloblastic, leukemia (AML). The table below presents the classes of acute non-lymphocytic leukemia according to the modified FAB scheme.

CLASSIFICATION OF ACUTE MYELOBLASTIC LEUKEMIAS (AML)

Class	Incidence (% of AML)	Features
M1: Myeloblastic leukemia without maturation	20	Myeloblasts predominant ($\approx$90%); nongranular; few Auer rods. 15% of patients show t (9;22) (q34;q11) Philadelphia (Ph) chromosome.
M2: Myeloblastic leukemia with maturation	35	Myeloblasts can range up to 90% but other myeloid cells, including polymorphonuclear leukocytes may be present. 20% of patients show t (8;21) (q22;q11), -y.
M3: Acute hypergranular promyelocytic leukemia	7	Mainly promyelocytes with distinct granules and numerous Auer rods; frequently associated with disseminated intravascular coagulation (DIC); some patients show t (15;17) (q22;q21).
M3V: Acute hypogranular promyelocytic leukemia	3	Promyelocyte granules not prominent; nucleus shows cleft.
M4: Myelomonocytic leukemia	16	Both myelocytic and monocytic differentiation; blasts greater than 30%; monocytes and promonocytes range between 20–80%.
M4-Eo: Myelomonocytic leukemia with eosinophilia	4	Increased abnormal marrow eosinophils; patients show inv(16) (p13;q22), del(16) (q22).
M5A: Monocytic leukemia without maturation	6	Monoblasts more than 80%; high incidence of tissue infiltration.
M5B: Monocytic leukemia with maturation	4	Monocytes and promonocytes account for 80%.
M6: Erythroleukemia	4	Erythroblasts more than 50% of marrow cells and show abnormal features (ie megaloblastoid, giant forms); nonerythroid blasts also present.
M7: Megakaryocytic leukemia	3	Megakaryoblasts predominant; many patients show myelofibrosis.

A 53-Year-Old
Woman With a
Lump in the
Breast

► **Clinical History and Presentation**

A 53-year-old woman was found, on routine physical examination, to have a lump in her breast. Except for some anxiety caused by this finding, the patient had no special complaints. Physical examination revealed a well-nourished female in no great distress. A pertinent finding was a palpable lump about 1 cm in diameter in the lower outer quadrant of the left breast. The overlying skin was not attached, and there was no discharge from the nipple, or history of such a discharge. There were no palpable lymph nodes in the axilla. Examination of the other breast was unremarkable. A mammogram was performed, followed by fine needle aspiration. The patient tolerated these procedures well.

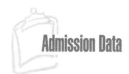 **Admission Data**

TABLE 24–1. HEMATOLOGY		
WBC	10.0 thousand/μL	(3.3–11.0)
Neut	83%	(44–88)
Band	0%	(0–10)
Lymph	10%	(12–43)
Mono	5%	(2–11)
Eos	1%	(0–5)
Baso	1%	(0–2)
RBC	4.37 million/μL	(3.9–5.0)
Hgb	12.4 g/dL	(11.6–15.6)
HCT	38.2%	(37.0–47.0)
MCV	87.5 fL	(79.0–99.0)
MCH	28.4 pg	(26.0–32.6)
MCHC	32.4 g/dL	(31.0–36.0)
Plts	247 thousand/μL	(130–400)

NOTES

TABLE 24–2. CHEMISTRY

Glucose	105 mg/dL	(65–110)
Creatinine	1.1 mg/dL	(0.7–1.4)
BUN	11 mg/dL	(7–24)
Uric acid	4 mg/dL	(3.0–7.5)
Cholesterol	200 mg/dL	(150–240)
Calcium	8.5 mg/dL	(8.5–10.5)
Protein	6.3 g/dL	(6–8)
Albumin	3.7 g/dL	(3.7–5.0)
LDH	179 U/L	(100–250)
Alk Phos	65 U/L	(0–120)
AST	22 U/L	(0–55)
GGTP	19 U/L	(0–50)
Bilirubin	0.4 mg/dL	(0.0–1.5)
Bilirubin, direct	0.13 mg/dL	(0.02–0.18)

TABLE 24–3. COAGULATION

PT	12 sec	(11–14)
aPTT	24 sec	(19–28)

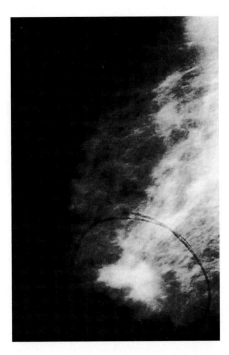 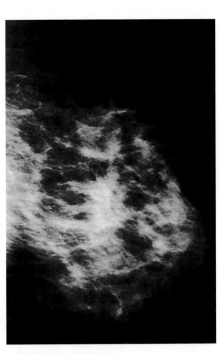

FIGURE 24–1. Mammograms of left and right breasts.

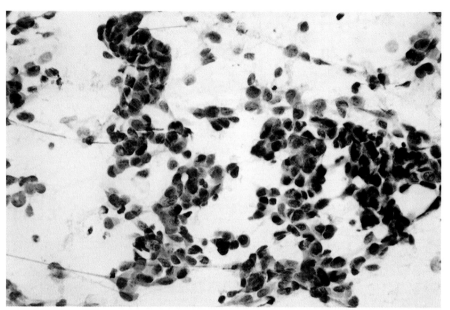

FIGURE 24–2. Left breast (fine needle aspiration). Papanicolaou stain. Original magnification ×78.

▶ Questions

On the basis of the preceding information, you can best conclude the following:

1. Figure 24–1 shows a radiographic density in the left breast. The approximate percentage of women with some irregular texture or density in the breast(s) on palpation or mammography is:
   a. more than 60%
   b. 40%
   c. 30%
   d. 20%

2. The cytologic appearance of the fine needle aspirate depicted in Figure 24–2:
   a. is insufficient for diagnosis
   b. shows evidence of cellulitis
   c. is diagnostic of carcinoma
   d. is diagnostic of fibroadenoma

3. Based on the cytological findings of Figure 24–2, you would recommend:
   a. re-examination in two months
   b. a repeated fine needle aspiration
   c. a surgical procedure with additional exploration
   d. antibiotic therapy

4. The most common site of lesions such as the one depicted in Figure 24–2 is:
   a. the lower outer quadrant
   b. the upper outer quadrant
   c. the subareolar area
   d. one of the inner quadrants

▶ Clinical Course

Following the fine needle aspiration, the patient was admitted to the hospital for surgery and exploration. The microscopic appearance of a section of breast tissue obtained at operation is shown in Figures 24–3, 24–4, and 24–5. The microscopic appearance of lymph node tissue obtained at the same time is shown in Figure 24–6. Two days after surgery, the patient was discharged to be followed on an out-patient basis. The additional tests done on the resected breast tissue are shown in Table 24–4 and Figures 24–7, 24–9, 24–10.

TABLE 24–4. SPECIAL TESTS	
c-erb-B2 oncogene amplification:	Negative

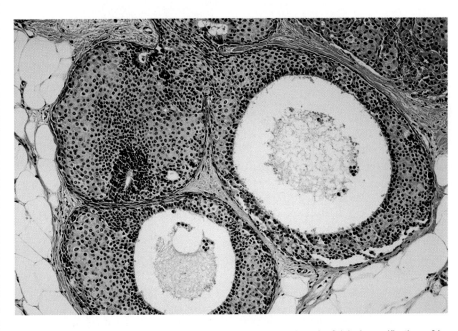

FIGURE 24–3. Left breast biopsy (frozen section). Hematoxylin–eosin stain. Original magnification ×31.

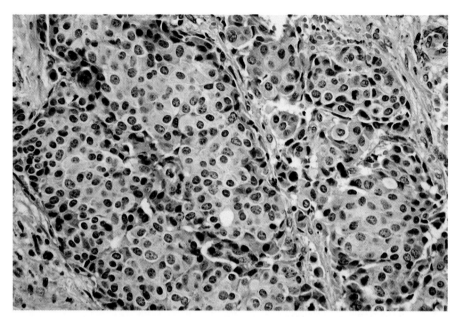

FIGURE 24–4. Left breast biopsy (frozen section). Hematoxylin–eosin stain. Original magnification ×78.

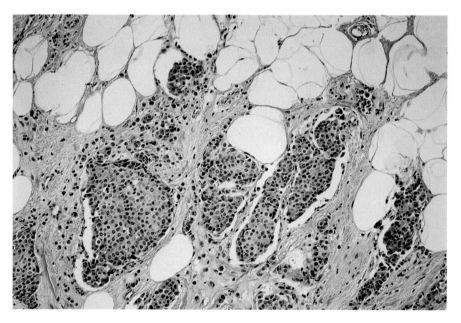

FIGURE 24–5. Left breast tissue. Hematoxylin–eosin stain. Original magnification ×31.

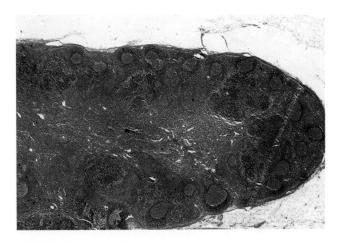

FIGURE 24–6. Lymph node from axillary dissection. Hematoxylin–eosin stain. Original magnification ×5.

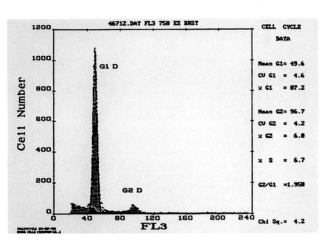

FIGURE 24–7. DNA ploidy/cell cycle analysis of patient.

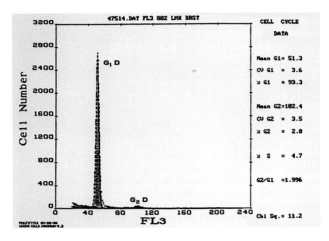

FIGURE 24–8. DNA ploidy/cell cycle analysis of normal breast.

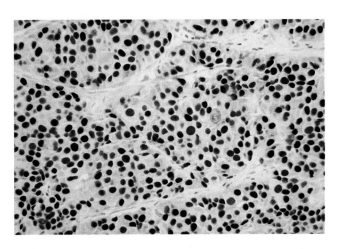

FIGURE 24–9. Left breast biopsy of patient. Immunoperoxidase stain for estrogen receptors. Original magnification ×78.

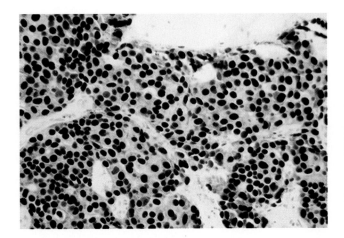

FIGURE 24–10. Left breast biopsy of patient. Immunoperoxidase stain for progesterone receptors. Original magnification ×78.

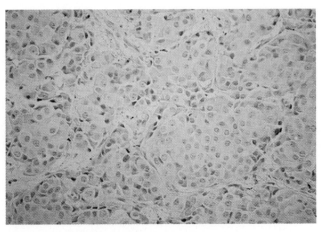

FIGURE 24–11. Negative control. Immunoperoxidase stain for estrogen receptors. Original magnification × 78.

▶ **Questions**

5. The lymph node section illustrated in Figure 24–6 shows:
   a. metastatic disease
   b. sinus histiocytosis
   c. mild follicular hyperplasia
   d. non-Hodgkin's follicular lymphoma
   e. multiple granulomas

6. Which of the data in Table 24–4 and Figures 24–6, 24–7, 24–9, and 24–10 is/are considered to be prognostically favorable?
   a. DNA ploidy status
   b. "S-phase" fraction value
   c. ER/PR positivity
   d. all of the above
   e. none of the above

7. The lesion shown in Figures 24–3, 24–4, and 24–5 is best described as:
   a. cystic change
   b. sclerosing adenosis
   c. invasive ductal carcinoma
   d. epithelial hyperplasia
   e. apocrine metaplasia

8. Among women with fibrocystic changes in the breast, the greatest risk of developing a breast cancer is seen among patients with:
   a. apocrine metaplasia
   b. fibrosis
   c. cystic changes
   d. sclerosing adenosis
   e. atypical ductal hyperplasia

9. The most important prognostic factor for patients with the disease depicted in Figures 24–3, 24–4, and 24–5 is:
   a. the DNA synthesis rate or the DNA ploidy status
   b. the estrogen receptor (ER) status of the tissue
   c. the progesterone receptor (PR) receptor status of the tissue
   d. the epidermal growth factor receptor (EGFR) status of the tissue
   e. the status of axillary lymph nodes

10. A predisposition to this patient's disease of the breast is associated with which of the following?
    a. the number of first degree relatives with the same disease
    b. the existence or history of the same disease in the contralateral breast
    c. the age at which a first child is born
    d. obesity
    e. all of the above

11. Which of the following genetic anomalies is considered likely to be useful in identifying women at risk for this patient's disease?
    a. amplification of the c-erb-B2 oncogene
    b. somatic mutation of the p53 tumor suppressor gene
    c. somatic mutation of the Rb (retinoblastoma) tumor suppressor gene
    d. inheritance of a mutation of the breast carcinoma 1 (BRCA1) tumor suppressor gene
    e. strong immunohistochemical staining for cathepsin D

NOTES

▶ Figure Descriptions

Figure 24–1. Mammograms of left and right breasts.

An irregular area of increased density is present in the lower outer quadrant of the left breast (left image). No microcalcifications are present. The right breast (right image) shows fibrocystic changes.

Figure 24–2. Left breast (fine needle aspiration). Papanicolaou stain. Original magnification ×78.

The aspiration smear shows increased cellularity with isolated tumor cells and various-sized cell clusters. The nuclei are enlarged, hyperchromatic, and have a coarse chromatin pattern. There is considerable variation in nuclear size. Cytoplasm is readily apparent. These cytologic features are sufficient for a diagnosis of carcinoma.

Figure 24–3. Left breast biopsy. Hematoxylin–eosin stain. Original magnification ×31.

This photomicrograph is from the tissue sent for frozen section analysis and shows several ducts containing tumor cells. Two of the ducts show central areas of necrosis (comedo pattern).

Figure 24–4. Left breast biopsy. Hematoxylin–eosin stain. Original magnification ×78.

The tumor cells are large, with relatively pale cytoplasm, enlarged, irregular nuclei, and focally prominent nucleoli. Mitotic figures are present.

Figure 24–5. Left breast biopsy. Hematoxylin–eosin stain. Original magnification ×31.

The edge of the tumor shows infiltration of the surrounding fatty breast tissue and lymphatics. Single cell invasion can also be identified in the fibrous stroma of the tumor. The histologic findings exhibited by Figures 24–2 through 24–5 define an intraductal and infiltrating duct carcinoma of the breast.

Figure 24–6. Lymph node from axillary dissection. Hematoxylin–eosin stain. Original magnification ×5.

This lymph node shows a mild follicular hyperplasia, but is negative for tumor, as were all the nodes retrieved in the resection.

Figure 24–7. DNA ploidy/Cell cycle analysis (patient).

The DNA histogram shows the presence of a diploid DNA peak only (G_1D). The G_2D population, however, is moderately increased, at 6.8% (reference range is <5.0%). The S phase fraction reflecting the proliferative activity of the cells is also slightly increased, at 6.7% (reference range is <6.0%). The absence of aneuploidy and of a high S phase fraction is known to correlate well with other favorable prognostic indicators. *See Chapters 9 and 10 for the explanation of the parameters in the DNA histograms.*

Figure 24–8. DNA ploidy/Cell cycle analysis (normal breast).

The histogram shows a diploid DNA peak and a small G_2D population (2.8 %), as well as a low S phase fraction (4.7%). *For the explanation of the parameters in the DNA histograms, see Chapters 9 and 10.*

Figure 24–9. Left breast biopsy. Immunoperoxidase stain for estrogen receptors. Original magnification ×78.

The patient's breast tumor was stained by the immunoperoxidase method using monoclonal antibodies for estrogen receptors and showed strong positivity.

Figure 24–10. Left breast biopsy. Immunoperoxidase stain for progesterone receptors. Original magnification ×78.

The tumor was positive for progesterone receptors using monoclonal antibodies for progesterone receptors.

Figure 24–11. Negative control. Immunoperoxidase stain for estrogen receptors. Original magnification ×78.

Breast tumor tissue (negative control) was stained by the immunoperoxidase method, using monoclonal antibodies for estrogen receptors. There is no evidence of nuclear staining.

▶ Answers

1. **(a)** In most cases, the radiographic densities in the breast reflect fibrocystic changes and do not necessarily indicate neoplasia, and would not lead to biopsy. The prevalence of irregular palpable breast texture or tissue density by mammography in women is very high, and is found in upwards of 60% of women.

2. **(c)** The fine needle aspirate shows cytologically malignant cells. The quality of the specimen is acceptable and sufficient for the identification of malignant cells. Cellulitis can be easily excluded by the absence of inflammatory cells. Fibroadenoma is a benign disease.

3. **(c)** Because of the malignant character of the aspirated cells, the only acceptable option is a surgical procedure with additional exploration. Waiting two months for a re-examination would only jeopardize the patient's prognosis. Repeated fine needle aspiration is unnecessary, since malignancy has already been established. Antibiotic therapy has no place in this patient's management, since the process is a malignant one and not of infectious etiology.

4. **(b)** About 50% of carcinomas of the breast arise in the upper outer quadrant, 20% in the central subareolar area, and 10% in each of the inner quadrants.

5. **(c)** This lymph node shows mild follicular hyperplasia and an essentially normal architecture. The sinusoids are not distended with the endothelial cells and prominent sinus histiocytes ("sinus histiocytosis") that are sometimes seen in axillary lymph nodes draining a breast carcinoma. The normal lymphoid architecture is intact and shows no evidence of metastatic disease or replacement by granulomas. The germinal centers are normal, with cuffs of small lymphocytes, and have not been replaced by the neoplastic nodules of non-Hodgkin's follicular lymphoma.

6. **(d)** The patient's diploid DNA status, low S-phase fraction, estrogen receptor (ER), and progesterone receptor (PR) positivity are all considered to be of favorable prognostic value. The tissue was also negative for the amplification of the c-erb-B2 oncogene, which is also a favorable prognostic factor.

7. (c) The lesion is characteristic of an intraductal and invasive ductal carcinoma, with cords of moderately hyperchromatic duct cells infiltrating the breast stroma. It goes beyond the pattern of epithelial ductular hyperplasia and exuberant fibrous tissue described as sclerosing adenosis, or the non-neoplastic proliferation of duct lining cells known as epithelial hyperplasia. There are no cysts.

8. (e) Fibrosis, apocrine metaplasia, and cystic changes carry no increased risk of breast carcinoma. Sclerosing adenosis is associated with a slightly increased risk of breast carcinoma. Atypical hyperplasia, whether of lobular or of ductal epithelium, however, carries a five-fold increase in risk. In addition, the risk is doubled in the presence of a family history. A family history of breast cancer also increases the risk of developing breast carcinoma with all fibrocystic changes.

9. (e) The most favorable prognostic factor is the absence of lymph node involvement. This has been associated with an 80% survival over a 5-year or even a 10-year period, especially in patients treated by radical or modified radical mastectomy. The presence of ER or PR indicates a better prognosis over a 10-year period, and a better response to endocrine therapy. Epidermal growth factor receptor (EGFR) positive tumors carry a worse prognosis than EGFR-negative tumors. The status of the S-phase fraction and ploidy is less certain; some studies suggest that an increased S-phase fraction or aneuploidy indicate a poorer prognosis. The test for amplification of the c-erb-B_2 oncogene is currently regarded as a research procedure.

10. (e) All of the factors listed contribute to the risk of carcinoma of the breast. The relative risk is approximately doubled for patients who have one first-degree relative with breast cancer, and increased four-fold for those with two affected relatives. Nulliparous women and women whose first child was born when they were over thirty years of age are at increased risk, as are women who have been treated for carcinoma of the contralateral breast. Obesity is associated with increased synthesis of estrogen in adipose tissue, which in turn increases the risk of breast cancer.

11. (d) Amplification of the c-erb-B2 oncogene and somatic mutations of the Rb tumor suppressor gene have been reported in sporadic cases of breast cancer, and germ-line mutations of the latter gene are responsible for rare cases of familial breast cancer. However, germ-line mutations of the BRCA1 gene are responsible for many cases of familial breast cancer, which often occur at an early age in these families. Additional susceptibility genes must exist to account for many other cases of familial breast cancer. Mutated BRCA1 genes are also associated with ovarian cancer.

▶ Final Diagnosis and Synopsis of the Case

• Carcinoma of the Breast

A 53-year-old woman was found, on routine physical examination, to have a lump in the lower, outer quadrant of her left breast. Mammography showed a suspicious area of increased density, without calcifications. Biopsy showed an infiltrating ductal carcinoma. Following discussion with the patient, she opted for restricted surgery ("lumpectomy") and local radiation therapy. The tumor was less than 1.0 cm in diameter, and its edges were well within the margins of the resected tissue. Six lymph nodes were identified after a limited axillary dissection and were free of metastatic tumor. Since the tumor was positive for estrogen receptors, the patient was placed on a course of adjuvant therapy with a drug which competes with estrogen for estrogen receptors, and was discharged for follow-up as an out-patient.

LAB TIPS

Prognostic Factors in Breast Cancer

There are a number of histologic features of carcinoma of the breast that have an influence on prognosis. The size of the primary tumor (<2.0 cm is favorable), metastatic disease in axillary lymph nodes (absence of metastatic disease is favorable), the number of lymph nodes involved (the fewer the better), the histologic type (intraductal is better than infiltrating duct, etc), and the tumor histologic and nuclear grade (well-differentiated tumors are more favorable than poorly differentiated tumors) are all important independent prognostic indicators. The more differentiated the tumor, the more likely it is to have estrogen and progesterone receptors, and the increased likelihood that the tumor will exhibit regression following antiestrogen therapy.

Listed below are a selection of other factors which have recently been suggested as influencing prognosis in patients with breast cancer. A number of these tests are currently for research purposes only.

FACTORS AFFECTING PROGNOSIS IN PATIENTS WITH BREAST CANCER

Test	Description/Method	Influence on prognosis
DNA ploidy	A measure of the total nuclear DNA content. Performed by flow cytometry.	Aneuploidy appears to be prognostically unfavorable.
Proliferation index (S–phase fraction)	Amount of active DNA synthesis which is an indication of the amount of cell proliferation. Calculation from flow cytometry analysis.	Increased S–phase fraction appears to be prognostically unfavorable.
C-*erb*–B2(Her–2/*neu*) oncogene amplification	One of the protooncogenes encoding for the epidermal growth factor (EGF). Immunohistochemistry can be used to identify the protein that is encoded by this gene.	The presence of C-*erb*–B2 amplification appears prognostically unfavorable.
Cathepsin D	An endoprotease found in lysosomes of mammalian cells. Can be identified by immunohistochemistry.	Strong immunohistochemical staining tumors may be prognostically unfavorable.
Ki–67	A nuclear protein expressed only during cell growth and thus correlating with mitotic activity. Performed by immunohistochemistry.	Positive Ki–67 staining appears prognostically unfavorable.

An 18-Year-Old Woman With Fever and Painful Cervical Lymph Nodes

▷ Clinical History and Presentation

An 18-year-old woman presented with a fever, sore throat and painful cervical adenopathy of about 10 day's duration, preceded by a few days of severe headache and general malaise. She also felt extremely tired and nauseous. She had been treated by her family physician unsuccessfully with antibiotics, but there had been no relief of her symptoms, and she came to the emergency room. She had no other significant medical or surgical history. She denied any contact with acutely ill persons in the last several weeks. Physical examination revealed an alert and oriented woman in mild distress due to her sore throat and nausea. Blood pressure was 100/70 mmHg, heart rate was 100 per minute and regular, temperature was 104.2° F and respiratory rate was 24 per minute. Pertinent physical findings included an erythematous oropharynx with exudate covering both tonsils. Bilateral tender cervical lymphadenopathy was noted. There was also some tenderness in both axillae. The rest of the physical examination was unremarkable.

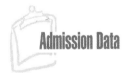

Admission Data

TABLE 25–1. HEMATOLOGY		
WBC	14.5 thousand/μL	(3.3–11.0)
Neut	35%	(44–88)
Band	0%	(0–10)
Lymph	45%	(12–43)
Mono	9%	(2–11)
Eos	1%	(0–5)
Baso	0%	(0–2)
Atyp. cells	10%	(0)
RBC	4.3 million/μL	(3.9–5.0)
Hgb	12.4 g/dL	(11.6–15.6)
HCT	36.8%	(37.0–47.0)
MCV	85.6 fL	(79.0–99.0)
MCH	28.8 pg	(26.0–32.6)
MCHC	33.6 g/dL	(31.0–36.0)
Plts	183 thousand/μL	(130–400)

TABLE 25–2. URINALYSIS

pH	6	(5.0–7.5)
Protein	Neg	(Neg)
Glucose	Neg	(Neg)
Ketone	Neg	(Neg)
Occult blood	Neg	(Neg)
Color	Yellow	(Yellow)
Clarity	clear	(Clear)
Sp. grav.	1.010	(1.010–1.035)
WBC	1–4/HPF	(0–5)
RBC	0/HPF	(0–2)

TABLE 25–3. CHEMISTRY

Glucose	105 mg/dL	(65–110)
Creatinine	0.9 mg/dL	(0.7–1.4)
BUN	11 mg/dL	(7–24)
Uric acid	6.1 mg/dL	(3.0–7.5)
Cholesterol	152 mg/dL	(150–240)
Calcium	8.5 mg/dL	(8.5–10.5)
Protein	7.0 g/dL	(6–8)
Albumin	3.7 g/dL	(3.7–5.0)
LDH	359 U/L	(100–250)
Alk Phos	197 U/L	(0–120)
AST	124 U/L	(0–55)
GGTP	89 U/L	(0–50)
Bilirubin	1.1 mg/dL	(0.0–1.5)
Bilirubin, direct	0.63 mg/dL	(0.02–0.18)

TABLE 25–4. ELECTROLYTES

Na	135 mEq/L	(134–143)
K	4.1 mEq/L	(3.5–4.9)
Cl	100 mEq/L	(95–108)
CO_2	22 mEq/L	(21–32)

TABLE 25–5. HETEROPHILE ANTIBODY TEST ("MONOSPOT")

Pending

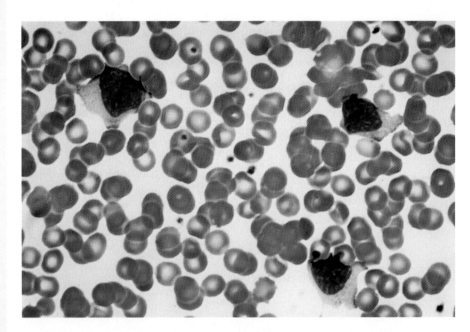

FIGURE 25–1. Admission peripheral blood smear. Wright/Giemsa stain. Original magnification ×252.

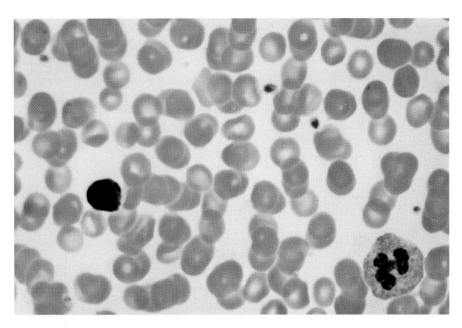

FIGURE 25–2. Normal peripheral blood smear. Wright/Giemsa stain. Original magnification ×315.

▶ **Questions**

On the basis of the preceding information, you can best conclude the following:

1. The abnormalities shown on this patient's routine chemistry panel are best explained by which of the following processes?
   a. acute hepatitis
   b. acute obstruction of the common bile duct by gallstones
   c. intravascular hemolysis
   d. none of the above

2. The findings on the peripheral blood smear in Figure 25–1 are most consistent with:
   a. the presence of atypical CD19 positive cells
   b. the presence of atypical CD8 positive cells
   c. the presence of band neutrophils
   d. the presence of red blood cell precursors
   e. the presence of none of the above

3. Which of the following tests would best support your diagnosis?
   a. blood culture
   b. liver biopsy
   c. flow cytometric immunophenotyping of peripheral blood
   d. "monospot" test
   e. antinuclear antibody (ANA) titer

4. Which of the following statements about this disease is INCORRECT?
   a. epithelial cells are involved in its pathogenesis
   b. B lymphocytes are involved in its pathogenesis
   c. splenomegaly is a common manifestation
   d. complete recovery from this condition is common
   e. the results of liver function tests are usually normal

▶ Clinical Course

The patient was admitted to the hospital and was started on intravenous antibiotics. All cultures and the "monospot" test that was performed on admission were negative. The "monospot" test was repeated and an Epstein-Barr virus antibody panel (see Table 25–2) was ordered. The antibiotic therapy was discontinued and the patient was discharged five days after admission. She was instructed to rest for two weeks before slowly returning to her normal activities. Her progress was to be followed by her family physician.

TABLE 25–6. EPSTEIN-BARR VIRUS (EBV) ANTIBODY PANEL

	Patient	Reference
EBV-VCA, IgM	110	0–90 EU
EBV-VCA, IgG	332	0–100 EU
EBV-EA	20	<10 EU
EBV-NA	0	0–47 EU

EBV-VCA = Antibody against EBV capsid antigens; EBV-EA = Antibody against EBV early antigens; EBV-NA = Antibody against EBV nuclear antigens; EU = ELISA unit.

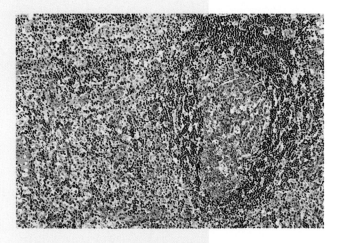

FIGURE 25–3. Lymph node from another patient with this disease. Hematoxylin–eosin stain. Original magnification ×31.

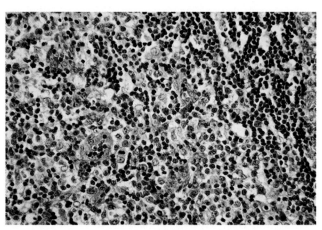

FIGURE 25–4. Lymph node from another patient with this disease. Hematoxylin–eosin stain. Original magnification ×100.

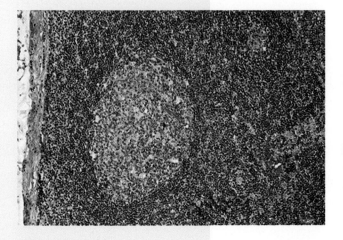

FIGURE 25–5. Normal lymph node. Hematoxylin–eosin stain. Original magnification ×31.

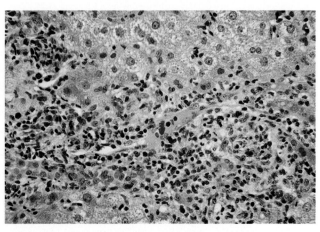

FIGURE 25–6. Liver biopsy from another patient with this disease. Hematoxylin–eosin stain. Original magnification ×78.

▶ Questions

5. The section of the lymph node in Figures 25–3 and 25–4 shows the presence of:
   a. numerous plasma cells
   b. numerous Reed-Sternberg (RS) cells
   c. numerous large, atypical lymphocytes
   d. granulomas
   e. none of the above

6. All of the following statements about the histological appearance of the liver at this stage of the disease are correct EXCEPT:
   a. it is similar to that of viral hepatitis except for the presence of large, atypical lymphocytes
   b. it shows an area of focal parenchymal necrosis
   c. it shows increased numbers of lymphocytes in the portal area
   d. it shows the formation of "bile lakes"
   e. it is consistent with fully reversible liver damage

7. This disease is known:
   a. to be of viral origin
   b. to affect patients in late adolescence or in young adulthood
   c. to be self-limited in most cases
   d. to elicit a specific immune response
   e. all of the above

8. This disease can be acquired by:
   a. kissing
   b. eating food contaminated with saliva of an infected person
   c. transplantation of tissue containing viable infected cells
   d. any of the above
   e. none of the above

9. The laboratory findings typical of the acute stage of this disease include all of the following EXCEPT:
   a. relative lymphocytosis
   b. absolute lymphocytosis
   c. the presence of heterophil antibodies
   d. a high titer of EBV-NA antibodies
   e. the presence of antibodies to EBV-EA

10. After recovery from the acute stage of this disease, one would expect to find all of the following EXCEPT:
    a. total elimination of the viral agent from the body
    b. immunity to subsequent reinfection
    c. serologic evidence of the infection
    d. fully functional humoral and cellular immune responses in the majority of patients

▶ Figure Descriptions

Figure 25–1. Admission peripheral blood smear. Wright/Giemsa stain. Original magnification ×252.

Several atypical lymphocytes are present in this photomicrograph. The cells are large, with abundant, pale blue, delicate cytoplasm. The nuclear chromatin is less dense and does not show the coarse clumping pattern seen in normal lymphocytes.

Figure 25–2. Normal peripheral blood smear. Wright/Giemsa stain. Original magnification ×315.

This photomicrograph shows a normal lymphocyte with typical scanty cytoplasm and a dense, coarse nuclear chromatin pattern. A neutrophil is also present.

Figure 25–3. Lymph node from another patient with this disease. Hematoxylin–eosin stain. Original magnification ×31.

This is a portion of a lymph node from another patient with this disease. It shows the characteristic features of infectious mononucleosis. The paracortex is markedly expanded and does not show the large numbers of small lymphocytes that are normally found in this region of the node. Instead, the paracortex appears to contain various sized "holes" which actually represent atypical, reactive lymphocytes with abundant cytoplasm and enlarged nuclei and prominent nucleoli. Small lymphocytes and occasional plasma cells are also present, but are not identifiable at this magnification. A germinal center is present on the right side of the image and its edges are somewhat irregular.

Figure 25–4. Lymph node from another patient with this disease. Hematoxylin–eosin stain. Original magnification ×100.

At higher magnification of the paracortex, we can clearly see the atypical, reactive lymphocytes with their enlarged vesicular nuclei and prominent nucleoli. These cells correspond to the atypical lymphocytes seen in the peripheral smear.

Figure 25–5. Normal lymph node. Hematoxylin–eosin stain. Original magnification ×31.

The cortex of a normal lymph node shows a well-defined germinal center and a paracortex with numerous small lymphocytes. The looseness of the paracortex seen in Figure 25–3 is not apparent in this lymph node.

Figure 25–6. Liver biopsy from another patient with this disease. Hematoxylin–eosin stain. Original magnification ×78.

A liver biopsy from another patient shows a portal area widened by an inflammatory infiltrate. While some of the lymphocytes appear small, many are large and atypical with abundant cytoplasm and large nuclei showing prominent nucleoli. These atypical lymphocytes can also be seen extending into the sinusoids adjacent to the portal area, surrounding some of the hepatocytes, and resulting in piecemeal necrosis.

▶ **Answers**

1. (**a**) The chemistry panel shows a moderate increase of alkaline phosphatase, aspartate aminotransferase (AST), glutamyl transferase (GGTP), lactate dehydrogenase (LDH) and a normal total bilirubin level with a relative increase of the direct bilirubin fraction. This pattern is typical of mild hepatitis. Acute obstruction of the common bile duct would lead to a marked elevation of serum alkaline phosphatase, AST, and an increase in total (mainly direct) bilirubin. Intravascular hemolysis would lead to an increase of total serum bilirubin (predominantly unconjugated) and to an increase of LDH.

2. (**b**) The peripheral blood smear (Figure 25–1) shows atypical (reactive) lymphocytes. These large cells have abundant cytoplasm, that is occasionally vacuolated (as is seen in one of the cells), and large pleomorphic nuclei and are suggestive of infectious mononucleosis. They are mostly of CD8 positive phenotype (cytotoxic/suppressor T cell). The CD19 positive phenotype denotes B lymphocytes. Reactive lymphocytes are distinct enough to be distinguished from band neutrophils and red blood cell precursors.

3. (**d**) Based on the patient's symptoms, laboratory results, and the presence of atypical lymphocytes in the peripheral smear, one can conclude that the patient has infectious mononucleosis. The presence of a positive "monospot" test (heterophil agglutination test) will strongly support the diagnosis. Blood cultures are expected to be negative (because of the patient's high fever, bacterial cultures have been performed to exclude other pathogens). Liver biopsy is not indicated, since in most cases there is some impairment of liver function, primarily in the form of a mild hepatitis. Flow cytometric immunophenotyping would serve to exclude lymphoma or leukemia, but is not used to diagnose infectious mononucleosis. Antinuclear antibody (ANA) could be falsely positive, but the test has no diagnostic value in infectious mononucleosis.

4. (**e**) Epstein-Barr virus (EBV) first infects epithelial cells of the oropharynx, then spreads to circulating B lymphocytes. Both types of cell have the EBV receptor (CD21). Infected B cells undergo polyclonal activation and proliferation and secrete antibodies (heterophil anti-sheep red blood cells antibody and specific anti-EBV antibodies). The proliferation of EBV infected B cells is controlled by T lymphocytes (CD8 positive subset) and by natural killer cells. This lymphoproliferation leads to enlargement of lymph nodes, spleen, and occasionally liver. Splenomegaly occurs in about 50% of cases. Liver function is almost always affected, but most otherwise healthy individuals are expected to fully recover.

5. (**c**) Figures 25–3 and 25–4 show lymph node morphology consistent with infectious mononucleosis, with numerous large, atypical (reactive) lymphocytes. The other options (plasma cells, Reed-Sternberg cells, and granulomas) are not obvious.

6. (**d**) The histologic appearance of the liver, combined with the laboratory findings, is consistent with infectious mononucleosis. Figure 25–6 shows an extensive lymphocytic infiltration of a portal area, with many of the lymphocytes being large and atypical. There is also focal parenchymal necrosis, and atypical lymphocytes are extending into the hepatic sinusoids The overall picture is similar to that of viral hepatitis. Such liver damage is fully reversible. There are no "bile lakes", suggestive of prolonged obstructive cholestasis, present in the liver.

7. (**e**) Infectious mononucleosis is caused by the Epstein-Barr virus (EBV), which is a herpes virus. The disease predominantly affects adolescents and young adults in developed countries and young children in the rest of the world. In young children the course is usually mild or clinically inapparent. In the majority of people with a normal immune response, it is self-limited in duration. The infection elicits a specific immune response; serologic evidence of EBV infection persists for years.

8. (**d**) Infectious mononucleosis is acquired by kissing, eating food contaminated with saliva of an infected person, and by transplantation of a tissue containing viable infected cells. Most of the primary Epstein-Barr virus (EBV) infections, however, do not result in a fully developed infectious mononucleosis syndrome.

9. (**d**) The acute stage of infectious mononucleosis lasts 2–3 weeks and is usually characterized by relative and/or absolute lymphocytosis, the presence of heterophil antibodies and by the presence of antibodies against EBV-EA (early antigen). Depending on the phase of the acute stage of mononucleosis, there is a high titer of EBV-VCA IgM antibody (which starts to fall by the third week) or EBV-VCA IgG antibody (which peaks with the clinical onset of the symptoms). The EBV-NA antibody is the last antibody to appear and is usually not found during the acute stage of the disease. The other clinical phases of infectious mononucleosis are the incubation phase, which lasts from 3–7 weeks, and the convalescent phase, which lasts from 4–8 weeks.

10. (**a**) After a patient recovers from infectious mononucleosis, the virus persists in a latent form within the infected B lymphocytes and oropharyngeal epithelial cells. The patient is immune to subsequent reinfection by the virus. The humoral and cellular immune responses become fully functional in the majority of patients. The serological evidence of the infection persists for years or for life.

► Final Diagnosis and Synopsis of the Case

- Infectious Mononucleosis
- Epstein-Barr Virus Hepatitis

This was a typical presentation and course of infectious mononucleosis in an 18-year-old woman. This previously healthy patient presented with a fever, pharyngitis, tender lymphadenopathy, and malaise that persisted in spite of several days of antibiotic treatment. The patient's CBC showed 45% lymphocytes and 10% atypical lymphocytes, identified on the peripheral blood smear. Her routine chemistry panel revealed abnormalities consistent with mild hepatitis. All these findings pointed to infectious mononucleosis. Her first "monospot" test, however, was negative. Since all cultures (blood, throat, and urine) were negative, antibiotic therapy was discontinued. The positive repeated "monospot" test, as well as the positivity for EBV-EA and EBV-VCA IgM and IgG antibodies, indicated an acute Epstein-Barr virus (EBV) infection. The patient's general status improved and she was expected to recover without complications. She will be immune to Epstein-Barr virus (EBV) reinfection and will be a carrier of Epstein-Barr virus (EBV), since the virus persists in a latent form within the infected B lymphocytes and oropharyngeal epithelial cells.

LAB TIPS

Heterophil Antibody ("Monospot") Test

This is the first and usually the only serologic test that should be performed when infectious mononucleosis is suspected. Patients with infectious mononucleosis produce IgM antibodies (heterophil antibodies) of uncertain origin that will agglutinate sheep or horse red blood cells. Unfortunately, patients with serum sickness and certain normal individuals produce a natural antibody (Forssmann antibody) which will also agglutinate sheep or horse red blood cells. The "monospot" slide test was developed to differentiate between these two antibodies. By dividing a glass slide into two sections, one can test for both antibodies on a single slide. Diagrammatic representation of the slide test is shown in the table below.

HETEROPHIL ANTIBODY ("MONOSPOT") TEST			
Side 1		**Side 2**	
Guinea pig kidney suspension[a] + Patient's serum + Sheep or horse red blood cells		Beef red blood cells[b] + Patient's serum + Sheep or horse red blood cells	
Examples			
Patient	**Side 1**	**Side 2**	**Conclusion**
A	Agglutination	No agglutination	Positive for heterophile antibodies of infectious mononucleosis
B	No agglutination	Agglutination	Positive for Forssmann antibodies and negative for heterophile antibodies
C	No agglutination	No agglutination	Negative for heterophile and Forssmann antibodies

[a]Absorbs (removes) Forssmann and serum sickness antibodies.
[b]Absorbs (removes) heterophile antibodies of infectious mononucleosis.

► Clinical History and Presentation

A 76-year-old woman with a long history of non-insulin dependent diabetes mellitus (NIDDM) was brought to the emergency room because of pain, swelling, and redness of her right foot. Two days previously, she had noticed pain and swelling around her toes, which prevented her from walking. The patient denied any significant medical history. She had been taking oral hypoglycemic agents and stated that her blood glucose level had been well controlled. Physical examination revealed an alert female in no acute distress. Blood pressure was 150/90 mmHg, temperature was 99° F, heart rate was 80 per minute, and respiratory rate was 18 per minute. Pertinent findings included a fungal rash under her breast and in the groin area and a very painful, hot, and edematous dorso-lateral aspect of her right foot around a deep fissure between the fourth and fifth toes.

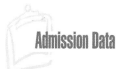

Admission Data

TABLE 26–1. HEMATOLOGY		
WBC	16.7 thousand/μL	(3.3–11.0)
Neut	34%	(44–88)
Band	0%	(0–10)
Lymph	61%	(12–43)
Mono	3%	(2–11)
Eos	1%	(0–5)
Baso	1%	(0–2)
RBC	3.59 million/μL	(3.9–5.0)
Hgb	11.2 g/dL	(11.6–15.6)
HCT	33.7%	(37.0–47.0)
MCV	93.8 fL	(79.0–99.0)
MCH	31.3 pg	(26.0–32.6)
MCHC	33.4 g/dL	(31.0–36.0)
Plts	165 thousand/μL	(130–400)

NOTES

TABLE 26–2. URINALYSIS

pH	6	(5.0–7.5)
Protein	Trace	(Neg)
Glucose	3+	(Neg)
Ketone	Neg	(Neg)
Occ. blood	Neg	(Neg)
Color	Pale Yellow	(Yellow)
Clarity	Clear	(Clear)
Sp. grav	1.020	(1.010–1.035)
WBC	4/HPF	(0–5)
RBC	0/HPF	(0–2)
Yeast	1+	(Neg)
Bacteria	Neg	(Neg)

TABLE 26–3. CHEMISTRY

Glucose	392 mg/dL	(65–110)
Creatinine	1.0 mg/dL	(0.7–1.4)
BUN	22 mg/dL	(7–24)
Uric acid	3.7 mg/dL	(3.0–7.5)
Cholesterol	155 mg/dL	(150–240)
Calcium	9.1 mg/dL	(8.5–10.5)
Protein	6.8 g/dL	(6–8)
Albumin	3.4 g/dL	(3.7–5.0)
LDH	225 U/L	(100–250)
Alk Phos	120 U/L	(0–120)
AST	18 U/L	(0–55)
GGTP	15 U/L	(0–50)
Bilirubin	0.4 mg/dL	(0.0–1.5)
Bilirubin, direct	0.06 mg/dL	(0.02–0.18)

TABLE 26–4. ELECTROLYTES

Na	134 mEq/L	(134–143)
K	3.9 mEq/L	(3.5–4.9)
Cl	100 mEq/L	(95–108)
CO_2	23 mEq/L	(21–32)

TABLE 26–5. GLYCOSYLATED HEMOGLOBIN

Patient's glycosylated hemoglobin	14.5 mg/dl
Reference values:	
Normal (nondiabetics)	4.0–7.0
Diabetics–good control	<9
Diabetics–fair control	9–12
Diabetics–poor control	>12

TABLE 26–6. MICROBIOLOGY

Blood cultures: pending
Wound culture (fissure of the foot): pending

▶ **Questions**

On the basis of the preceding information, you can best conclude the following:

1. The CBC shows:
   a. relative lymphocytosis
   b. absolute lymphocytosis
   c. leukocytosis
   d. all of the above
   e. none of the above

2. All of the following statements about cutaneous candidiasis are true EXCEPT:
   a. *Candida* is a normal inhabitant of the human skin
   b. moisture of the skin weakens its resistance to fungus infection
   c. patients with diabetes mellitus are susceptible to cutaneous candidiasis
   d. patients with hematologic malignancies are susceptible to cutaneous candidiasis
   e. patients with leukocytosis are susceptible to cutaneous candidiasis

3. Which of the following factors is/are likely to contribute to this patient's hyperglycemia?
   a. insulin deficiency
   b. insulin resistance
   c. accelerated hepatic glucose production
   d. all of the above
   e. none of the above

4. The lesion of the patient's right foot is most likely:
   a. due to an acute arterial occlusion
   b. due to thromboangiitis obliterans
   c. of infectious etiology
   d. none of the above

NOTES

▶ Clinical Course

The patient was admitted to the hospital for treatment of her right foot problem and control of her hyperglycemia. The hospital course was uncomplicated. Her foot lesion responded to intravenous antibiotics (wound culture was positive for *Staphylococcus aureus*). Her hyperglycemia came under control with a change of the oral hyperglycemic agent. The candidiasis lesions were treated topically and showed improvement. The repeated CBC values and a peripheral blood smear are shown in Figure 26–1. A bone marrow aspiration and biopsy were performed (Figures 26–2 and 26–3). The patient was discharged on oral antibiotics and was to be followed on an outpatient basis.

TABLE 26–7. HEMATOLOGY

WBC	13.1 thousand/μL	(3.3–11.0)
Neut	40%	(44–88)
Band	0%	(0–10)
Lymph	56%	(12–43)
Mono	2%	(2–11)
Eos	1%	(0–5)
Baso	1%	(0–2)
RBC	3.93 million/μL	(3.9–5.0)
Hgb	12.1 g/dL	(11.6–15.6)
HCT	36.6%	(37.0–47.0)
MCV	93.2 fL	(79.0–99.0)
MCH	30.8 pg	(26.0–32.6)
MCHC	33.0 g/dL	(31.0–36.0)
Plts	218 thousand/μL	(130–400)

TABLE 26–8. FLOW CYTOMETRIC ANALYSIS OF THE PATIENT'S PERIPHERAL BLOOD

Cluster Designation		Percent of Positive Cells Lymphoid Cluster
CD45	(Pan-leukocytic)	98
CD14	(Monocytic)	1.5
CD2	(Pan-T cell)	14.4
CD3	(T-cell receptor)	12.3
CD5	(T-cell/B-cell subset)	94.9
CD4	(T-cell; helper)	5.6
CD8	(T-cell; suppressor)	6.6
CD19	(Pan-B cell)	88.4
CD5/CD19	(B-cells co-expressing CD5)	86.7
CD10	(CALLA, Early B-cell)	0.0
Kappa light chain	(Mature B-cell)	0.1
Lambda light chain	(Mature B-cell)	84.8
MLA-DR	(B-cells; activated T-cells; macrophages)	92.3

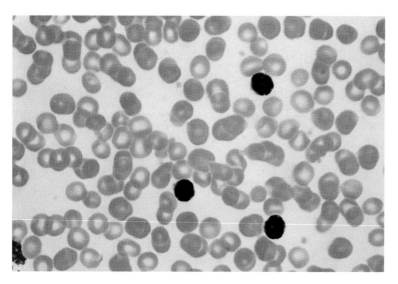

FIGURE 26–1. Peripheral blood smear (patient). Wright/Giemsa stain. Original magnification ×252.

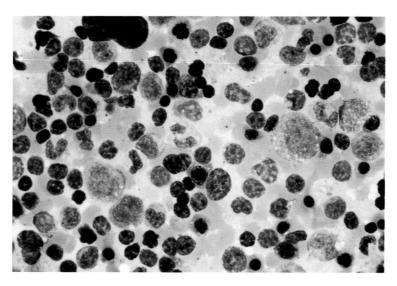

FIGURE 26–2. Bone marrow aspirate (patient). Wright/Giemsa stain. Original magnification ×197.

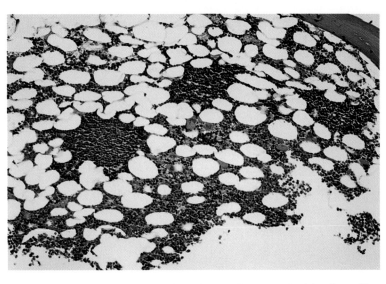

FIGURE 26–3. Bone marrow biopsy (patient). Hematoxylin–eosin stain. Original magnification ×31.

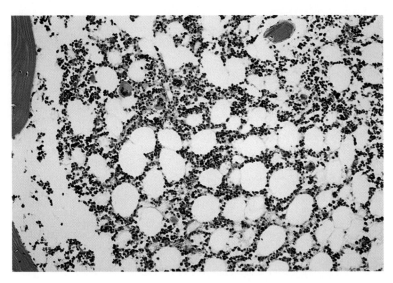

FIGURE 26–4. Normal bone marrow biopsy from another patient. Hematoxylin–eosin stain. Original magnification ×31.

▶ **Questions**

5. Which of the following statements about the flow cytometric analysis in this patient is INCORRECT?
   a. the relative proportions of T and B lymphocytes are within the normal range
   b. the B cells show a mature phenotype
   c. the B cells are of restricted clonality
   d. the T lymphocyte subsets show an abnormal ratio of CD4+ to CD8+ cells
   e. the relative proportions of Kappa and Lambda light chain-expressing cells are abnormal

6. The peripheral blood smear in Figure 26–1 shows:
   a. an increased proportion of lymphocytes
   b. blast cells
   c. megaloblasts
   d. band neutrophils
   e. all of the above

7. The bone marrow biopsy depicted in Figure 26–3 shows:
   a. a diffuse infiltrate of the bone marrow
   b. scattered lymphoid nodules
   c. marked hypocellularity
   d. metastatic carcinoma
   e. none of the above

8. Based on the hematologic and flow cytometric findings in this patient, it can be concluded that:
   a. this patient has a chronic inflammatory disease
   b. the patient shows a polyclonal proliferation of B cells
   c. the patient has an acute lymphoblastic leukemia (ALL)
   d. the patient has a chronic lymphocytic leukemia (CLL)
   e. the patient has none of the above

9. As this patient progresses through the course of her hematological disease, she could develop:
   a. anemia
   b. thrombocytopenia
   c. hypersplenism
   d. lymphadenopathy
   e. all of the above

10. All of the following statements about this patient are correct EXCEPT:
    a. the patient is in the early stage of her hematological disease
    b. the treatment of her hematological problem can be postponed
    c. the immune system of this patient is likely to be abnormal
    d. this patient is in an atypical age category for the development of her hematological disease

▶ Figure Descriptions

Figure 26–1. Peripheral blood smear (patient). Wright/Giemsa stain. Original magnification ×252.

Several normal-appearing, small lymphocytes are present in this photomicrograph. No blasts are present and the erythrocytes are unremarkable.

Figure 26–2. Bone marrow aspiration (patient). Wright/Giemsa stain. Original magnification ×197.

This photomicrograph shows an increased number of lymphocytes in the bone marrow. Occasional normoblasts and cells of the myeloid series are present.

Figure 26–3. Bone marrow biopsy (patient). Hematoxylin–eosin stain. Original magnification ×31.

In this low power photomicrograph of the patient's bone marrow biopsy, several nodules of lymphocytes are present with normal intervening marrow. The marrow architecture is intact. This is the nodular pattern of bone marrow involvement in chronic lymphocytic leukemia.

Figure 26–4. Normal bone marrow biopsy. Hematoxylin–eosin stain. Original magnification ×31.

The bone marrow biopsy is normocellular and shows heterocellular hematopoietic cells and no lymphoid infiltrate.

▶ **Answers**

1. (**d**) The CBC of this patient shows leukocytosis (a WBC count of more than 11,000/μL), absolute lymphocytosis (more than 4000 lymphocytes/μL), and a relative lymphocytosis (lymphocytes representing more than 43% of WBC).

2. (**e**) An increased WBC count is not per se associated with increased susceptibility to candidiasis: neutrophils and lymphocytes play important roles in the host defense against *Candida,* which is a normal inhabitant of the human skin. Certain conditions, such as moisture and traumatization of skin, diabetes mellitus, and/or hematological malignancies, increase the susceptibility of the skin to fungal infection and inflammation.

3. (**d**) The majority of patients with non-insulin-dependent diabetes mellitus (NIDDM) are insulin-deficient and insulin-resistant. Insulin deficiency is most apparent following oral glucose intake, while fasting insulin levels can be normal or even elevated. Insulin resistance is predominantly due to a post-binding defect rather than an insulin-binding defect, which is, however, also present in most patients. The hepatic glucose production rate is increased, and this increase is proportional to the degree of fasting hypoglycemia.

4. (**c**) The lesion was most likely one of infectious etiology. It was hot, red, painful, and swollen. The deep fissure on the right foot most likely served as a point of entry for bacteria. Thromboangiitis obliterans is typically a disease of young, heavy-smoking males and causes ischemia of the extremities due to inflammatory and proliferative lesions of medium and small arteries and veins of the limbs. Acute arterial occlusion leads to cyanosis or pallor, decrease in skin temperature, and a loss of sensation.

5. (**a**) Flow cytometric analysis of this patient's peripheral blood shows findings typical of chronic lymphocytic leukemia (CLL). The majority of lymphocytes show a B cell phenotype (CD19+) of restricted clonality (virtually all cells express the Lambda light chain, and normally the Kappa to Lambda ratio is 2 to 1). The expression of surface immunoglobulin light chains and the absence of CD10 (CALLA) antigen on the surface of B lymphocytes characterize these cells as mature B lymphocytes. There is a co-expression of CD5 (T cell) antigen on leukemic CD19+ cells (B cells), a finding characteristic of CLL. The T lymphocyte subsets show a decreased CD4+ to CD8+ ratio (normally the CD4 to CD8 ratio is 2–3 to 1). In normal peripheral blood, the majority of lymphocytes are of T cell phenotype (about 80% of all lymphocytes).

6. (**a**) The peripheral blood smear shows an increased proportion of fairly uniform, small-to-medium size lymphocytes. No blasts, megaloblasts, or band neutrophils are present.

7. (**b**) The bone marrow biopsy shows scattered nodules of lymphoid tissue with normal intervening marrow (see description of Figure 26–3). There is no diffuse infiltration of the marrow with lymphoid or other neoplastic cells. The bone marrow is not hypocellular.

8. (**d**) The patient has chronic lymphocytic leukemia (CLL), which is a neoplastic process. Inflammatory causes of lymphocytosis would not show restriction of B cell clonality. Acute lymphoblastic leukemia (ALL) would show blasts characterized by an immature B cell phenotype (CD19+, CD10+, and SIg–).

9. (**e**) Anemia, thrombocytopenia, hypersplenism, and lymphadenopathy are all features of chronic lymphocytic leukemia (CLL), especially in the more advanced stages.

10. **(d)** Chronic lymphocytic leukemia (CLL) is a disease of an elderly population (over 60 years of age). This patient's hemoglobin and platelet count are almost within the normal range. The lymphocytosis is relatively low ($<15,000$ /μL), and there is no splenomegaly or lymphadenopathy. The treatment in these patients is usually delayed, since early treatment with alkylating agents is associated with an increased risk of the development of secondary malignancies. The immune system of this patient is likely to be abnormal because of her diabetes mellitus and her chronic lymphocytic leukemia (CLL).

▶ Final Diagnosis and Synopsis of the Case

- Poorly Controlled Diabetes Mellitus
- Cellulitis
- Candidiasis
- Chronic Lymphocytic Leukemia

An elderly female with a long history of non-insulin-dependent diabetes mellitus (NIDDM) was admitted to the hospital for the treatment of cellulitis in her right foot and better control of her hyperglycemia. Subsequently, she was found to have an absolute lymphocytosis, which was then diagnosed as chronic lymphocytic leukemia. The patient had no peripheral adenopathy, splenomegaly, significant anemia, or thrombocytopenia. The lymphocytic infiltration pattern of her bone marrow was prognostically favorable (focal lymphocytic aggregates). This represents an early stage of CLL, for which chemotherapeutic therapy is usually not indicated. The patient was treated with antibiotics for her acute infectious problem, her blood glucose level was stabilized, and she was to be followed on an outpatient basis.

LAB TIPS

Bone Marrow Infiltration Pattern

The histologic pattern of infiltration of the bone marrow in chronic lymphocytic leukemia is a major prognostic factor for survival. The proportion of lymphocytes present in the marrow in this disease may range from 30%–100%, and four patterns of infiltration are recognized:

CHRONIC LYMPHOCYTIC LEUKEMIA: BONE MARROW INFILTRATION PATTERN	
Bone Marrow Pattern on Biopsy	**Description**
Interstitial (infiltrative) pattern (See Figure 26–5.)	Architecture of bone marrow preserved and cellularity is nearly normal. Tumor cells are intermixed with normal hematopoietic cells. Accounts for 30% of cases and is associated with early stages of disease and a good prognosis.
Nodular pattern (See Figure 26–3.)	Scattered nodules of lymphocytes with normal intervening marrow. This pattern is also seen predominantly in early stages of disease and carries a good prognosis. It is seen in about 15% of cases.
Mixed nodular and infiltrative pattern (See Figure 26–6.)	It is a combination of the above two patterns and is seen in about 30% of cases.
Diffuse pattern (See Figure 26–7.)	Marked hypercellularity, and decreased fat cells and decreased numbers of normal hematopoietic elements, is present with the tumor cells diffusely infiltrating the marrow. Found in about 35% of cases, it is usually associated with advanced stage of disease. Carries the poorest prognosis, regardless of stage.

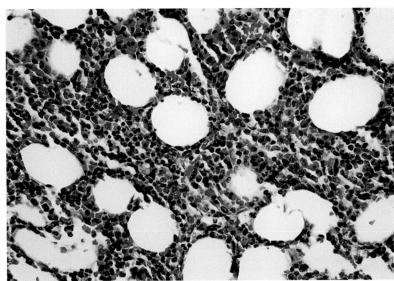

FIGURE 26–5. Bone marrow biopsy from another patient. Hematoxylin–eosin stain. Original magnification ×78. This is the interstitial pattern of bone marrow involvement in chronic lymphocytic leukemia. The marrow is normocellular, and although it is heterocellular with numerous normal hematopoietic elements, increased numbers of lymphocytes are apparent. The marrow architecture is intact.

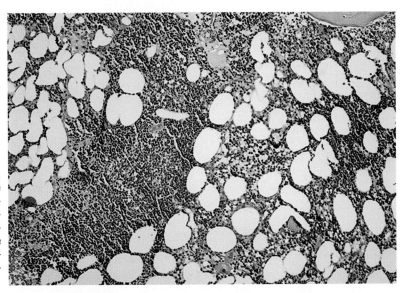

FIGURE 26–6. Bone marrow biopsy from another patient. Hematoxylin–eosin stain. Original magnification ×31. In the mixed pattern of bone marrow involvement in chronic lymphocytic leukemia, there is both interstitial and nodular involvement of the marrow. Note that the marrow adjacent to the lymphoid nodule does not show the heterocellularity that may be seen in Figure 26–5. Increased numbers of leukemic lymphocytes are present in both the nodule and the intervening marrow, but the marrow architecture is still mainly intact.

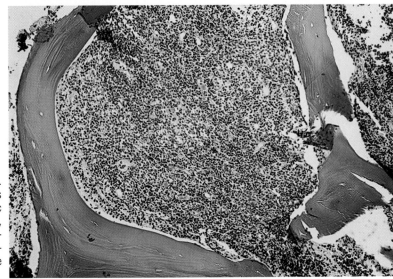

FIGURE 26–7. Bone marrow biopsy from another patient. Hematoxylin–eosin stain. Original magnification ×31. This is the diffuse pattern of bone marrow involvement in chronic lymphocytic leukemia. The marrow is markedly hypercellular, with distortion of the normal architecture (marrow fat is absent). Normal hematopoietic elements are significantly reduced in numbers, with most of the cells visible in this image being leukemic lymphocytes.

27
Chapter

A 29-Year-Old
Woman With
Premature
Rupture of
Membranes

▶ Clinical History and Presentation

A 29-year-old primigravida, at term, was admitted several hours after she experienced a copious escape of watery fluid from her vagina. Physical examination revealed a febrile patient (temperature was 100° F) in no acute distress. Blood pressure was 130/90 mmHg and heart rate was 90 per minute. The uterus was globular and term size. Contractions were occurring every 3 minutes, each lasting approximately 45 seconds. There was no edema. The uterine cervix was dilated 2 cm and the membranes were ruptured.

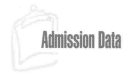

Admission Data

TABLE 27–1. HEMATOLOGY		
WBC	7.5 thousand/μL	(3.3–11.0)
Neut	54%	(44–88)
Band	0%	(0–10)
Lymph	38%	(12–43)
Mono	5%	(2–11)
Eos	2%	(0–5)
Baso	1%	(0–2)
RBC	4.11 million/μL	(3.9–5.0)
Hgb	12.4 g/dL	(11.6–15.6)
HCT	36.4%	(37.0–47.0)
MCV	88.6 fL	(79.0–99.0)
MCH	30.2 pg	(26.0–32.6)
MCHC	34.1 g/dL	(31.0–36.0)
Plts	189 thousand/μL	(130–400)

TABLE 27–2. CHEMISTRY

Glucose	84 mg/dL	(65–110)
Creatinine	1.1 mg/dL	(0.7–1.4)
BUN	12 mg/dL	(7–24)
Uric acid	5.3 mg/dL	(3.0–7.5)
Cholesterol	160 mg/dL	(150–240)
Calcium	8.4 mg/dL	(8.5–10.5)
Protein	6.1 g/dL	(6–8)
Albumin	3.1 g/dL	(3.7–5.0)
LDH	203 U/L	(100–250)
Alk Phos	200 U/L	(0–120)
AST	25 U/L	(0–55)
GGTP	23 U/L	(0–50)
Bilirubin	0.4 mg/dL	(0.0–1.5)
Bilirubin, direct	0.13 mg/dL	(0.02–0.18)

TABLE 27–3. COAGULATION

PT	13.5 sec	(11–14)
aPTT	25 sec	(19–28)

TABLE 27–4. URINALYSIS

Within normal limits

TABLE 27–5. ALPHA-FETOPROTEIN[a]

Within normal range for gestational age

[a]Done at week 12 of pregnancy

▶ **Questions**

On the basis of the preceding information, you can best conclude the following:

1. The patient has an increased serum alkaline phosphatase. Most of this increase is due to:
   a. placenta
   b. liver
   c. bone
   d. none of the above

2. Pre-term premature rupture of membranes (PROM) has been associated with:
   a. polyhydramnios
   b. twin pregnancies
   c. amniocentesis
   d. incompetent uterine cervix
   e. all of the above

3. Premature rupture of membranes (PROM) occurs in 10% of all pregnancies. What proportion of these occur at term?
   a. $\frac{4}{5}$
   b. $\frac{3}{5}$
   c. $\frac{2}{5}$
   d. $\frac{1}{5}$

4. Complications of premature rupture of membranes (PROM) include:
   a. premature labor
   b. maternal infection
   c. fetal infection
   d. prolapse of the cord
   e. all of the above

5. Apparently normal maternal α-fetoprotein levels tend to exclude:
   a. open defects of the fetal neural tube
   b. recent fetal death
   c. Down's syndrome
   d. incorrect estimation of gestational age
   e. all of the above

▶ Clinical Course

The patient was observed for the onset of active labor. Twelve hours after the rupture of the membranes, she was given a soap-suds enema. Fifteen hours after the rupture, the oxytocin stimulation of labor was begun. Progress was slow. Twenty-six hours after membrane rupture, the cervix was 5 cm dilated and the patient's temperature was 101° F. The patient was not progressing as expected, and she was scheduled for caesarean section. She tolerated the surgery well, and a live baby boy was delivered. The placenta was sent for histological examination (Figures 27–1 and 27–3). Bacterial cultures of the patient's blood and placenta were ordered. The cultures were reported positive for group B streptococci. A post-delivery smear of the patient's peripheral blood is shown in Figure 27–4 and her CBC is shown below.

TABLE 27–6. HEMATOLOGY

WBC	17.2 thousand/μL	(3.3–11.0)
Neut	35%	(44–88)
Band	49%	(0–10)
Lymph	9%	(12–43)
Mono	5%	(2–11)
Eos	1%	(0–5)
Baso	1%	(0–2)
RBC	3.02 million/μL	(3.9–5.0)
Hgb	9.1 g/dL	(11.6–15.6)
HCT	26.2%	(37.0–47.0)
MCV	86.7 fL	(79.0–99.0)
MCH	30.1 pg	(26.0–32.6)
MCHC	34.7 g/dL	(31.0–36.0)
Plts	132 thousand/μL	(130–400)

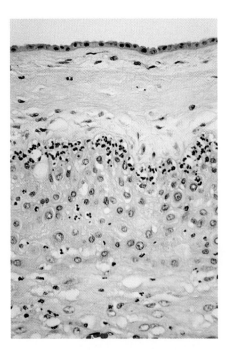 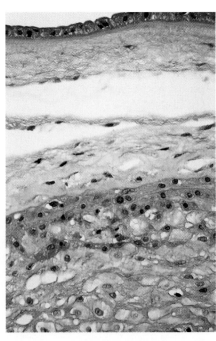

FIGURE 27–1. Placental membranes (patient). Hematoxylin–eosin stain. Original magnification ×78.

FIGURE 27–2. Normal placental membranes. Hematoxylin–eosin stain. Original magnification ×78.

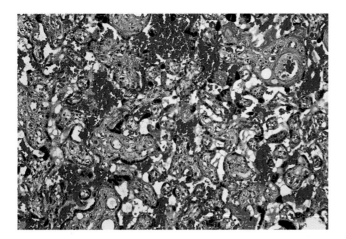

FIGURE 27–3. Portion of placental villi (patient). Hematoxylin–eosin stain. Original magnification ×31.

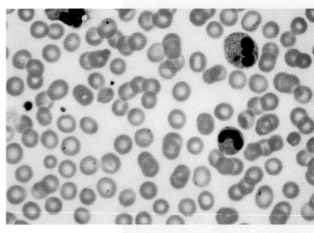

FIGURE 27–4. Post-delivery peripheral blood smear (patient). Wright/Giemsa stain. Original magnification ×252.

▶ Questions

6. The sections of the patient's placenta in Figures 27–1 and 27–3 show:
   a. edematous placental villi
   b. hyperplasia of trophoblast
   c. acute inflammation
   d. all of the above

7. The organisms LEAST likely to be associated with lesions similar to that shown in Figure 27–1 are:
   a. group B streptococci
   b. enterococci
   c. lactobacilli
   d. *Clostridium* species
   e. *E. coli*

8. The patient's peripheral blood smear (Figure 27–4) shows which of the following?
   a. "band" forms
   b. Döhle body
   c. "toxic granulations"
   d. all of the above

9. An increased risk of intra-amniotic infection is associated with:
   a. lengthy duration of membrane rupture
   b. amniocentesis
   c. cervical cerclage
   d. all of the above situations

10. Assays of maternal serum human chorionic gonadotropin (hCG) are useful in the diagnosis of:
    a. normal pregnancy
    b. ectopic pregnancy
    c. threatened abortion
    d. hydatidiform mole
    e. all of the above

Figure Descriptions

Figure 27–1. Placental membranes (patient). Hematoxylin–eosin stain. Original magnification ×78.

The amnion, with its single cell layer of cuboidal cells, is present at the top of the image. At the junction of the amnion and the chorion, a band of neutrophils is present. Isolated neutrophils extend toward the surface of the amnion and down into the chorion. This is an example of acute chorioamnionitis.

Figure 27–2. Normal placental membranes. Hematoxylin–eosin stain. Original magnification ×78.

The amnion is present at the top of the photomicrograph and the chorion is at the bottom. No inflammatory cells are present.

Figure 27–3. Portion of placental villi (patient). Hematoxylin–eosin stain. Original magnification ×31.

This is the histologic picture of a normal term placenta showing a number of chorionic villi, some of which have syncytial knots, and intervillous spaces. Only rare inflammatory cells can be seen, and they are in the vessels of the villi.

Figure 27–4. Post-delivery peripheral blood smear (patient). Wright/Giemsa stain. Original magnification ×252.

The smear shows a normocytic, normochromic anemia and three band leukocytes. All show toxic granulations, and one shows a large, oval, bluish, cytoplasmic inclusion (Döhle body), while another shows cytoplasmic vacuolation. These features may all be found in infections or toxic conditions.

Answers

1. **(a)** In pregnancy, maternal serum alkaline phosphatase is increased up to four-fold over the upper reference range limit. Most of the additional alkaline phosphatase is from the placenta, though a lesser proportion is from bone. If the liver were a source of increased alkaline phosphatase, an accompanying increase in gamma glutamyl transferase (GGTP) would be expected.

2. **(e)** All of the factors listed (ie, polyhydramnios, twin pregnancy, amniocentesis, and incompetent cervix) have been causally associated with pre-term premature rupture of the membranes (PROM). Abruptio placentae has also been associated with PROM, but it is not clear which comes first.

3. **(a)** About 10% of all pregnancies are complicated by premature rupture of the membranes (PROM). About ⅘ of these occur in term patients. Prolonged rupture of the membranes, which means that the membranes have been ruptured for more than 24 hours, poses an increased risk of infection for the neonate and mother. It poses a special risk at term, both for the neonate and for the mother who delivers by caesarean section.

4. (**e**) Maternal and fetal infections, premature labor and delivery, and fetal hypoxia due to compression or prolapse of the cord are complications of premature rupture of the membranes (PROM). Infections are particularly likely with long, latent periods in term PROM. In pre-term pregnancy, the incidence of fetal or maternal infection does not appear to increase, regardless of the duration of the latency period. (The delay between rupture of the membranes and delivery is termed the latency period).

5. (**e**) All of the options listed can be excluded by a normal level of maternal α-fetoprotein. Down's syndrome is associated with significantly lower levels of circulating maternal α-fetoprotein: about 20% of cases of Down's syndrome are associated with maternal α-fetoprotein levels below a level of 0.5 × (median level for gestational age). Apparently elevated levels of circulating maternal α-fetoprotein are associated with open fetal neural tube defects, recent fetal death, and twin pregnancies. α-fetoprotein levels may also appear elevated in cases of incorrect estimation of gestational age.

6. (**c**) The section of the patient's placenta shows chorioamnionitis. Note the acute inflammatory cells in the chorioamnion depicted in Figure 27–1. Edematous villi and hyperplasia of the trophoblast, not evident in Figure 27–3, are features of hydatidiform moles.

7. (**c**) The placenta of this patient showed chorioamnionitis (Figure 27–1). In prolonged premature rupture of the membranes (PROM), chorioamnionitis is seen in 3%–15% of all cases. Intra-amniotic infection, which may lead to chorioamnionitis and later to endometritis, is usually polymicrobial. Infection with low-virulence organisms, which include lactobacilli, diphtheroids, and *Staphylococcus epidermidis,* are seldom associated with chorioamnionitis. Highly virulent organisms, often associated with chorioamnionitis, include group B streptococci (eg, the *Streptococcus agalactiae,* found in this case), *Staphylococcus aureus, E. coli,* and *Clostridium* species).

8. (**d**) This peripheral blood smear (Figure 27–4) shows a "shift to the left" of granulocyte maturation (an increase in the number of "band" neutrophils), the presence of granulocytes with "toxic granulations," Döhle bodies, and vacuolated cytoplasm.

9. (**d**) Intact fetal membranes and the cervical mucus plug are not an absolute barrier to the ascent of microorganisms from the lower genital tract into the uterus during labor. Blood-borne infection can also occur. An increased risk of infection is associated with factors such as long duration of membrane rupture and obstetric procedures such as amniocentesis or cervical cerclage.

10. (**e**) During the first four weeks of pregnancy, the maternal serum level of human chorionic gonadotropin (hCG) approximately doubles every two days, reaching about 500 mIU/mL about 16 days after conception. Ectopic pregnancy and abortion follow the same pattern up to a point at which the rise in hCG levels is interrupted. Multiple pregnancies and trophoblastic tumors (hydatidiform moles and choriocarcinomas) give rise to higher levels of hCG than normal.

NOTES

▶ Final Diagnosis and Synopsis of the Case

- Term Pregnancy
- Premature and Prolonged Rupture of the Membranes
- Dysfunctional Labor
- Acute Chorioamnionitis

A 29-year-old primigravida was admitted at term for premature rupture of the membranes. Labor was induced fifteen hours after membrane rupture. Progress was slow due to dysfunctional labor. Twenty-six hours after rupture of the membranes, the patient was scheduled for caesarean section. At this time, her temperature was noted to be 101° F. After delivery of a live baby boy by caesarean section, her hemoglobin dropped from 12.4 to 9.1 g/dL, and her white cell count increased from 7500/μL to over 17,000/μL with a pronounced shift to the "left." This pattern coincided with her fever of 101° F. Postoperatively, the patient was placed on intravenous fluids and antibiotics. Histological examination of the placenta revealed chorioamnionitis, and a bacteriological report of the culture showed a group B streptococcus (*Streptococcus agalactiae*). The patient responded well to treatment, and was discharged after her antibiotic treatment was switched from intravenous to oral.

LAB TIPS

Placental Alkaline Phosphatase

Alkaline phosphatase (ALP) is present in a number of human tissues in distinct forms with varying chemical properties. These isozymes are named for their main tissue of origin, and in the normal individual the total serum alkaline phosphatase includes isozymes from liver, bone, placenta, and intestine. A number of diseases affecting these organs may lead to elevations of total serum alkaline phosphatase and techniques are available (heat fractionation, phenylalanine inhibition, and electrophoretic mobility) to identify the different isozymes to help determine the source of the elevation. Cholestatic lesions of the liver and a number of different bone lesions are frequent causes of elevation of the serum alkaline phosphatase, and this enzyme plays an important role in aiding in the diagnosis of diseases of bone and the hepatobiliary system. It is also important in patients with malignancies, where it may be elevated due to metastases to bone (bone isozyme), liver (liver isozyme), or production of the enzyme (tumor-associated isozyme) by the tumor itself.

During the first and second trimester of pregnancy, the alkaline phosphatase isozyme derived from the placenta begins to rise and reaches a peak during the third trimester, where as much as two-thirds of the total serum alkaline phosphatase may be due to this isozyme. Since its level is related to cytotrophoblast maturity, serum levels of ALP are lower in pregnant diabetics because of decreased growth of the cytotrophoblast. Serum levels approach normal levels about one month following delivery. A distinguishing characteristic of this isozyme in normal individuals is its heat stability. Since many of the tumor-associated isozymes of alkaline phosphatase (Regan isozyme, Nagao isozyme, etc) are also heat stable, the elevation of the placental isozyme in the heat fractionation of alkaline phosphatase in a non-pregnant individual raises the suspicion that a malignancy may be present. A significant number of patients with ovarian or testicular cancer will show elevations of the placental isozyme, but it has also been found to be elevated, in smaller numbers, in other tumors, including carcinomas of the breast and lungs. Note that smokers may have a 5 to 10-fold increase in the level of this isozyme.

Alpha-Fetoprotein (AFP)

Produced in the fetal liver and yolk sac, AFP is a glycoprotein found in fetal serum, amniotic fluid (by fetal urination), and maternal serum (by transfer across the placental barrier). It is believed to play a role as a carrier protein, similar to that played by albumin. After peaking around the 15th to 16th week of gestation, the level of amniotic fluid AFP declines during the remainder of the pregnancy. Maternal serum AFP, on the other hand, rises during pregnancy, beginning at about the 12th to 14th week, and reaches a peak near the end of the third trimester. Fetal serum AFP peaks at approximately the 12th to 13th week of gestation, then falls, reaching the normal adult level by the 8th month post-delivery. *(Continued)*

NOTES

Lab Tips (continued)

Elevated levels of maternal serum AFP during pregnancy may be due to the presence of an open neural tube defect, such as anencephaly or spina bifida, and the serum AFP is used as a screen for these conditions. If a repeat test is elevated, ultrasonography is performed to confirm gestational age, rule out a multiple pregnancy, and to identify a gross neural tube defect. If the cause of the elevation is still not determined, an amniocentesis is performed to measure the amniotic fluid AFP. False positive elevations of maternal serum AFP may occur in a number of conditions, including twin pregnancies, gestational age underestimation, fetal distress or death, fetomaternal hemorrhage, and maternal AFP-producing tumors. Low levels of maternal serum AFP have been associated with several chromosomal abnormalities, especially trisomy 21 (Down's syndrome), and it is a justified screening procedure for these conditions. Obesity and maternal insulin-dependent diabetes mellitus may falsely decrease the maternal serum AFP.

In the non-pregnant patient, serum AFP levels are markedly elevated in primary cancer of the liver and certain germ cell tumors.

28

Chapter

A 55-Year-Old
Woman With
Shortness of
Breath and
Lightheadedness

▶ Clinical History and Presentation

A 55-year-old woman presented at the emergency room complaining of shortness of breath on exertion and lightheadedness. She had a history of heartburn, for which she had been taking medications, and a chronic cough and wheezing, for which she had been using inhalers. Physical examination revealed a pale, well-developed woman. Blood pressure was 130/80 mmHg supine, and 115/75 mmHg in the standing position. Heart rate was 80 per minute. She was alert and oriented, and in no acute distress. The chest was clear on auscultation. The abdomen was soft, without masses, hepatomegaly, or splenomegaly. Bowel sounds were present. The stool was negative for occult blood. She was admitted for evaluation and treatment.

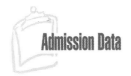

Admission Data

TABLE 28–1. HEMATOLOGY		
WBC	5.4 thousand/μL	(3.3–11.0)
Neut	78%	(44–88)
Band	0%	(0–10)
Lymph	12%	(12–43)
Mono	6%	(2–11)
Eos	3%	(0–5)
Baso	1%	(0–2)
RBC	1.73 million/μL	(3.9–5.0)
Hgb	5.6 g/dL	(11.6–15.6)
HCT	15.2%	(37.0–47.0)
MCV	86.8 fL	(79.0–99.0)
MCH	32.3 pg	(26.0–32.6)
MCHC	37.3 g/dL	(31.0–36.0)
Plts	301 thousand/μL	(130–400)

TABLE 28–2. CHEMISTRY

Glucose	105 mg/dL	(65–110)
Creatinine	1.0 mg/dL	(0.7–1.4)
BUN	15 mg/dL	(7–24)
Uric acid	3.1 mg/dL	(3.0–7.5)
Cholesterol	158 mg/dL	(150–240)
Calcium	9.1 mg/dL	(8.5–10.5)
Protein	6.8 g/dL	(6–8)
Albumin	4.3 g/dL	(3.7–5.0)
LDH	501 U/L	(100–250)
Alk Phos	90 U/L	(0–120)
AST	35 U/L	(0–55)
GGTP	16 U/L	(0–50)
Bilirubin	2.1 mg/dL	(0.0–1.5)
Bilirubin, direct	0.36 mg/dL	(0.02–0.18)

TABLE 28–3. COAGULATION

PT	12 sec	(11–14)
aPTT	25 sec	(19–28)

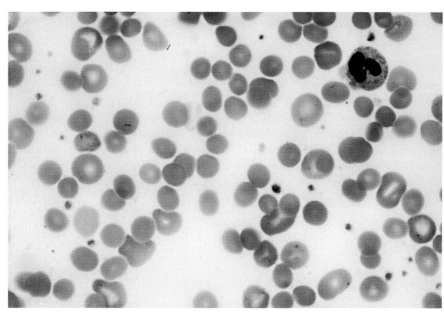

FIGURE 28–1. Admission peripheral blood smear. Wright/Giemsa stain. Original magnification ×252.

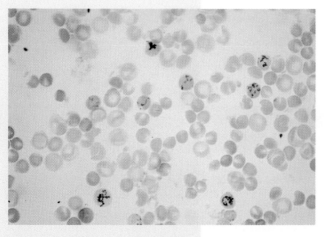

FIGURE 28–2. Admission peripheral blood smear. New methylene blue stain. Original magnification ×252.

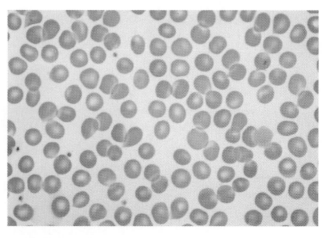

FIGURE 28–3. Normal peripheral blood smear. Wright/Giemsa stain. Original magnification ×252.

▶ **Questions**

On the basis of the preceding information, you can best conclude the following:

1. The CBC results in this patient are most compatible with which of the following diagnoses?
   a. severe iron deficiency
   b. vitamin B$_{12}$ deficiency
   c. folate deficiency
   d. hemoconcentration due to blood loss
   e. hemolytic anemia

2. The patient's total LDH serum level most likely reflects:
   a. liver disease
   b. myocardial infarction
   c. iron deficiency anemia
   d. hemolysis
   e. none of the above

3. The increase in the LDH and direct and total bilirubin levels in this patient most likely indicate:
   a. mild intrahepatic biliary obstruction
   b. viral hepatitis
   c. chronic systemic infection
   d. none of the above

4. The LEAST helpful test to support your diagnosis at this stage would be:
   a. an antiglobulin (Coombs') test
   b. a reticulocyte count
   c. a viral hepatitis panel
   d. determination of serum LDH isoenzymes

5. Figures 28–1 and 28–2 represent smears of the patient's peripheral blood. They show all of the following EXCEPT:
   a. anisocytosis
   b. reticulocytosis
   c. hypochromic, microcytic erythrocytes
   d. erythrocytes showing polychromasia

▶ Clinical Course

The patient was transfused with two units of packed red blood cells and was begun on corticosteroid therapy. Her condition improved, additional laboratory tests were performed, and she was discharged to be followed as an outpatient.

TABLE 28–4. SPECIAL HEMATOLOGY

Reticulocytes	20.9%	(0.1–2.0)
Vitamin B_{12}	262 pg/mL	(200–950)
Folate	15.4 ng/mL	(3.0–17.0)
Haptoglobin	10 mg/dL	(40–270)

TABLE 28–5. IMMUNOHEMATOLOGY

Direct Coombs' Test		
Polyspecific IgG, C3d	3+	(Neg)
Monospecific IgG	3+	(Neg)
C3d (complement)	+/−	(Neg)

TABLE 28–6. LDH ISOENZYMES

LDH	437 U/L	(100–225)
LDH_1	33%	(17–27)
LDH_2	45%	(28–38)
LDH_3	12%	(18–28)
LDH_4	5%	(5–15)
LDH_5	6%	(5–15)

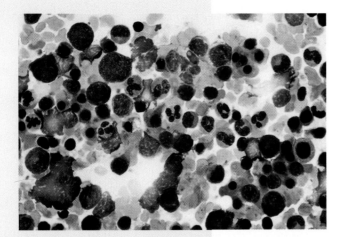

FIGURE 28–4. Bone marrow aspiration (patient). Wright/Giemsa stain. Original magnification ×252.

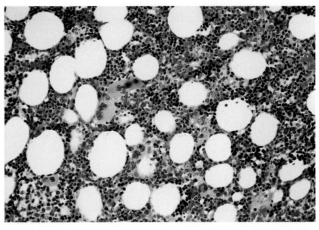

FIGURE 28–5. Bone marrow biopsy (patient). Hematoxylin–eosin stain. Original magnification ×50.

▶ **Questions**

6. In general, an increased reticulocyte count can be a feature of all of the following diseases EXCEPT:
   a. hereditary spherocytosis
   b. sickle cell anemia
   c. uncomplicated and untreated iron deficiency anemia
   d. autoimmune hemolytic anemia
   e. treated megaloblastic anemia

7. From the photomicrographs of the bone marrow biopsy and aspirate (Figures 28–4 and 28–5), you can conclude:
   a. there is an infiltrate of extrinsic cells
   b. there is an excess of lymphoid cells
   c. there is an excess of megakaryocytes
   d. there is an abnormal myeloid to erythroid ratio

8. The LDH isoenzyme pattern of the patient is best interpreted as evidence of:
   a. liver disease
   b. hemolysis
   c. lung disease
   d. myocardial ischemia
   e. none of the above

9. Reduced or absent serum haptoglobin levels are found in patients with all of the following conditions EXCEPT:
   a. hemolytic anemia
   b. a congenital lack of haptoglobin
   c. megaloblastic anemia
   d. acute myocardial infarction

10. The direct antiglobulin (Coombs') test is useful in investigating or diagnosing:
    a. hemolytic transfusion reactions
    b. drug-induced hemolytic anemias
    c. autoimmune hemolytic anemias
    d. hereditary spherocytosis
    e. all of the above

NOTES

▶ Figure Descriptions

Figure 28–1. Admission peripheral blood smear. Wright/Giemsa stain. Original magnification ×252.

The red blood cells exhibit a number of abnormal features. In addition to being reduced in numbers, there is moderate anisocytosis and poikilocytosis, marked polychromasia, diffuse basophilic stippling, and spherocytosis. This picture is very suggestive of a hemolytic anemia.

Figure 28–2. Admission peripheral blood smear. New methylene blue stain. Original magnification ×252.

The new methylene blue stain reacts with residual ribosomal RNA and clearly shows that a number of red blood cells in this patient's peripheral smear are immature. These immature erythrocytes appear polychromatophilic with the Wright/Giemsa stain.

Figure 28–3. Normal peripheral blood smear. Wright/Giemsa stain. Original magnification ×252.

The red blood cells are fairly uniform in size, shape, and color. Spherocytes are not present.

Figure 28–4. Bone marrow aspiration (patient). Wright/Giemsa stain. Original magnification ×252.

Although the photomicrograph illustrates a heterocellular marrow population, there are increased numbers of normoblasts.

Figure 28–5. Bone marrow biopsy (patient). Hematoxylin–eosin stain. Original magnification ×50.

The erythroblastic hyperplasia of the bone marrow is easily seen in this image. Numerous masses of cells with small, dark nuclei and very little apparent cytoplasm are scattered throughout the photomicrograph. They represent islands of normoblasts.

▶ Answers

1. **(e)** In terms of hemoglobin levels and the hematocrit value, the patient had a severe anemia. However, the elevated mean cell hemoglobin concentration (MCHC) rules out iron deficiency, and even if a smear showed some microcytes, the normal mean cell volume (MCV) excludes microcytosis and vitamin B_{12} or folate deficiency. This leaves hemolytic anemia as the best interpretation of the CBC.

2. **(d)** Liver disease and myocardial infarction would be expected to show an increase in aspartate aminotransferase (AST) and lactate dehydrogenase (LDH). Iron deficiency anemia should be without effect on the total LDH level. Erythrocytes, however, contain lactate dehydrogenase (LDH), which is released on hemolysis.

3. **(d)** The patient showed an increase in serum LDH and total bilirubin levels. The increase in bilirubin was mainly due to the unconjugated fraction. This combination is typically found in hemolytic anemias. In biliary obstruction or hepatitis, the LDH and bilirubin levels are also increased, but hyperbilirubinemia is predominantly of the conjugated type. The LDH is also increased in many other conditions, including chronic infectious diseases, but these are not characteristically accompanied by hyperbilirubinemia.

4. **(c)** The aspartate aminotransferase (AST), lactate dehydrogenase (LDH), and bilirubin levels do not suggest hepatic disease. Accordingly, a viral hepatitis panel is not indicated. The patient has a hemolytic disease, and here a reticulocyte count, antiglobulin (Coombs') test, and LDH isoenzyme test would all be relevant in supporting the diagnosis.

5. **(c)** It is clear from the MCH that the erythrocytes are not hypochromic. They are not microcytic, on the average, though some microcytes might be seen on a smear. Polychromasia, some reticulocytosis, and anisocytosis are to be expected.

6. **(c)** Reticulocytes are erythrocytes newly released from the bone marrow. They are still able to synthesize hemoglobin. It takes them 1–2 days to mature fully in the peripheral blood. The reticulocyte count rises upon erythropoietin stimulation of a normally functioning bone marrow. This occurs in anemias such as sickle cell anemia, hemolytic anemias, acquired or hereditary hemolytic anemias (spherocytosis), or in treated megaloblastic anemia. A reticulocytosis does not occur in untreated iron deficiency anemias, since in the absence of an adequate iron supply erythrocyte formation is impaired.

7. **(d)** The normal bone marrow myeloid to erythroid ratio should be about 2–4.5 to 1. In this case, the myeloid to erythroid ratio was 1 to 2, indicating marked erythroid hyperplasia. The increased cells are not extrinsic to the marrow and are not lymphocytes. The number of megakaryocytes is normal.

8. **(b)** The rise in LDH_1, considered alone, could be attributed to hemolysis, or to myocardial ischemia with infarction. However, in the latter case, the aspartate aminotransferase (AST) would be increased. A pulmonary embolus or infarction would tend to increase LDH_3, and a liver disease to increase LDH_5. This leaves hemolysis as the best interpretation of the patient's LDH isoenzyme pattern.

9. **(d)** Haptoglobin is an alpha-2 globulin which binds free hemoglobin. Accordingly, it tends to be depleted in the presence of hemolysis, whether in hemolytic anemias, or anemias such as megaloblastic anemias with a hemolytic tendency. It is congenitally absent in 3% of African-Americans, and in 1%–2% of Europeans. However, it is also an acute phase reactant, and is therefore increased, not decreased, in acute myocardial infarction.

10. **(e)** The direct antiglobulin test is useful in all situations listed. It detects immunoglobulin attached to red blood cells in hemolytic transfusion reactions, and in drug-induced and autoimmune hemolytic anemias. It demonstrates the absence of such antibodies in hereditary spherocytosis, a condition due to an inherited defect in one of the structural proteins of the erythrocyte membrane cytoskeleton, usually spectrin.

▶ Final Diagnosis and Synopsis of the Case

• Autoimmune Hemolytic Anemia of Undetermined Origin

A 55-year-old woman was admitted to the hospital because of shortness of breath on exertion and lightheadedness due to severe anemia. Laboratory findings included a positive Coombs' test (IgG antibody) and a bone-marrow biopsy that excluded a possible lymphoproliferative disorder. The patient was begun on corticosteroid therapy, to which she responded well. She was discharged for follow-up as an outpatient.

NOTES

LAB TIPS

Lactate Dehydrogenase (LDH)

This enzyme is found in many mammalian tissues, especially muscle, liver, kidney, and myocardium. It is elevated in a number of conditions, with marked serum levels in megaloblastic anemia and widespread metastatic disease. Moderate elevations are seen in myocardial infarction, acute leukemia, chronic myelocytic leukemia, pulmonary infarction, hemolytic anemia, Hodgkin's disease, and infectious mononucleosis, while minimal increases are seen in hepatitis, cirrhosis, obstructive liver disease, and chronic renal disease. With electrophoresis, normal serum LDH can be separated into five chemically and serologically distinct isozymes, each of which is a tetramer of two different subunits (H for heart polypeptide chain and M for skeletal muscle polypeptide chain). In normal serum, the relative concentrations of the isozymes are $LDH_2 > LDH_1 > LDH_3 > LDH_4 > LDH_5$, with the subscripts representing their electrophoretic mobility. LDH_1 is the most anodic.

THE ISOZYMES OF LACTATE DEHYDROGENASE

Name	Composition	Main location	Elevated mainly in
LDH_1	HHHH	Myocardium, red blood cell	Myocardial infarction, megaloblastic anemia, hemolytic anemia, muscular dystrophy
LDH_2	HHHM	Myocardium, red blood cell, brain	Myocardial infarction, carcinomatosis, myelocytic leukemia, pancreatitis, megaloblastic anemia, hemolytic anemia, muscular dystrophy
LDH_3	HHMM	Brain, kidney, lung	Pancreatitis, carcinomatosis, myelocytic leukemia, pulmonary infarction
LDH_4	HMMM	Liver, skeletal muscle, brain, kidney	Hepatitis, congestive heart failure, pulmonary infarction, cirrhosis
LDH_5	MMMM	Liver, skeletal muscle	Hepatitis, congestive heart failure, pulmonary infarction, cirrhosis

ANTIGLOBULIN TESTS (COOMBS' TESTS)

Procedure	Significance
Direct antiglobulin test Patient or donor red blood cells are washed, mixed with an antihuman globulin reagent, and visually inspected for agglutination	Detects the presence of immunoglobulin and/or complement bound, in vivo, to a patient's red blood cells. Used in the diagnosis of immune hemolytic anemias (autoimmune hemolytic anemia [AIHA], isoimmune hemolytic anemia, and drug-induced hemolytic anemia) and transfusion reactions.
Indirect antiglobulin test Patient or donor serum is mixed with reference red blood cells, washed to remove unbound globulins, mixed with an antihuman globulin reagent, and visually inspected for agglutination	Detects the presence of free serum antibodies to red blood cells; used for detection and identification of serum red blood cell antibodies, red blood cell antigen typing, and compatibility testing

Clinical History and Presentation

A 23-year-old man was brought to the emergency room with a chief complaint of bloody, mucoid diarrhea, fever and general weakness of 10 days' duration. The patient initially attributed his symptoms to food poisoning from an undercooked hamburger. When symptoms persisted for 5 days, the patient was seen by his family physician and was started on antibiotics. In the next five days there was no improvement and the patient was brought to the emergency room. The patient had no other significant medical history, and had no known allergies. The family history was noncontributory. Physical examination revealed an alert, ill-appearing male. Blood pressure was 120/90 mmHg, temperature was 102.7° F, heart rate was 118 per minute and respiratory rate was 20 per minute. The rest of the physical examination was unremarkable, including the examination of the abdomen, which was soft and nontender. No splenomegaly was apparent, and bowel sounds were normal. A rectal examination showed normal sphincter tone, no tenderness, and no palpable mass. Fresh blood was noted on the examining glove.

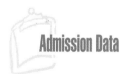

Admission Data

TABLE 29–1. HEMATOLOGY		
WBC	11.28 thousand/µL	(3.3–11.0)
Neut	69%	(44–88)
Band	22%	(0–10)
Lymph	4%	(12–43)
Mono	3%	(2–11)
Eos	1%	(0–5)
Baso	1%	(0–2)
RBC	4.76 million/µL	(3.9–5.0)
Hgb	14.1 g/dL	(11.6–15.6)
HCT	43.1%	(37.0–47.0)
MCV	90.4 fL	(79.0–99.0)
MCH	29.6 pg	(26.0–32.6)
MCHC	32.8 g/dL	(31.0–36.0)
Plts	280 thousand/µL	(130–400)

TABLE 29–2. URINALYSIS

pH	6	(5.0–7.5)
Protein	Neg	(Neg)
Glucose	Neg	(Neg)
Ketone	Trace	(Neg)
Occ. blood	Neg	(Neg)
Color	Yellow	(Yellow)
Clarity	Clear	(Clear)
Sp. grav	1.028	(1.010–1.035)
WBC	0/HPF	(0–5)
RBC	0/HPF	(0–2)
Bacteria	Neg	(Neg)
Urobilinogen	Neg	(Neg)

TABLE 29–3. STOOL EXAMINATION

	Patient	Reference
Stool Leukocytes	12 WBC/HPF Mainly neut.	(<5)
Blood (Hemoccult)	Positive	(Neg)
Ova and Parasites	Negative	(Neg)
Culture & Sensitivity for Common Enteric Pathogens and Campylobacter	Pending	
Clostridium Difficile Toxin	Pending	

TABLE 29–4. CHEMISTRY

Glucose	100 mg/dL	(65–110)
Creatinine	1.4 mg/dL	(0.7–1.4)
BUN	7 mg/dL	(7–24)
Uric acid	6.2 mg/dL	(3.0–7.5)
Cholesterol	151 mg/dL	(150–240)
Calcium	8.6 mg/dL	(8.5–10.5)
Protein	6.2 g/dL	(6–8)
Albumin	3.4 g/dL	(3.7–5.0)
LDH	176 U/L	(100–250)
Alk Phos	77 U/L	(0–120)
AST	12 U/L	(0–55)
GGTP	15 U/L	(0–50)
Bilirubin	0.7 mg/dL	(0.0–1.5)
Bilirubin, direct	0.15 mg/dL	(0.02–0.18)
Amylase	24 U/L	(23–85)

TABLE 29–5. MICROBIOLOGY	
Blood culture	Pending

TABLE 29–6. ELECTROLYTES		
Na	136 mEq/L	(134–143)
K	3.5 mEq/L	(3.5–4.9)
Cl	95 mEq/L	(95–108)
CO_2	32 mEq/L	(21–32)

TABLE 29–7. ERYTHROCYTE SEDIMENTATION RATE		
E.S.R.	20 mm/hr	(0–15)

▷ Questions

On the basis of the preceding information, you can best conclude the following:

1. The LEAST likely cause of this patient's acute problem was:
   a. bacteria
   b. a viral agent
   c. inflammatory bowel disease
   d. antibiotic associated colitis

2. Which of the following bacteria would LEAST likely cause this patient's symptoms and laboratory abnormalities?
   a. shigella
   b. *Campylobacter jejuni*
   c. entero-toxigenic *E. coli*
   d. *Yersinia enterocolitica*

3. Which of the following non-infectious conditions would MOST likely cause this patient's symptoms and findings?
   a. irritable bowel syndrome
   b. celiac sprue
   c. ulcerative colitis
   d. exocrine pancreatic insufficiency
   e. carcinoid syndrome

4. If the patient's condition was not symptomatically treated, one would have expected the development of which of the following changes?
   a. weight loss
   b. anemia
   c. electrolyte imbalance
   d. dehydration
   e. all of the above

▶ Clinical Course

The patient was admitted to the hospital and started on intravenous fluids. A colonoscopy was performed with multiple biopsies of the rectum, the sigmoid, and the descending colon. Figures 29–1 and 29–3 show the microscopic appearance of the colonic mucosa. The blood and stool cultures, as well as the *Clostridium difficile* toxin analysis, were reported as negative. The patient was started on specific treatment. His symptoms subsided and his diet was slowly advanced. The CBC performed before the patient's discharge is shown below.

TABLE 29–8. HEMATOLOGY

WBC	17.28 thousand/μL	(3.3–11.0)
Neut	80%	(44–88)
Band	5%	(0–10)
Lymph	5%	(12–43)
Mono	3%	(2–11)
Eos	7%	(0–5)
Baso	0%	(0–2)
RBC	5.17 million/μL	(3.9–5.0)
Hgb	15.7 g/dL	(11.6–15.6)
HCT	47.1%	(37.0–47.0)
MCV	91.1 fL	(79.0–99.0)
MCH	30.3 pg	(26.0–32.6)
MCHC	33.2 g/dL	(31.0–36.0)
Plts	434 thousand/μL	(130–400)

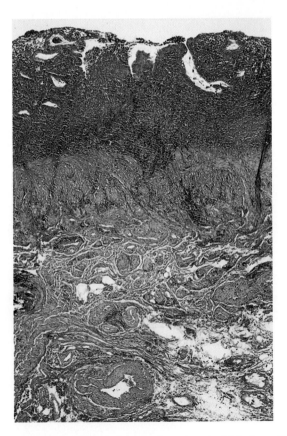

FIGURE 29–1. Colonic biopsy (patient). Hematoxylin–eosin stain. Original magnification ×12.

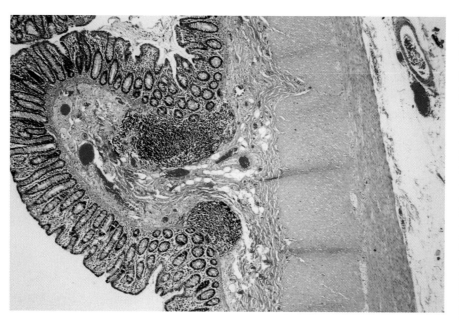

FIGURE 29–2. Portion of normal colon. Hematoxylin–eosin stain. Original magnification ×8.

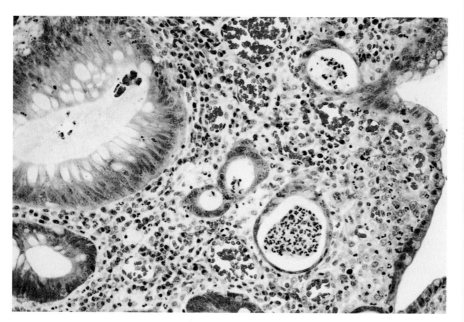

FIGURE 29–3. Colonic biopsy (patient). Hematoxylin–eosin stain. Original magnification ×50.

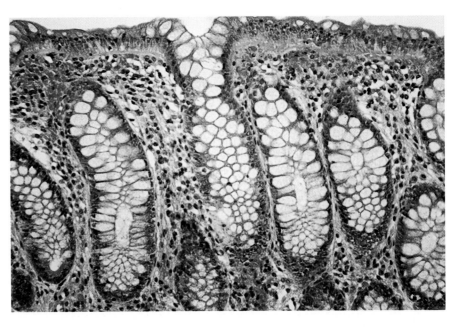

FIGURE 29–4. Normal colonic mucosa. Hematoxylin–eosin stain. Original magnification ×50.

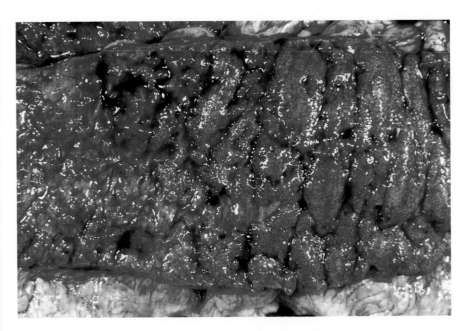

FIGURE 29–5. Portion of colon from another patient with this disease.

► **Questions**

5. Pathological changes in the colon as depicted in Figures 29–1 and 29–3 show:
   a. inflammatory infiltrate
   b. crypt abscess formation
   c. distortion of glandular architecture
   d. all of the above
   e. none of the above

6. The lesion depicted in Figure 29–3 demonstrates:
   a. a high grade dysplasia of epithelial cells
   b. a granuloma
   c. the presence of *Entamoeba histolytica* trophozoites
   d. all of the above
   e. none of the above

7. The pathological changes depicted in Figure 29–1 and 29–3 are most consistent with:
   a. carcinoid tumor
   b. ulcerative colitis
   c. adenocarcinoma
   d. villous adenoma
   e. none of the above

8. Characteristic features of this patient's disease include all of the following EXCEPT:
   a. colonic involvement typically affecting only the mucosa and submucosa
   b. it is a systemic disease
   c. an onset peaking in the third decade of life
   d. discontinuous colonic involvement is producing "skip lesions"
   e. it is a relapsing disorder

9. Before discharging the patient from the hospital, the attending physician was asked to explain some facts to the patient. He should have avoided which of the following statements?
   a. the patient should consider himself to be cured after he finishes his course of therapy
   b. the patient's disease carries an increased risk of the development of colon cancer
   c. as a manifestation of the same disease, the patient could develop symptoms other than intestinal ones
   d. an increased WBC count after the improvement of his acute condition would most likely be caused by the treatment

▶ **Figure Descriptions**

Figure 29–1. Colonic biopsy (patient). Hematoxylin–eosin stain. Original magnification ×12.

This is a cross-section of part of the colonic wall in a patient with ulcerative colitis. An area of ulceration is present in the top center of the photomicrograph. The tubular glands are distorted, there is a significant decrease in the number of goblet cells and a crypt abscess is present. Inflammatory cells (lymphocytes, plasma cells, and neutrophils) diffusely infiltrate the lamina propria and involve and widen the underlying muscularis mucosae. The inflammation does not extend into the richly vascularized submucosa seen in the bottom half of the image.

Figure 29–2. Portion of normal colon. Hematoxylin–eosin stain. Original magnitication ×8.

The tubular glands are straight, with numerous goblet cells. No inflammatory infiltrate is present. The muscularis mucosae is thin and the submucosa contains numerous vessels. Note the lymphoid follicles. The muscularis propria contains an inner circular layer and a longitudinal external layer. The serosa can be seen at the right of the photomicrograph.

Figure 29–3. Colonic biopsy (patient). Hematoxylin–eosin stain. Original magnification ×50.

The colonic mucosa shows a neutrophilic infiltrate with crypt abscesses. The crypt pattern is distorted and some of the lining cells show goblet cell depletion.

Figure 29–4. Normal colonic mucosa. Hematoxylin–eosin stain. Original magnification ×50.

No inflammatory infiltrate is present. The tubular glands are straight, show no distortion or branching, and are lined by numerous goblet cells.

Figure 29–5. Portion of colon from another patient with this disease.

This is the gross appearance of active ulcerative colitis. There are multiple areas of ulceration on the mucosal surface. The intact mucosa between the ulcers is markedly hemorrhagic and appears granular.

▶ **Answers**

1. **(b)** Viruses are the most common cause of non-inflammatory diarrhea. The presence of more than five polymorphonuclear leukocytes per high power field in the stool of patients with acute diarrhea suggests that the disease is probably inflammatory, and the cause of inflammation should be determined. All other options should be considered (bacteria, inflammatory bowel disease, and antibiotic associated colitis) as possible causes of this patient's symptoms and laboratory findings.

2. **(c)** Entero-toxigenic *E. coli* has the capacity to adhere to small bowel epithelial cells and to produce diarrheagenic toxins, which will induce a secretory, non-inflammatory diarrhea. It is the most common cause of "traveler's diarrhea," in which fecal leukocytes are typically absent. All other options should be considered. *Shigella* is one of the principal causes of dysentery and should be considered in patients presenting with bloody diarrhea. *Campylobacter jejuni* causes patchy destruction of the mucosa in the small and large intestine and may cause inflammatory diarrhea, fever, and abdominal pain. *Yersinia enterocolitica* is another important invasive enteric bacterial pathogen capable of producing a similar clinical picture.

3. (c) The patient's symptoms and laboratory findings are most consistent with the diagnosis of ulcerative colitis in the acute stage. Diarrhea, fever, and abdominal pain combined with leukocytosis and a "left" shift, increased erythrocyte sedimentation rate, and the presence of fecal leukocytes and red blood cells in the stool establish the inflammatory character of the diarrhea. Celiac sprue is a disease characterized by malabsorption resulting from injury of villous epithelial cells in the small intestine by gluten. Patients suffer from non-inflammatory diarrhea which characteristically produces greasy, malodorous stools and other signs and symptoms of malabsorption. The symptoms usually appear in infancy, disappear in late childhood, and reappear in the third decade of life or later and usually respond well to withdrawal of gluten from the diet. Irritable bowel syndrome is characterized by cramping abdominal pain and altered bowel habits. The diarrhea is not of an inflammatory character and is not bloody. The diagnosis of irritable bowel syndrome requires, however, exclusion of other organic diseases. Exocrine pancreatic insufficiency causes a malabsorption syndrome with steatorrhea and other symptoms, and does not manifest itself as an inflammatory diarrhea. Carcinoid syndrome is characterized by a history of flushing and diarrhea, which is most likely due to serotonin secretion. There is a markedly increased urinary excretion of 5-hydroxyindoleacetic acid. The syndrome is usually associated with an ileal carcinoid tumor that has metastasized to the liver. The diarrhea is not of an inflammatory character.

4. (e) Weight loss and anemia secondary to intestinal bleeding, electrolyte imbalance due to diarrhea, and dehydration due to diarrhea and fever are all features of active inflammatory bowel disease.

5. (d) Figures 29–1 and 29–3 show the typical microscopic appearance of the colon during an acute attack of ulcerative colitis. There is a distortion of the mucosal and glandular architecture with crypt abscess formation and an inflammatory cell infiltrate.

6. (e) None of the features mentioned (high grade dysplasia of epithelial cells, granuloma, or the presence of *Entamoeba histolytica* trophozoites) are present in Figure 29–3.

7. (b) The pathological changes depicted in Figures 29–1 and 29–3 are most consistent with ulcerative colitis. Features characteristic of carcinoid tumor, adenocarcinoma, and villous adenoma are not present.

8. (d) The patient had ulcerative colitis, which is an inflammatory bowel disease of unknown etiology. It is also a systemic disease. The colonic involvement is continuous (no skip lesions) and it may affect the entire colon in severe cases. The onset of ulcerative colitis peaks between the ages of 20–25 years, but is not limited to this age category. The disease is typically a relapsing disorder. The severity and duration of the disease are the main prognostic indicators.

9. (a) Ulcerative colitis typically presents as recurrent attacks of bloody, mucoid diarrhea. Between the attacks, patients may be asymptomatic for months or years. Patients rarely present with only one attack. Cancer is considered to be the most feared complication of ulcerative colitis; the risk of cancer increases with the duration of the disease. Intestinal symptoms dominate in ulcerative colitis, but the disease is a systemic disorder and may be associated with symptoms of migratory polyarthritis, ankylosing spondylitis, uveitis, and other symptoms. The treatment of acute diarrheal attacks in ulcerative colitis consists of the administration of anti-inflammatory agents and adrenal glucocorticoids or ACTH. Glucocorticoids cause a polymorphonuclear leukocytosis, which is due to release of leukocytes from the bone marrow and also due to the inhibition of their egress through the capillary wall.

NOTES

▶ Final Diagnosis and Synopsis of the Case

• Ulcerative Colitis

A 23-year-old man developed bloody diarrhea and fever, which he attributed to food poisoning. His symptoms persisted and were not relieved by antibiotics. Subsequent work-up showed mild leukocytosis with "left" shift (an increased proportion of band neutrophils), an increased erythrocyte sedimentation rate, and the presence of fecal leukocytes and erythrocytes. Stool and blood cultures were negative. Colonoscopy revealed an acute inflammation of the rectum and severe inflammatory changes in the descending colon. Because of the degree of inflammation, colonoscopy beyond the junction of the descending colon and the sigmoid was abandoned. Multiple biopsies were obtained and microscopic examination revealed changes consistent with ulcerative colitis. The patient was started on an anti-inflammatory drug (mesolamine) and intravenous ACTH. This was the likely cause of the patient's leukocytosis. His diarrhea and fever subsided in a few days. The patient's appetite improved and he was able to resume an oral diet. The patient was discharged to be followed up on an outpatient basis. One year later the patient was admitted with a similar episode.

LAB TIPS

THE LABORATORY ANALYSIS OF STOOL[a]

Test	Method	Reference Range	Comments
Amount, consistency, form, color	Visual inspection	100–200 g brown, formed stool/day	Watery—diarrhea Black, tarry—upper GI bleeding Small, firm stool—constipation Bulky, foul-smelling—steatorrhea Clay color—decreased bile Red color—lower GI bleeding, beets, tomatoes Mucus—spastic constipation, inflammatory process, neoplasm
Fecal fat, qualitative	Microscopic examination	<100 stained droplets/high power field	Increase—steatorrhea, mineral, or castor oil ingestion
Fecal fat, quantitative	Chemical	<7 g/24 hrs[a]	The definitive test for malabsorption Increase—chronic pancreatitis, high fiber diet
Fecal leukocytes	Microscopic examination	Leukocytes not predominant	Neutrophils predominant—Salmonellosis, shigellosis, ulcerative colitis, antibiotic-associated colitis Neutrophils absent—toxigenic bacterial infection, viral diarrhea, parasitic infestations
Fecal urobilinogen, quantitative	Chemical	40–200 mg/24 hr	A measure of the total excretion of bile pigments Increase—hemolytic anemia Decrease—obstructive jaundice, severe liver disease, oral broad-spectrum antibiotics, severe malnutrition
Stool culture	Aerobic culture	Negative for bacterial pathogens	Indications—acute onset diarrhea, bloody diarrhea, fever, fecal leukocytes Used for diagnosis of Salmonella infection, bacillary dysentery, enteric fever, typhoid fever, etc.
Stool parasitology	Microscopic examination (Direct wet mounts, stained smears)	No parasites seen	Used to establish the diagnosis of parasitic infection. Cysts often found in formed stool; trophozoites often found in loose stool; *Giardia lamblia,* Cryptosporidium, and *Entamoeba histolytica* in stool of patients with AIDS.

[a]Based on a 3-day sample of stool from a patient on a 60–100 g/day fat diet.

▶ Clinical History and Presentation

A 37-year-old woman was seen in her physician's office complaining of post-coital vaginal bleeding. The patient had noticed the problem two weeks prior to her office visit. She had had two normal pregnancies. The patient's family history was unremarkable. Physical examination revealed a slightly overweight female in no acute distress. Blood pressure was 120/85 mmHg, heart rate was 85 per minute and regular, temperature was 98° F. Chest and abdominal examination were unremarkable. Colposcopy revealed white patches on the cervix following the application of acetic acid, as well as a distinct vascular punctuation pattern. A Papanicolaou (PAP) smear was obtained and sent to Pathology. Her previous PAP smear, (Figure 30–1), performed a year before, was reviewed.

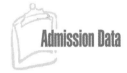

Admission Data

No laboratory tests were ordered at this time.

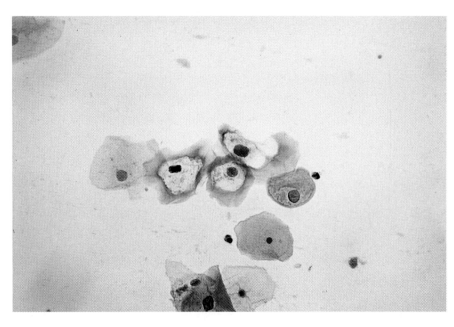

FIGURE 30–1. Pap smear from this patient one year ago. Papanicolaou stain. Original magnification ×78.

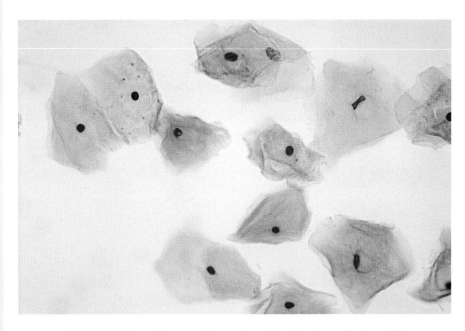

FIGURE 30–2. Normal Pap smear. Papanicolaou stain. Original magnification ×125.

▶ **Questions**

On the basis of the preceding information, you can best conclude the following:

1. The cytological changes depicted in Figure 30–1 represent:
   a. squamous cell carcinoma
   b. koilocytic atypia
   c. adenocarcinoma
   d. changes normally seen in the secretory phase of the menstrual cycle
   e. none of the above

2. The most likely etiological agent(s) associated with the changes seen in Figure 30–1 is/are:
   a. human papilloma virus (HPV)
   b. cytomegalovirus (CMV)
   c. herpes virus
   d. all of the above
   e. none of the above

3. Acetic acid is applied to the cervix before colposcopy to:
   a. accentuate the difference between normal and abnormal epithelium
   b. remove excess cellular debris
   c. remove excess mucus
   d. do all of the above
   e. none of the above

4. All of the following statements about the putative causative agent of the lesion depicted in Figure 30–1 are correct EXCEPT:
   a. certain types have the ability to transform cells in culture
   b. all infected individuals will develop a malignant growth
   c. it may inactivate the tumor suppressor gene p53
   d. types 16 and 18 of this agent are associated with a high risk of the development of cervical carcinoma

▶ Clinical Course

One week later, the patient was called to the physician's office to discuss the result of her recent Papanicolaou (PAP) smear (Figure 30–3) and of viral typing studies that had been performed a year earlier (Figure 30–4). She was scheduled for cervical biopsy for the following week. The microscopic appearance of this biopsy is depicted in Figure 30–5.

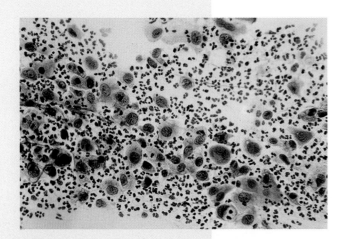

FIGURE 30–3. Patient's current Pap smear. Papanicolaou stain. Original magnification ×78.

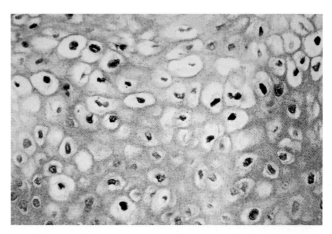

FIGURE 30–4. Cervical biopsy. HPV *in situ* hybridization. Original magnification ×78. (This test was performed one year ago by the patient's physician).

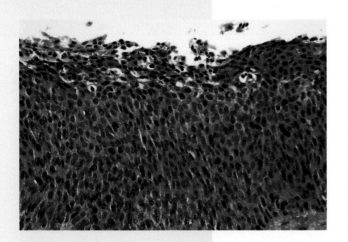

FIGURE 30–5. Cervical biopsy (patient). Hematoxylin–eosin stain. Original magnification ×78.

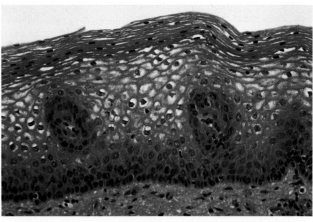

FIGURE 30–6. Normal cervical mucosa. Hematoxylin–eosin stain. Original magnification ×78.

▶ **Questions**

5. Changes shown on the current Papanicolaou (PAP) smear (Figure 30–3) are:
   a. identical to those seen one year before (Figure 30–1)
   b. typical of acute inflammatory changes
   c. metaplastic changes
   d. neoplastic changes

6. The most likely diagnosis of the lesion seen in Figure 30–5 is:
   a. mild cervical intraepithelial neoplasia (CIN I)
   b. adenocarcinoma
   c. carcinoma in situ (CIS)
   d. acute cervicitis

7. The recommended treatment for this patient at this stage should be:
   a. cervical cone biopsy
   b. total abdominal hysterectomy
   c. chemotherapy
   d. pelvic radiation therapy
   e. antibiotic therapy

8. The lesion seen in Figure 30–5 usually arises from:
   a. endocervical glandular epithelium
   b. squamous epithelium of the cervix
   c. endometrial glandular epithelium
   d. lymphocytes

9. Predisposing factors for the lesion seen in Figure 30–5 include all of the following EX-CEPT:
   a. early age at the first intercourse
   b. multiple sexual partners
   c. a male partner with multiple previous sexual partners
   d. atypical endometrial hyperplasia
   e. cigarette smoking

▶ Figure Descriptions

Figure 30–1. Pap smear from the patient one year ago. Papanicolaou stain. Original magnification ×78.

Several koilocytes are seen in this photomicrograph. They are mature squamous cells, each showing a large perinuclear, lightly-stained area. The surrounding peripheral cytoplasm stains much more intensely. The chromatin appears relatively normal. These changes are characteristic of human papillomavirus (HPV) infection. Another common finding in HPV infections, but not seen here, is dyskeratocytes which are keratinized squamous cells.

Figure 30–2. Normal Pap smear. Papanicolaou stain. Original magnification ×125.

Several normal mature squamous cells with small pyknotic nuclei and no perinuclear halo are present. The yellow color is due to cytoplasmic glycogen, a normal finding in some cervical squamous cells.

Figure 30–3. Current Pap smear from patient. Papanicolaou stain. Original magnification ×78.

One of the first observations that can be made in this photomicrograph is the high nuclear/cytoplasmic (N/C) ratio. Also apparent are a marked variation in nuclear size (anisokaryosis), irregular nuclear membranes, and hyperchromatic nuclei with coarse chromatin patterns. These changes would be classed as severe dysplasia or carcinoma in situ (CIN III, or cervical intraepithelial neoplasia). In the Bethesda system the terminology would be high-grade squamous intraepithelial lesion (HGSIL).

Figure 30–4. Cervical biopsy. Human papilloma virus in situ hybridization. Original magnification ×78.

Many of the nuclei in this portion of the cervical biopsy show a dark purple precipitate indicating the site of hybridization between the target and probe DNA, which in this case was for human papilloma virus (HPV) types 16 and 18.

Figure 30–5. Cervical biopsy (patient). Hematoxylin–eosin stain. Original magnification ×78.

The tissue section reflects the changes noted on the Pap smear. The squamous epithelium shows no evidence of maturation, there is a loss of cell polarity, and the nuclei are hyperchromatic and vary in size. These histologic findings are consistent with severe dysplasia or carcinoma in situ.

Figure 30–6. Normal cervical mucosa. Hematoxylin–eosin stain. Original magnification ×78.

The normal cervical mucosa shows normal maturation with hyperchromatic basal cells and flattened squamous surface cells. The cleared cytoplasm in some of the cells represents glycogen deposition.

▶ Answers

1. **(b)** Figure 30–1 shows superficial squamous epithelium with sharply demarcated extensive perinuclear cytoplasmic clearing and slightly enlarged abnormal nuclei. These changes are consistent with koilocytic atypia. No "secretory" changes (predominantly intermediate cells with folding of the cytoplasm) are seen. No malignant cells (squamous or glandular) are seen in Figure 30–1.

2. **(a)** Koilocytic atypia is due to the cytopathic effects of the human papilloma virus (HPV). This Papanicolaou (PAP) smear does not show the nuclear inclusion bodies seen with herpes virus or cytomegalovirus (CMV).

3. **(d)** The cervix is routinely cleansed with 3% acetic acid before colposcopy in order to remove excess cellular debris and mucus. This will help grossly to differentiate between normal and abnormal epithelium.

4. **(b)** The causative agent of the lesion depicted in Figure 30–1 is the human papilloma virus (HPV), which is a double stranded DNA virus. HPV types 6, 11, 42 and 44 are associated with the development of benign condylomas (low risk), and types 16, 18, 31 and 33 are associated with the development of cervical carcinoma (high risk). The oncoprotein E6 of the HPV types 16 and 18 transforms cells in culture by binding to and inactivating the human suppressor gene p53. Immunohistocytochemical and in-situ hybridization techniques can detect HPV in histological sections and in cytological preparations. The large majority of low-grade cervical intraepithelial lesions (CIN 1) exhibit features of HPV infection. However, only a small percentage of women infected with HPV develop cervical carcinoma. HPV is not the only factor predisposing to cervical carcinoma; about 15% of cervical carcinomas do not show evidence of HPV infection.

5. **(d)** Figure 30–3 depicts changes consistent with severe cervical intraepithelial neoplasia (CIN III)*(see Figure description).* There are no inflammatory or metaplastic changes and the PAP smear is clearly different from the one done a year ago.

6. **(c)** The cervical biopsy shown in Figure 30–5 demonstrates loss of epithelial maturation and severe nuclear atypia consistent with cervical carcinoma in situ (CIS). The presence of intact basement membrane rules out invasive squamous cell carcinoma. There is no atypical glandular epithelium to suggest adenocarcinoma nor severe inflammatory cell infiltrate and reactive changes of the cervical epithelium to suggest acute cervicitis.

7. **(a)** The treatment of choice for this patient at this stage (carcinoma in situ) is cervical cone biopsy. In addition, the cervical cone biopsy will further help to establish the extent of the lesion. At this stage, there is no indication for total abdominal hysterectomy, chemotherapy or pelvic radiation therapy.

8. **(b)** Carcinoma in situ (CIS) arises from the squamous cell epithelium of the cervix.

9. **(d)** Atypical endometrial hyperplasia is a predisposing factor for endometrial carcinoma, but not for cervical carcinoma. Early age at first intercourse, multiple sexual partners, and a male partner with multiple previous sexual partners are well established predisposing factors for cervical carcinoma. In addition, cigarette smoking, the use of oral contraceptives, the lack of circumcision in the male partner, and a family history may increase the risk of developing cervical carcinoma.

▶ **Final Diagnosis and Synopsis of the Case**

• Carcinoma In Situ of the Cervix Associated With
Human Papilloma Virus (HPV) Infection

A 37-year-old woman presented with post-coital vaginal bleeding. Colposcopic examination revealed white cervical patches following the application of acetic acid, as well as a distinct vascular punctuation pattern characteristic of cervical intraepithelial neoplasia (CIN). The patient's previous Papanicolaou (PAP) smear, done about one year before, had shown koilocytic atypia, a cytopathic effect associated with human papilloma virus (HPV) infection. In-situ hybridization studies performed at that time revealed the presence of HPV type 16 and/or 18 DNA in the cervical squamous cell epithelium. Infection with human papilloma virus (HPV) of these types has been associated with a high risk of developing cervical carcinoma. The biopsy of the current cervical lesion showed changes consistent with squamous cell carcinoma in situ (CIS). The patient underwent a cervical cone biopsy and was to be followed on an outpatient basis. About 1 in 500 patients with treated CIN III will develop an invasive carcinoma later. This case demonstrates the importance of Papanicolaou (PAP) smear screening as a powerful tool in detecting early cervical carcinoma.

LAB TIPS

Bethesda System of Nomenclature for Reporting Cervical/Vaginal
Cytologic Diagnoses

Since Dr. George Papanicolaou proposed the five classes of changes in the cervical squamous epithelium, a number of other systems have been suggested in order to keep up with the advances in diagnostic cytology. The Bethesda system is the latest of these systems of nomenclature for cervical/vaginal cytology. A full description is beyond the function of this Lab Tip, but several points should be emphasized:

1. It is solely for use in cervical and vaginal cytology.

2. The cytopathology report should contain a statement on the adequacy of the specimen for diagnostic evaluation, (ie, satisfactory for interpretation, less than optimal, or unsatisfactory).

3. The cytopathology report should include a general categorization of the diagnosis: within normal limits or other (see descriptive diagnosis).

4. The cytopathology report should contain a descriptive diagnosis: infection (type), reactive and reparative changes, epithelial cell abnormalities, or hormonal evaluation (vaginal smears only).

In-Situ Hybridization

This is a method which is used to detect the presence of specific nucleotide sequences in cytological preparations or tissue sections. It is based on hybridization of a labeled (biotinylated) oligonucleotide probe, specific to the nucleic acid sequence in question. When a biotinylated probe is used, a positive reaction is detected by the binding of avidin-linked enzyme molecules to the biotinylated probe, which will cause a color change in the presence of an added chromogen. The chromogen serves as a substrate for the enzyme used. The sensitivity of the reaction can be amplified by the polymerase chain reaction technique (PCR).

A-P view	Anterior-posterior view
ACE	Angiotensin coverting enzyme
ACTH	Adrenocorticotropic hormone
AFB	Acid-fast bacilli
AFP	α(Alpha)-fetoprotein
AG	Anion gap
AIDS	Acquired immunodeficiency syndrome
Alk Phos	Alkaline phosphatase
ALL	Acute lymphoblastic leukemia
ALP	Alkaline phosphatase
ALT (SGPT)	Alanine aminotransferase (glutamic-pyruvic transaminase)
AML	Acute myeloblastic leukemia.
ANA	Anti-nuclear antibodies
ApoA	Apolipoproteins A
ApoB	Apolipoproteins B
ApoC	Apolipoproteins C
ApoE	Apolipoproteins E
aPTT	Activated partial thromboplastin time
AST (SGOT)	Aspartate aminotransferase (glutamic-oxaloacetic transaminase)
Baso	Basophil
BJ proteinuria	Bence Jones proteinuria
BRCA1	Breast carcinoma 1, tumor suppressor gene
BUN	Blood urea nitrogen
C3b	Complement component, fragment C3b
C3d	Complement component, fragment C3d
C5a	Complement component, fragment C5a
CA-125	Tumor marker
CALLA	Common acute lymphoblastic leukemia antigen
CAT; CT scan	Computed axial tomography; computed tomography scan
CBC	Complete blood count
CCU	Critical care unit
CD	Cluster designation
CDC	Centers for Disease Control and Prevention
CEA	Carcinoembryonic antigen
CFU	Colony-forming units
CHD	Coronary heart disease
CIN-I	Mild cervical intraepithelial neoplasia

CIN-II	Moderate cervical intraepithelial neoplasia
CIN-III	Severe cervical intraepithelial neoplasia
CIS	Carcinoma in situ
CK (CPK)	Creatine kinase
CK MB	Creatine kinase, MB fraction
Cl	Chloride
CLL	Chronic lymphocytic leukemia
CML	Chronic myelogenous leukemia
CMV	Cytomegalovirus
CNS	Central nervous system
CO_2	Carbon dioxide
CSF	Cerebrospinal fluid
CSF	Colony stimulating factor
DIC	Disseminated intravascular coagulation
DIC microscopy	Differential interference contrast microscopy
DJD	Degenerative joint disease
DNA	Deoxyribonucleic acid
E coli	*Escherichia coli*
EBV	Epstein-Barr virus
EBV-EA	Antibody against EBV early antigens
EBV-NA	Antibody against EBV nuclear antigens
EBV-VCA	Antibody against EBV capsid antigens
ECM	Erythema chronicum migrans
EDTA	Ethylene diamine tetraacetic acid
EGFR	Epidermal growth factor receptor
EKG	Electrocardiogram
ELISA	Enzyme-linked immunosorbent assay
Eos	Eosinophil
ER	Estrogen receptor
ESR	Erythrocyte sedimentation rate
ETOH	Alcohol
EU	ELISA unit
FAB	French-American-British Co-operative Group (classification system for acute leukemias)
FDP	Fibrin degradation products
FNAB	Fine needle aspiration biopsy
GGTP (GGT)	Gamma glutamyl transpeptidase (transferase)
GI bleeding	Gastrointestinal bleeding
g/dL	grams per deciliter
GMS stain	Grocott-Gomori's methenamine silver stain
H&E	Hematoxylin and eosin stain
HA Ab	Antibody to hepatitis A virus
HAV	Hepatitis A virus
HBc Ab	Antibody to hepatitis B core antibody
HBc Ag	Hepatitis B core antigen
HBs Ab	Antibody to hepatitis B surface antigen
HBs Ag	Hepatitis B surface antigen
HBV	Hepatitis B virus
HC Ab	Antibody to hepatitis C virus
hCG	Human chorionic gonadotropin
HCO_3	Bicarbonate
HCT	Hematocrit
HCV	Hepatitis C virus
HDL	High density lipoproteins

HDV	Hepatitis D virus "delta agent"
Hg	Mercury
HgB	Hemoglobin
Hgb A	Adult hemoglobin
Hgb F	Fetal hemoglobin
Hgb S	Hemoglobin S
Hgb A_{1c}	Glycosylated hemoglobin
Hgb A_2	Hemoglobin A_2
HgbC	Hemoglobin C
HGPRT	Hypoxanthine guanine phosphoribosyl transferase
HIV	Human immunodeficiency virus
HLA-DR	Class II major histocompatibility gene complex product
HPF	High power field
HPV	Human papilloma virus
IDDM	Insulin-dependent diabetes mellitus
IgA	Immunoglobulin A
IgD	Immunoglobulin D
IgE	Immunoglobulin E
IgG	Immunoglobulin G
IgM	Immunoglobulin M
IL-2	Interleukin-2
IL-4	Interleukin-4
IL-6	Interleukin-6
ISC	Irreversibly sickled cells
IVP	Intravenous pyelogram
K	Potassium
Ki-67	A nuclear protein expressed only during cell growth (an indicator for proliferative activity)
L	Liter
LB_4	Leukotriene B_4; an arachidonic acid metabolite
LDH	Lactate dehydrogenase
LDL	Low-density lipoproteins
LFB/PAS stain	Luxol fast blue/periodic acid-Schiff stain
Lyme Ab	Antibodies to *Borrelia burgdorferi* (ELISA)
lymph	Lymphocytes
M1	Myeloblastic leukemia without maturation
M2	Myeloblastic leukemia with maturation
M3	Acute hypergranular promyelocytic leukemia
M3V	Acute hypogranular promyelocytic leukemia
M4	Myelomonocytic leukemia
M4-Eo	Myelomonocytic leukemia with eosinophilia
M5A	Monocytic leukemia without maturation
M5B	Monocytic leukemia with maturation
M6	Erythroleukemia
M7	Megakaryocytic leukemia
MAI	*Mycobacterium avium-intracellulare*
MBP	Myelin basic protein
MCH	Mean corpuscular hemoglobin
MCHC	Mean corpuscular hemoglobin concentration
MCV	Mean corpuscular volume
MEN	Multiple endocrine neoplasia
mEq	Milliequivalent
mg/dL	milligrams per deciliter
min	Minute

mL	Milliliter
mm^3	Cubic millimeter
mono	Monocytes
MRI	Magnetic resonance imaging
MS	Multiple sclerosis
Na	Sodium
Neut; poly	Neutrophils
ng	Nanogram
NIDDM	Non-insulin-dependent diabetes mellitus
NPH insulin	Intermediate insulin (lente)
NSAID	Nonsteroidal anti-inflammatory drugs
O$_2$	Oxygen
O$_2$ sat.	Oxygen saturation
Occ. blood	Blood, occult
p53	Tumor suppressor gene
PAP stain	Papanicolaou stain
PAS	Periodic acid-Schiff stain
PCO$_2$	Carbon dioxide partial pressure
PCR	Polymerase chain reaction
pg	Picogram
Plts	Platelets
PO$_2$	Oxygen partial pressure
Poly; neut	Neutrophils
PPD	Purified protein derivative (tuberculin test)
PR	Progesterone receptor
PROM	Premature rupture of membranes
PSA	Prostate specific antigen
PSAP (PAP)	Prostate-specific acid phosphatase
PT	Prothrombin time
R.A.	Rheumatoid arthritis
RA	Refractory anemia
Rb	Retinoblastoma tumor suppressor gene
RBC	Red blood cell
Retic	Reticulocyte
RF	Rheumatoid factor
RPR	Rapid plasma reagin
SLE	Systemic lupus erythematosus
TH protein	Tamm-Horsfall glycoprotein
TIBC	Total iron binding capacity
TNF-B	Tumor necrosis factor-B
Transf. sat.	Transferrin saturation
U	Unit
μL	Microliter
UTI	Urinary tract infection
VLDL	Very low density lipoproteins
W/G stain	Wright/Giemsa stain
WBC	White blood cells

	Convention	Conversion	SI
ACTH, serum (adrenocorticotrophic hormone)	pg/mL	0.22	pmol/L
ALT (alanine amino transferase)	U/L	1	U/L
aPTT (activated partial thromboplastin time)	seconds		seconds
AST (aspartate amino transferase)	U/L	1	U/L
Acetaminophen (Tylenol)	μg/mL	6.62	μmol/L
Albumin	g/dL	10	gm/L
Albumin cerebrospinal fluid	mg/dL	10	mg/L
Aldosterone serum	ng/dL	0.0277	nmol/L
Alkaline Phosphatase	U/L	1	U/L
Amylase serum (DuPont aca)	U/L	0.017	uKat/L
Amylase urinary (DuPont aca)	U/hr	1	U/hr
Angiotensin-1-converting enzyme	U/L	0.017	uKat/L
Apoprotein A-1 (apolipoprotein A-1)	mg/dL	0.01	g/dL
Apoprotein B100 (apolipoprotein B)	mg/dL	0.01	g/dL
BUN (blood urea nitrogen)	mg/dL	0.357	mmol/L
Bands blood (band neutrophils)	%	0.01	fraction
Base excess	mEq/L	1	mmol/L
Baso blood (basophils)	%	0.01	fraction
Bilirubin direct	mg/dL	17.1	μmol/L
Bilirubin total	mg/dL	17.1	μmol/L
CA-125 (cancer antigen 125)	AU/mL	1	kAU/L
CEA (carcinoembryonic antigen)	μg/L	1	μg/L
CK (creatine kinase)	U/L	1	U/L
CO_2 venous whole blood (carbon dioxide)	mEq/L	1	mmol/L
CPK MB (creatine kinase MB isoenzyme)	%	.01	fraction
CPK MM (creatine kinase MM isoenzyme)	%	.01	fraction
Calcium total	mg/dL	0.2500	mmol/L
Cholesterol	mg/dL	0.02586	mmol/L
Cl (chloride)	mEq/L	1	mmol/L
Cortisol serum	μg/dL	27.59	nmol/L
Creatinine	mg/dL	88.40	μmol/L
ETOH (ethanol)	mg/dL	0.217	mmol/L
Eos blood (eosinophils)	%	0.01	fraction
Ferritin	ng/mL	1	μg/L
Fibrin degradation products (FDP)	μg/mL	1	mg/L
Fibrinogen	mg/dL	0.01	g/L
Folate	ng/mL	2.265	nmol/L
GGTP (gamma glutamyl transferase)	U/L	1	U/L
Glucose blood	mg/dL	0.05551	mmol/L
Glucose cerebrospinal fluid	mg/dL	0.05551	mmol/L
Glycosylated hemoglobin	%	.01	fraction

(Continued)

	Convention	Conversion	SI
HCO₃, arterial whole blood (carbon dioxide content)	mEq/L	1	mmol/L
HDL (high-density lipoprotein cholesterol)	mg/dL	0.0259	mmol/L
Haptoglobin	mg/dL	10	mg/L
Hct (hematocrit)	%	0.01	fraction
Hgb (hemoglobin)	g/dL	10	g/L
IgG cerebrospinal fluid (immunoglobulin G)	mg/dL	10	mg/L
Iron total	μg/dL	0.1791	μmol/L
Iron-binding capacity total	μg/dL	0.1791	μmol/L
K (potassium)	mEq/L	1	mmol/L
LDH (lactate dehydrogenase)	U/L	1	U/L
LDH₁, LDH₂, LDH₃, LDH₄, LDH₅	%	.01	fraction
LDL (low-density lipoprotein cholesterol)	mg/dL	0.0259	mmol/L
Lipase serum	U/L	0.017	uKat/L
Lymph blood (lymphocytes)	%	0.01	fraction
Lymph cerebrospinal fluid (lymphocytes)	%	0.01	fraction
MCH (mean corpuscular hemoglobin)	pg	1	pg
MCHC (mean corpuscular hemoglobin concentration)	%	0.01	fraction
MCV (mean corpuscular volume)	μm³	1	fL
Monos, blood (monocytes)	%	0.01	fraction
Myelin basic protein, cerebrospinal fluid	ng/mL	1	μg/L
Na (sodium)	mEq/L	1	mmol/L
Neuts, blood	%	0.01	fraction
Neuts, synovial fluid (neutrophils)	%	0.01	fraction
O₂ saturation (arterial whole blood)	%	0.01	fraction
PCO₂, arterial whole blood (CO₂ partial pressure)	mmHg	0.1333	kPa
PO₂, arterial whole blood (oxygen pressure)	mmHg	0.1333	kPa
PT (prothrombin time)	seconds	1	seconds
Plt (platelets)	thou/μL	1,000,000	10⁹/L
Prostate specific antigen (PSA)	ng/mL	1	μg/L
Prostatic acid phosphatase (PAP)	ng/mL	1	μg/L
Protein, cerebrospinal fluid	mg/dL	10	mg/L
Protein total	g/dL	10	g/L
RBC, blood (red cell count)	mill/μL	1,000,000	10¹²/L
RBC, cerebrospinal fluid (red cell count)	cells/μL	1,000,000	cells/L
RF (rheumatoid factor)	U/mL	1	kU/L
Reticulocytes	%	0.01	fraction
Transferrin saturation	%	0.01	fraction
Triglycerides	mg/dL	0.01129	mmol/L
Uric acid	mg/dL	0.05948	mmol/L
Vitamin B12	pg/mL	0.7378	pmol/L
WBC, blood (total white cell count)	thou/μL	1,000,000	10⁹/L
WBC, cerebrospinal fluid (total white cell count)	cells/μL	1,000,000	cells/L
WBC, synovial fluid (total white cell count)	cells/μL	1,000,000	cells/L

III
Appendix

Final Diagnoses

IV

Appendix

Lab Tips